Advances in Experimental Medicine and Biology

Volume 1433

Advances in Experimental Medicine and Biology provides a platform for scientific contributions in the main disciplines of the biomedicine and the life sciences. This series publishes thematic volumes on contemporary research in the areas of microbiology, immunology, neurosciences, biochemistry, biomedical engineering, genetics, physiology, and cancer research. Covering emerging topics and techniques in basic and clinical science, it brings together clinicians and researchers from various fields.

Advances in Experimental Medicine and Biology has been publishing exceptional works in the field for over 40 years, and is indexed in SCOPUS, Medline (PubMed), EMBASE, BIOSIS, Reaxys, EMBiology, the Chemical Abstracts Service (CAS), and Pathway Studio.

2022 CiteScore: 6.2

Qin Yan
Editor

Targeting Lysine Demethylases in Cancer and Other Human Diseases

Springer

Editor
Qin Yan
Department of Pathology
Yale Cancer Center
Yale Stem Cell Center
Yale Center for Immuno-Oncology
Yale Center for Research on Aging
Yale School of Medicine
New Haven, CT, USA

ISSN 0065-2598 ISSN 2214-8019 (electronic)
Advances in Experimental Medicine and Biology
ISBN 978-3-031-38175-1 ISBN 978-3-031-38176-8 (eBook)
https://doi.org/10.1007/978-3-031-38176-8

This Springer imprint is published by the registered company Springer Nature Switzerland AG
The registered company address is: Gewerbestrasse 11, 6330 Cham, Switzerland

Preface

Epigenetics mechanisms, which do not involve changes of the underlying DNA sequences, have major impact on cell fate and behavior. Histone methylation is a major epigenetic mechanism that play critical roles in pathogenesis of cancer and other diseases. This covalent modification was once considered irreversible until the discovery of two classes of lysine demethylases in 2004 and 2005. This book aims to provide a comprehensive summary of the history of their discovery and the progress made in understanding lysine demethylases over the past two decades. We express our gratitude to the leaders in this field who have contributed to the chapters of this book and the research presented within. Chapter 1 provides an overview of these enzymes, while Chaps. 2, 3, 4, 5, 6, 7, and 8 delve into specific major families of lysine demethylases, covering aspects such as their protein structures, mechanisms of action, roles in development and diseases, development of diagnostic and therapeutic strategies, and future directions for further unraveling their functions and translating these findings into clinical applications.

New Haven, USA | Qin Yan Ph.D.

Contents

Lysine Demethylation in Pathogenesis

1

Jian Cao and Qin Yan

Abstract

Epigenetics has major impact on normal development and pathogenesis. Regulation of histone methylation on lysine and arginine residues is a major epigenetic mechanism and affects various processes including transcription and DNA repair. Histone lysine methylation is reversible and is added by histone lysine methyltransferases and removed by histone lysine demethylases. As these enzymes are also capable of writing or erasing lysine modifications on non-histone substrates, they were renamed to lysine demethylases (KDMs) in 2007. Since the discovery of the first lysine demethylase LSD1/KDM1A in 2004, eight more subfamilies of lysine demethylases have been identified and further characterized. The joint efforts by academia and industry have led to the development of potent and specific small molecule inhibitors of KDMs for treatment of cancer and several other diseases. Some of these inhibitors have already entered clinical trials since 2013, less than 10 years after the discovery of the first KDM. In this chapter, we briefly summarize the major roles of histone demethylases in normal development and human diseases and the efforts to target these enzymes to treat various diseases.

Keywords

Histone methylation · Histone demethylase · Lysine demethylase · KDM · LSD1 · Amine oxidase · JmjC · Hydroxylase · KDM inhibitor · Cancer

1.1 Epigenetic Regulation and Human Health

Although different cell types in a multicellular organism carry the identical genome, they present remarkable differences on morphology, function, and behavior. Interestingly, the cell type-specific phenotypes determined by the previous

J. Cao (✉)
Rutgers Cancer Institute of New Jersey, New Brunswick, NJ 08901, USA
e-mail: jian.cao@rutgers.edu

J. Cao
Department of Medicine, Robert Wood Johnson Medical School, Rutgers, The State University of New Jersey, New Brunswick, NJ 08901, USA

Q. Yan (✉)
Department of Pathology, Yale Cancer Center, Yale Stem Cell Center, Yale Center for Immuno-Oncology, Yale Center for Research on Aging, Yale School of Medicine, New Haven, CT 06520, USA
e-mail: qin.yan@yale.edu

Q. Yan (ed.), *Targeting Lysine Demethylases in Cancer and Other Human Diseases*, Advances in Experimental Medicine and Biology 1433, https://doi.org/10.1007/978-3-031-38176-8_1

developmental history of the cell, known as cell identity, are largely stable, even through successive rounds of DNA replication and cell division (Probst et al. 2009). The biological processes bridging genotype and phenotype and maintaining the heritable phenotypes have been defined by "epigenetics", which literally means "above" or "on top of" genetics (Goldberg et al. 2007; Bird 2007).

The molecular basis of epigenetics has been studied in a variety of organisms, leading to the establishment of three major layers of chromatin-related regulation, including chromatin structure, DNA methylation, and histone posttranslational modifications. Hundreds of epi-genes, or genes encoding the epigenetic regulators, including "writers", "erasers", and "readers" of these epigenetic events, have been identified. In fact, they form one of the largest functional groups of genes in our genome. It is not surprising that dysregulation of these epi-genes and the epigenetic pathways leads to diverse types of human diseases, including developmental abnormalities, psychological disorders, aging-related diseases, and cancers.

1.2 Histone and Histone Methylation

Histones are among the most conserved and redundant proteins in the eukaryotic cells. Two copies of each core histones H2A, H2B, H3, and H4 form an octamer, which is wrapped around by DNA double helix to form chromatin (Luger et al. 1997). However, histones are not just the packing material for eukaryotic nuclear DNA, but also regulatory platforms for chromatin-related functions. Core histones are heavily modified by posttranslational modifications, including methylation, acetylation, phosphorylation, ubiquitination, and sumoylation (Cao and Yan 2012). These modifications either alter the charge and/or the conformation of chromatin, or act as the platform to recruit protein factors to facilitate transcription regulation, DNA repair, DNA replication, X chromosome inactivation, and other chromatin-related activities (Jenuwein and Allis 2001; Kouzarides 2007).

Methylation is among the most important posttranslational modifications on histones (Greer and Shi 2012). Histone can be methylated at lysine and arginine and rarely at histidine (Paik et al. 2007). Canonical core histones have 57 lysine residues (13, 20, 13, and 11 for H2A, H2B, H3, and H4, respectively) and 50 arginine residues (13, 8, 18, and 11 for H2A, H2B, H3, and H4, respectively) (Makalowska et al. 1999). However, like other histone post-transcriptional modifications, the majority of the known histone methylation are located within the highly basic N-terminal tail domains (Fig. 1.1) (Tan et al. 2011). The complexity of histone methylation is further increased by the multiple modification degrees and types in lysine and arginine residues. Lysine can be mono-, di-, or tri-methylated (Schneider et al. 2004) (Fig. 1.2). Arginine only allows mono- and di-methylation, but di-methylation on arginine can be symmetrical or asymmetrical (Fig. 1.2) (Bedford and Clarke 2009). The most extensively studied histone methylation sites include histone H3

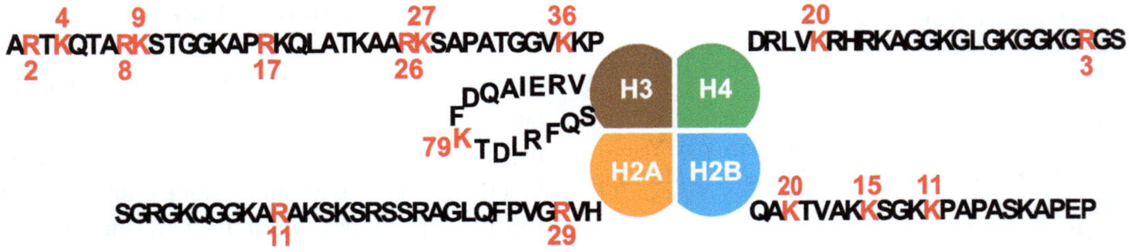

Fig. 1.1 Reported major methylation sites on core histones

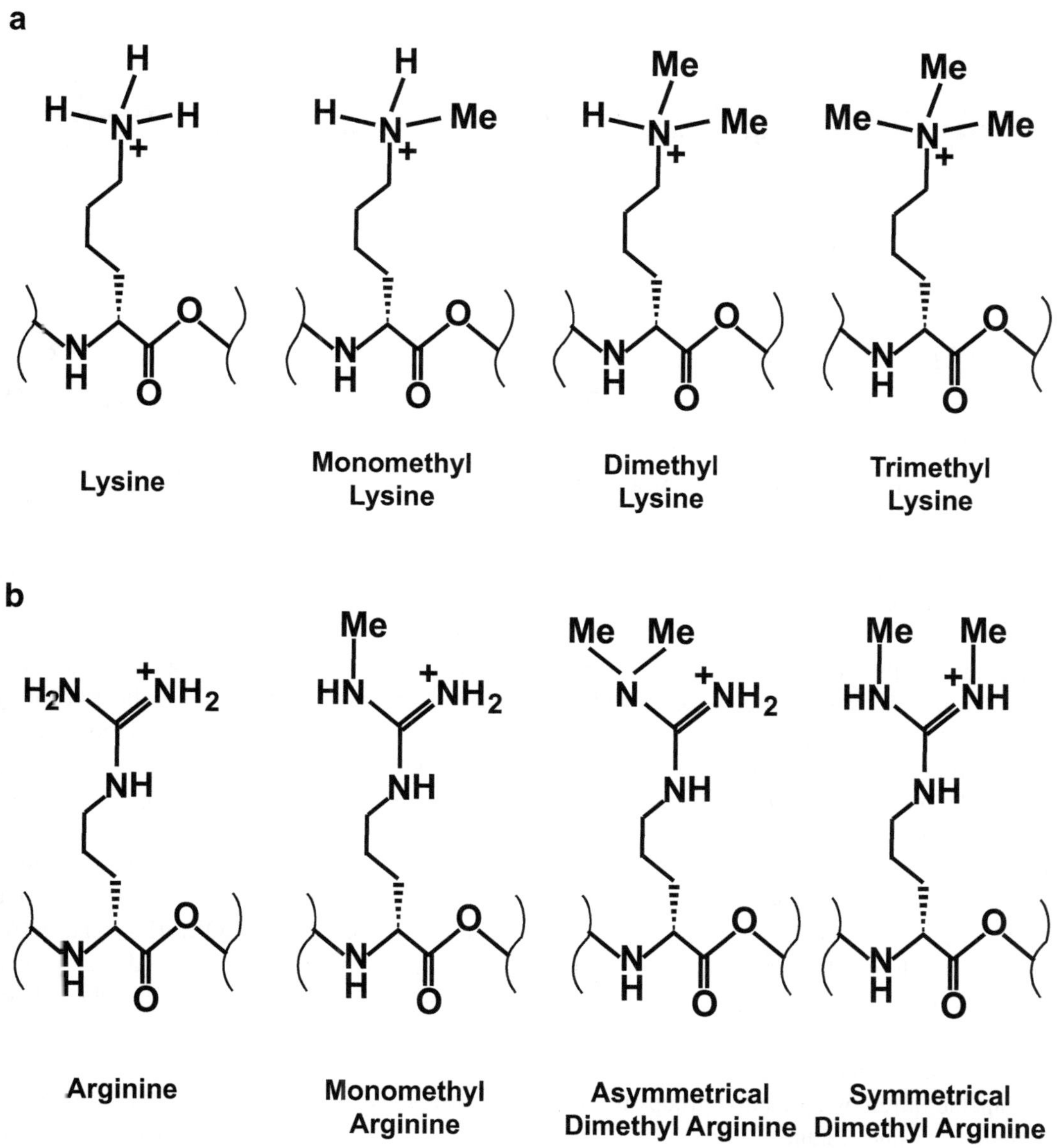

Fig. 1.2 **Lysine and arginine methylation**. Shown are structures of unmethylated and methylated forms of lysine (**a**) and arginine (**b**)

lysine 4 (H3K4), H3K9, H3K27, H3K36, H3K79, H4K20, histone H3 arginine 2 (H3R2), H3R8, H3R17, H3R26, and H4R3 (Greer and Shi 2012).

1.3 Histone Demethylases

As histone methylation is a relatively stable modification, it was once considered as a non-reversible modification that was only removed by histone exchange or diluted during DNA replication. This has changed when Yang Shi's group discovered lysine-specific demethylase 1A (LSD1, also known as KDM1A) in 2004 (Shi et al. 2004). However, KDM1A and its homolog KDM1B (LSD2) are flavin-dependent amine oxidases, which require a protonated nitrogen to form an imine intermediate (Fig. 1.3). Therefore, these demethylases cannot catalyze the removal of methyl groups from

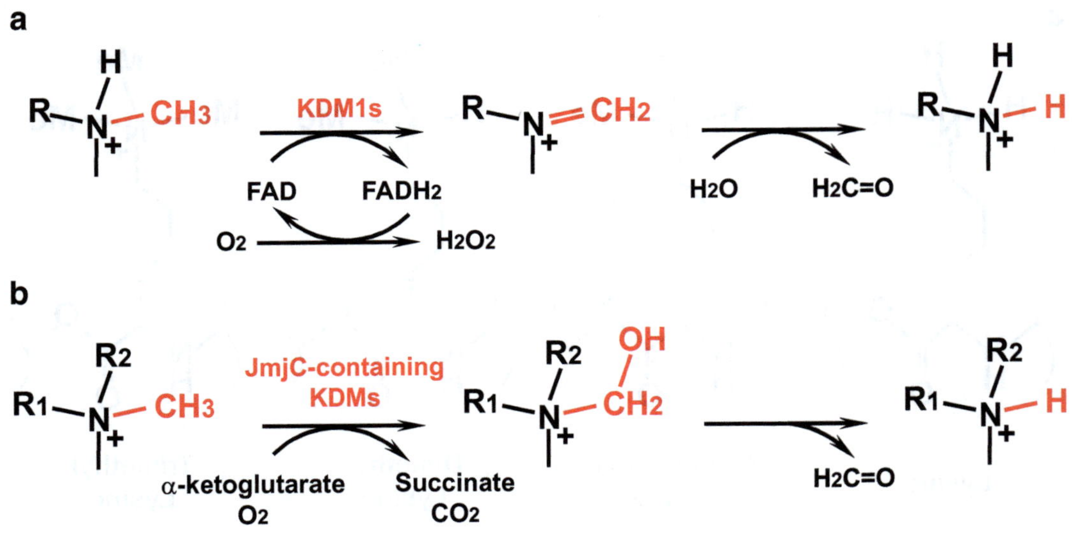

Fig. 1.3 Lysine and arginine demethylation. The proposed demethylation reactions catalyzed by KDM1s (**a**) and JmjC domain-containing KDMs (**b**)

lysine at a fully methylated state (tri-methylated). In 2005, Trewick and coworkers predicted a second class of histone demethylases that contain a Jumonji C (JmjC) domain and catalyze demethylation through iron and 2-oxoglutarate-dependent hydroxylation of methylated lysine residues (Fig. 1.3) (Trewick et al. 2005). Around the same time, Yi Zhang's group independently purified several histone demethylases and found them to be JmjC domain-containing proteins (Tsukada et al. 2006). With a different catalytic mechanism, compared to KDM1 family demethylases, JmjC domain-containing demethylases are capable of removing methyl groups from trimethylated lysine residues. More than 30 genes were predicted to contain JmjC domain in the human genome (Klose et al. 2006a). About two dozen of them were subsequently identified as histone demethylases by biochemical or cell-based assays (Fig. 1.4; Table 1.1).

Based on a new nomenclature introduced in 2007, the identified histone demethylases were renamed as KDMs (lysine demethylases) (Allis et al. 2007) to reflect the fact that they can also demethylate non-histone substrates. They can be separated into two major groups: the LSD1-like, flavin-dependent amine oxidases, including KDM1A and KDM1B, and the JmjC domain-containing, 2-oxoglutarate-dependent hydroxylases, comprised of the remaining KDMs. Based on JmjC domain homology, the second group were further divided into seven subfamilies, KDM2-KDM9 (Fig. 1.5) (Allis et al. 2007; Nowak et al. 2016; Brejc et al. 2017). Two additional JmjC domain-containing ribosomal oxygenases NO66/RIOX1 (Sinha et al. 2010) and MINA/RIOX2 (Lu et al. 2009) were also identified as histone demethylases, but were not named as KDMs and their demethylase function has been challenged (Fig. 1.5) (Williams et al. 2014).

Comprised of multiple domains for demethylation activity, substrate recognition, cofactor binding, and protein–protein interaction, most of KDMs are large proteins with more than 1,000 amino acid residues. The structures of most KDMs have now been solved or at least partially solved (Horton et al. 2017). It is worth mentioning that many structures were solved by the Structural Genomics Consortium (SGC), supported by both academia and industry. The crystal structures of the human KDM1A and KDM1B define a new subfamily of FAD-dependent oxidases with a remarkable substrate-binding cavity with a highly negative electrostatic potential (Chen et al. 2006, 2013).

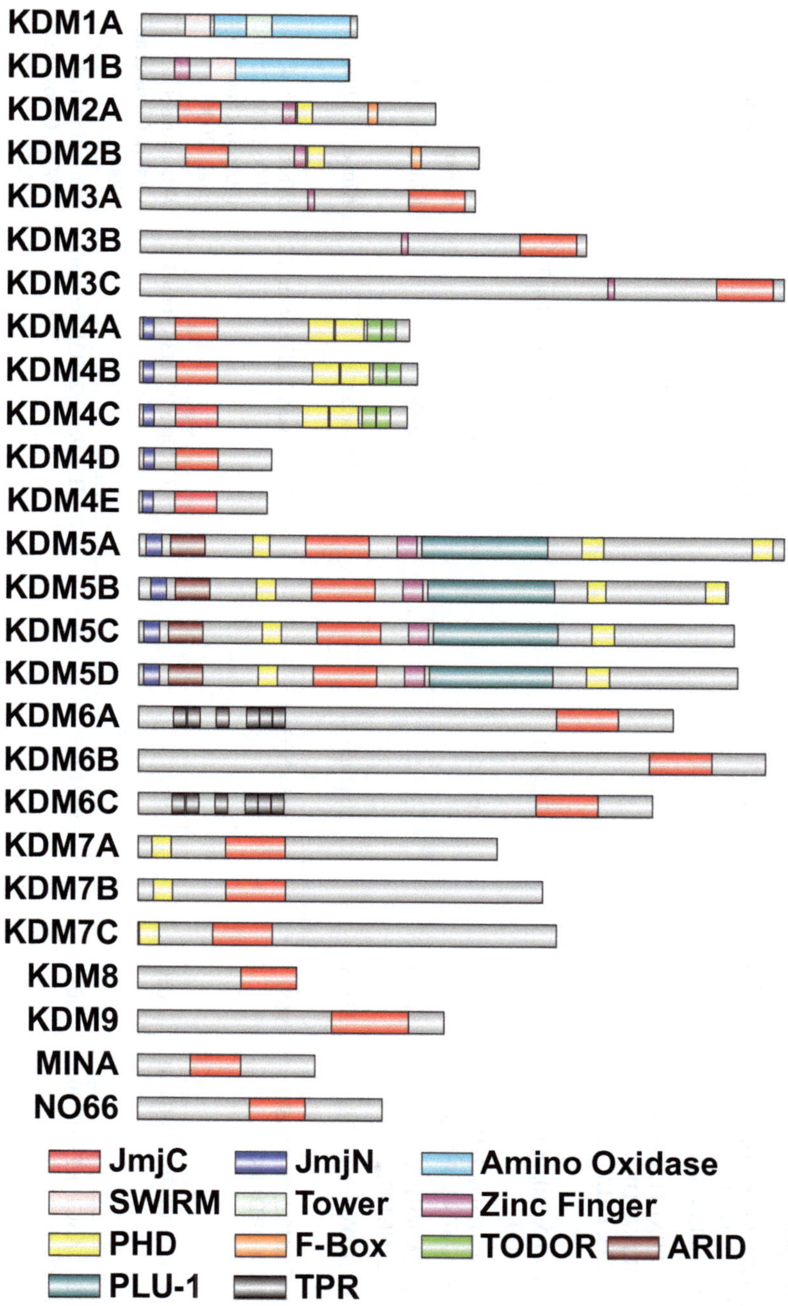

Fig. 1.4 Domain structures of KDMs. The protein sequences of the major isoforms were identified in the UniProt database. Prediction was performed with PROSITE and NCBI conserved domains. The prediction of jmjC domain in KDM9, from the original report, was below a common threshold

Table 1.1 Lysine demethylases in mammalian genome and their substrates

Gene symbol	Aliases	Gene ID	Chromosome location	Substrate specificity	Demethylase activity first identified
KDM1A	LSD1, AOF2, KDM1, KIAA0601, BHC110, CPRF	23028	1p36.12	H3K4me2/1, H3K9me2/1	Shi et al. (2004)
KDM1B	LSD2, AOF1, C6orf193, FLJ34109, FLJ33898, dJ298J15.2, bA204B7.3, FLJ43328	221656	6p22.3	H3K4me2/1	Karytinos et al. (2009)
KDM2A	JHDM1A, FBXL11, KIAA1004, FBL11, LILINA, DKFZP434M1735, FBL7, FLJ00115, CXXC8	22992	11q13.2	H3K36me2/1	Tsukada et al. (2006)
KDM2B	JHDM1B, FBXL10, PCCX2, CXXC2, Fbl10	84678	12q24.31	H3K36me2/1, H3K4me3	He et al. (2008)
KDM3A	JHDM2A, JMJD1A, JMJD1, TSGA, KIAA0742, JHMD2A	55818	2p11.2	H3K9me2/1	Yamane et al. (2006)
KDM3B	JHDM2B, JMJD1B, C5orf7, KIAA1082, NET22, 5qNCA	51780	5q31.2	H3K9me2/1	Kim et al. (2012)
KDM3C[a]	JMJD1C, JHDM2C, TRIP8, TRIP-8	221037	10q21.3	H3K9me2/1	Kim et al. (2010)
KDM4A	JMJD2A, JMJD2, KIAA0677, JHDM3A, TDRD14A	9682	1p34.2-p34.1	H3K9me3/2, H3K36me3/2	Whetstine et al. (2006), Klose et al. (2006b), Cloos et al. (2006)
KDM4B	JMJD2B, KIAA0876, TDRD14B	23030	19p13.3	H3K9me3/2, H3K36me3/2	Whetstine et al. (2006), Cloos et al. (2006)
KDM4C	JMJD2C, GASC1, KIAA0780, TDRD14C, JHDM3C	23081	9p24.1	H3K9me3/2, H3K36me3/2	Whetstine et al. (2006), Cloos et al. (2006)
KDM4D	JMJD2D, FLJ10251	55693	11q21	H3K9me3/2/1	Whetstine et al. (2006)

(continued)

Table 1.1 (continued)

Gene symbol	Aliases	Gene ID	Chromosome location	Substrate specificity	Demethylase activity first identified
KDM4E	JMJD2E, KDM4DL, KDM5E	390245	11q21	H3K9me3, H3K56me3	Sakurai et al. (2010)
KDM5A	JARID1A, RBP2, RBBP-2, RBBP2	5927	12p13.33	H3K4me3/2/1	Klose et al. (2007), Christensen et al. (2007), Iwase et al. (2007)
KDM5B	JARID1B, PLU-1, PLU-1, RBB-P2H1A, CT31, PPP1R98, PUT1, RBP2-H1	10765	1q32.1	H3K4me3/2/1	Iwase et al. (2007), Yamane et al. (2007), Christensen et al. (2007), Seward et al. (2007)
KDM5C	JARID1C, SMCX, MRX13, DXS1272E, XE169, MRXJ, MRX-SCJ, MRXSJ	8242	Xp11.22	H3K4me3/2	Christensen et al. (2007), Iwase et al. (2007), Tahiliani et al. (2007)
KDM5D	JARID1D, SMCY, HYA, HY, KIAA0234	8284	Yq11.223	H3K4me3/2	Lee et al. (2007a), Iwase et al. (2007)
KDM6A	UTX, KABUK2, bA386N14.2	7403	Xp11.3	H3K27me3/2	Agger et al. (2007), Lee et al. (2007b), Lan et al. (2007), Hong et al. (2007)
KDM6B	JMJD3, KIAA0346	23135	17p13.1	H3K27me3/2	Agger et al. (2007), De Santa et al. (2007), Lan et al. (2007), Hong et al. (2007)
KDM6C[a]	UTY, KDM6AL, UTY1	7404	Yq11.221	H3K27me3/2	Walport et al. (2014)
KDM7A	KIAA1718, JHDM1D	80853	7q34	H3K9me2/1, H3K27me2, H4K20me1	Horton et al. (2010)
KDM7B[a]	PHF8, ZNF422, KIAA1111, JHDM1F, MRXSSD	23133	Xp11.22	H3K9me2/1, H3K27me2, H4K20me1	Loenarz et al. (2010), Horton et al. (2010)

(continued)

Table 1.1 (continued)

Gene symbol	Aliases	Gene ID	Chromosome location	Substrate specificity	Demethylase activity first identified
KDM7C[a]	PHF2, KIAA0662, JHDM1E, CENP-35, GRC5	5253	9q22.31	H3K9me2/1, H4K20me3	Wen et al. (2010)
KDM8[b]	JMJD5, FLJ13798	79831	16p12.1	H3K36me2	Hsia et al. (2010)
KDM9	RSBN1, ROSBIN	54665	1p13.2	H4K20me2	Brejc et al. (2017)
NO66[c]	RIOX1, ROX, NO66, JMJD9, MAPJD, URLC2, hsNO66, C14orf169	79697	14q24.3	H3K4me3, H3K36me3	Sinha et al. (2010)
MINA[c]	RIOX2, ROX, MDIG, NO52, JMJD10, MINA53,	84864	3q11.2	H3K9me3	Lu et al. (2009)

[a] KDM6C, KDM7B, KDM7C, KDM8, and KDM9 were discovered after publication of (Allis et al. 2007)
[b] Whether KDM8 is a bona fide demethylase has been challenged
[c] Not included in the KDM nomenclature and whether NO66 and MINA are bona fide demethylases has been challenged

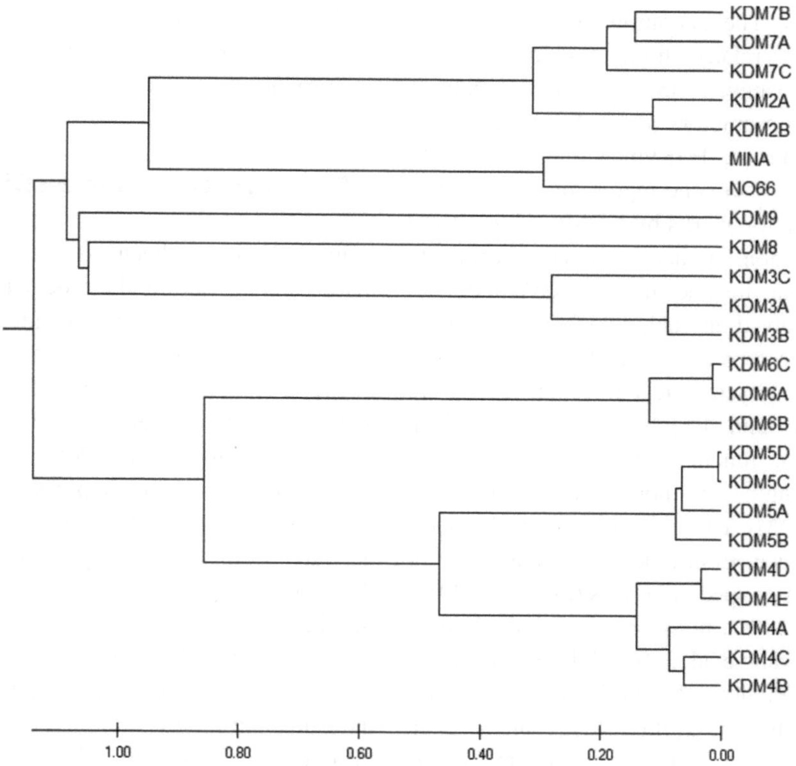

Fig. 1.5 A phylogenetic tree of JmjC domain-containing KDMs. The phylogenetic analysis was based on JmjC domain sequences. The phylogenetic tree was generated with MEGA-X software using ClustalW alignment and minimal evaluation settings

The JmjC domains in KDMs are conserved across species in eukaryotes (Tsukada et al. 2006) and share a double-stranded β-helical structure. It contains two groups of four-stranded antiparallel β-sheets to form a sandwich-like structure (Horton et al. 2017; Klose et al. 2006a). A highly conserved motif (His-X-(Asp/Glu)-Xn-His) provides three chemical groups to chelate the Fe(II) cofactor (Horton et al. 2017).

Beyond the catalytic domains, KDMs usually carry multiple chromatin binding domains, e.g., Tudor and PHD domains. These domains recognize modified or unmodified histone tails; therefore, these erasers of histone methylation are also readers of epigenetic marks at the same time (Lee et al. 2008). The cross talks between different histone modifications suggest complexity of epigenetic regulatory networks.

1.4 Functions of Histone Demethylases

The effects of KDMs can be broadly divided into three layers. Firstly, the biochemical function of KDMs is, by definition, to remove methyl groups from histones, as well as a limited number of non-histone proteins. Secondly, through modulating the level and localization of histone methylation, KDMs are involved in the regulation of chromatin-dependent processes. Thirdly, these KDM-dependent molecular changes contribute to the ultimate biological phenotypes.

Accordingly, the most KDM studies are to explore their roles at these three levels. When manipulating a KDM by genetic or chemical approaches, the increase of its substrate and the decrease of its product are the direct consequences. The alteration of histone marks then modulates related chromatin-dependent processes. For example, H3K4me3 and H3K4me1 define active promotors and enhancers, respectively. In contrast, H3K9me3 and H3K27me3 are correlated with gene repression. Removal of these methylation marks by KDMs led to altered gene expression. Other chromatin-dependent processes that histone methylation/demethylation are involved in include DNA replication, DNA damage repair, and X chromosome inactivation. The physiological roles of KDMs are very diverse and largely context dependent. Many of these functions were discovered using genetically engineered mouse models. Depletion of some KDMs causes developmental abnormalities in mice, from a developmental delay or abnormalities of specific tissues (Zou et al. 2014; Okada et al. 2007), to embryotic lethal (Boulard et al. 2015; Wang et al. 2007). Additionally, adult mice with deletion of KDMs display various phenotypes, including infertility (Sankar et al. 2017; Okada et al. 2007), metabolism defects (Tateishi et al. 2009), failure of gene imprinting (Ciccone et al. 2009), or behavioral abnormalities (Klose et al. 2007). Due to the functional redundancy of each KDM subfamily, combined deletion of several or all subfamily members is necessary to fully reveal the normal functions of these KDMs (Cao et al. 2016).

Epigenetic regulation is unique, compared to other regulatory mechanisms, such as phosphorylation-mediated signal transduction, because it is largely DNA locus dependent. The functional consequence is dictated by the locations of KDM binding sites, the changes of histone methylation marks, and recruitment of epigenetic regulators and transcription factors at these locations. Such information can be obtained by chromatin immunoprecipitation (ChIP) or CUT and RUN/Tag with specific antibodies. ChIP grade antibodies are available for the most known human KDMs and for major histone methylation marks with specificities for both methylation sites, such as H3K4, and degrees, such as tri-methylation. ChIP followed with high-throughput sequencing techniques, also known as ChIP-seq, is commonly used in KDM studies to determine their genomic occupancy and global changes of their histone substrates and products.

1.5 KDMs and Human Diseases

Some KDMs have been associated with various diseases long before their demethylase activities were discovered. For example, mutations in KDM5C and KDM7B were found to cause inherited X-linked mental retardation (Tzschach et al. 2006; Jensen et al. 2005; Siderius et al. 1999; Laumónnier et al. 2005); and KDM8 was identified as a tumor suppressor gene (Suzuki et al. 2006). Most of these discoveries were derived from genetic population analyses; therefore, the molecular mechanism underlying these diseases was poorly understood at that time. Since the discovery of histone demethylase activities of KDMs, compelling evidence indicates that methylation and demethylation of histones play essential roles in differentiation and development, response to environmental and metabolic agents, neural and cognitive function, and diseases. In the last decade, new technologies, such as next-generation sequencing, have dramatically advanced our understanding of epigenetic regulation. Whole-genome sequencing (WGS), whole-exome sequencing (WES), and transcriptome sequencing (RNA-seq) studies of multiple cancer types have revealed that genes encoding for epigenetic regulators, including histone demethylases, are frequently mutated or dysregulated (Feinberg et al. 2016; You and Jones 2012). However, we are still far away from fully understanding the roles of histone demethylases in human diseases.

1.6 Targeting KDMs in Human Diseases

Emerging evidence shows that histone demethylases are attractive drug targets (Hojfeldt et al. 2013). Because epigenetic changes in disease conditions are reversible, targeting histone demethylases may reprogram the epigenetic states

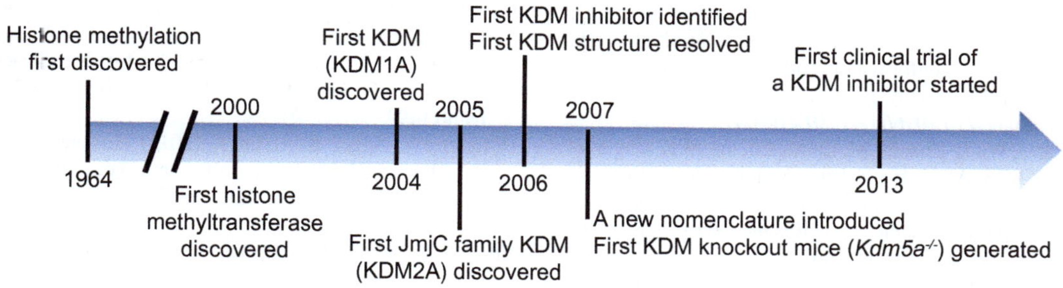

Fig. 1.6 Timeline of major discoveries in the field of histone demethylation

back to normal conditions. Since the discovery of KDM1A, the first identified histone lysine demethylases, tremendous effects have been devoted to developing small molecular inhibitors against these demethylases. Many research teams employed high-throughput methods to screen for KDM inhibitors. The commonly used methods include FDH-coupled assay, AlphaScreen, LANCE Ultra, DELFIA, and multiplexed RapidFire mass spectrometry (Gale and Yan 2015). The JmjC catalytic domains are highly conservative, and α-KG and Fe(II) are required as cofactors for all JmjC-containing KDMs in the demethylation reaction. Therefore, the most identified small molecular inhibitors of KDMs are α-KG-competitive and coordinate to Fe (II) in the catalytic site and usually hit multiple enzymes in or between subfamilies. With many solved three-dimensional structures, rational drug design and computational modeling were used to improve the specificity of inhibitors against desired demethylase without affecting their homologs.

Many KDM inhibitors have entered in clinical trials, including KDM1A inhibitors TCP, ORY-1001, and GSK2879552 (Morera et al. 2016). It only took nine years from the discovery of KDM1A to the first clinical trial targeting KDM1A (Fig. 1.6). Moreover, highly potent and selective inhibitors against JmjC domain-containing histone demethylases have been developed, but most of these are still examined in pre-clinical studies. Thus, targeting key KDMs in human diseases, particularly in cancers, is one of the fast evolving fields in epigenetics.

1.7 Conclusion

KDMs are a group of enzymes responsible for demethylation of histones and non-histone substrates. About two dozen of known KDMs in human genome have been discovered. The number of KDMs will likely increase in the next few years. The known KDMs are flavin-dependent amine oxidases or 2-oxoglutarate-dependent hydroxylases and can be categorized into nine subfamilies. In this book, we will review our current knowledge on the biological functions of KDM1-7 subfamilies and their roles in cancer and other diseases. We will also discuss strategies of targeting them to treat human diseases.

References

Agger K, Cloos PA, Christensen J, Pasini D, Rose S, Rappsilber J et al (2007) UTX and JMJD3 are histone H3K27 demethylases involved in HOX gene regulation and development. Nature 449(7163):731–734. https://doi.org/10.1038/nature06145

Allis CD, Berger SL, Cote J, Dent S, Jenuwien T, Kouzarides T et al (2007) New nomenclature for chromatin-modifying enzymes. Cell 131(4):633–636. https://doi.org/10.1016/j.cell.2007.10.039

Bedford MT, Clarke SG (2009) Protein arginine methylation in mammals: who, what, and why. Mol Cell 33(1):1–13. https://doi.org/10.1016/j.molcel.2008.12.013

Bird A (2007) Perceptions of epigenetics. Nature 447(7143):396–398. https://doi.org/10.1038/nature05913

Boulard M, Edwards JR, Bestor TH (2015) FBXL10 protects Polycomb-bound genes from hypermethylation. Nat Genet 47(5):479–485. https://doi.org/10.1038/ng.3272

Brejc K, Bian Q, Uzawa S, Wheeler BS, Anderson EC, King DS et al (2017) Dynamic control of X chromosome conformation and repression by a histone H4K20 demethylase. Cell 171(1):85–102.e23. https://doi.org/10.1016/j.cell.2017.07.041

Cao J, Wu L, Zhang SM, Lu M, Cheung WK, Cai W et al (2016) An easy and efficient inducible CRISPR/Cas9 platform with improved specificity for multiple gene targeting. Nucleic Acids Res 44(19):e149. https://doi.org/10.1093/nar/gkw660

Cao J, Yan Q (2012) Histone ubiquitination and deubiquitination in transcription, DNA damage response, and cancer. Front Oncol 2:26. https://doi.org/10.3389/fonc.2012.00026

Chen F, Yang H, Dong Z, Fang J, Wang P, Zhu T et al (2013) Structural insight into substrate recognition by histone demethylase LSD2/KDM1b. Cell Res 23(2):306–309. https://doi.org/10.1038/cr.2013.17

Chen Y, Yang Y, Wang F, Wan K, Yamane K, Zhang Y et al (2006) Crystal structure of human histone lysine-specific demethylase 1 (LSD1). Proc Natl Acad Sci USA 103(38):13956–13961. https://doi.org/10.1073/pnas.0606381103

Christensen J, Agger K, Cloos PA, Pasini D, Rose S, Sennels L et al (2007) RBP2 belongs to a family of demethylases, specific for tri-and dimethylated lysine 4 on histone 3. Cell 128(6):1063–1076. https://doi.org/10.1016/j.cell.2007.02.003

Ciccone DN, Su H, Hevi S, Gay F, Lei H, Bajko J et al (2009) KDM1B is a histone H3K4 demethylase required to establish maternal genomic imprints. Nature 461(7262):415–418. https://doi.org/10.1038/nature08315

Cloos PA, Christensen J, Agger K, Maiolica A, Rappsilber J, Antal T et al (2006) The putative oncogene GASC1 demethylates tri- and dimethylated lysine 9 on histone H3. Nature 442(7100):307–311. https://doi.org/10.1038/nature04837

De Santa F, Totaro MG, Prosperini E, Notarbartolo S, Testa G, Natoli G (2007) The histone H3 lysine-27 demethylase Jmjd3 links inflammation to inhibition of polycomb-mediated gene silencing. Cell 130(6):1083–1094. https://doi.org/10.1016/j.cell.2007.08.019

Feinberg AP, Koldobskiy MA, Gondor A (2016) Epigenetic modulators, modifiers and mediators in cancer aetiology and progression. Nat Rev Genet 17(5):284–299. https://doi.org/10.1038/nrg.2016.13

Gale M, Yan Q (2015) High-throughput screening to identify inhibitors of lysine demethylases. Epigenomics 7(1):57–65. https://doi.org/10.2217/epi.14.63

Goldberg AD, Allis CD, Bernstein E (2007) Epigenetics: a landscape takes shape. Cell 128(4):635–638. https://doi.org/10.1016/j.cell.2007.02.006

Greer EL, Shi Y (2012) Histone methylation: a dynamic mark in health, disease and inheritance. Nat Rev Genet 13(5):343–357. https://doi.org/10.1038/nrg3173

He J, Kallin EM, Tsukada Y, Zhang Y (2008) The H3K36 demethylase Jhdm1b/Kdm2b regulates cell proliferation and senescence through p15(Ink4b). Nat Struct Mol Biol 15(11):1169–1175. https://doi.org/10.1038/nsmb.1499

Hojfeldt JW, Agger K, Helin K (2013) Histone lysine demethylases as targets for anticancer therapy. Nat Rev Drug Discov 12(12):917–930. https://doi.org/10.1038/nrd4154

Hong S, Cho YW, Yu LR, Yu H, Veenstra TD, Ge K (2007) Identification of JmjC domain-containing UTX and JMJD3 as histone H3 lysine 27 demethylases. Proc Natl Acad Sci U S A 104(47):18439–18444. https://doi.org/10.1073/pnas.0707292104

Horton JR, Gale M, Yan Q, Cheng X (2017) The molecular basis of histone demethylation. In Kaneda A, Tsukada Y-I (eds) DNA and histone methylation as cancer targets. Springer International Publishing, Cham, pp 151–219. https://doi.org/10.1007/978-3-319-59786-7_7

Horton JR, Upadhyay AK, Qi HH, Zhang X, Shi Y, Cheng X (2010) Enzymatic and structural insights for substrate specificity of a family of jumonji histone lysine demethylases. Nat Struct Mol Biol 17(1):38–43. https://doi.org/10.1038/nsmb.1753

Hsia DA, Tepper CG, Pochampalli MR, Hsia EY, Izumiya C, Huerta SB et al (2010) KDM8, a H3K36me2 histone demethylase that acts in the cyclin A1 coding region to regulate cancer cell proliferation. Proc Natl Acad Sci USA 107(21):9671–9676. https://doi.org/10.1073/pnas.1000401107

Iwase S, Lan F, Bayliss P, de la Torre-Ubieta L, Huarte M, Qi HH et al (2007) The X-linked mental retardation gene SMCX/JARID1C defines a family of histone H3 lysine 4 demethylases. Cell 128(6):1077–1088. https://doi.org/10.1016/j.cell.2007.02.017

Jensen LR, Amende M, Gurok U, Moser B, Gimmel V, Tzschach A et al (2005) Mutations in the JARID1C gene, which is involved in transcriptional regulation and chromatin remodeling, cause X-linked mental retardation. Am J Hum Genet 76(2):227–236. https://doi.org/10.1086/427563

Jenuwein T, Allis CD (2001) Translating the histone code. Science 293(5532):1074–1080. https://doi.org/10.1126/science.1063127

Karytinos A, Forneris F, Profumo A, Ciossani G, Battaglioli E, Binda C et al (2009) A novel mammalian flavin-dependent histone demethylase. J Biol Chem 284(26):17775–17782. https://doi.org/10.1074/jbc.M109.003087

Kim JY, Kim KB, Eom GH, Choe N, Kee HJ, Son HJ et al (2012) KDM3B is the H3K9 demethylase involved in transcriptional activation of lmo2 in leukemia. Mol Cell Biol 32(14):2917–2933. https://doi.org/10.1128/MCB.00133-12

Kim SM, Kim JY, Choe NW, Cho IH, Kim JR, Kim DW et al (2010) Regulation of mouse steroidogenesis by WHISTLE and JMJD1C through histone methylation

balance. Nucleic Acids Res 38(19):6389–6403. https://doi.org/10.1093/nar/gkq491
Klose RJ, Kallin EM, Zhang Y (2006a) JmjC-domain-containing proteins and histone demethylation. Nat Rev Genet 7(9):715–727. https://doi.org/10.1038/nrg1945
Klose RJ, Yamane K, Bae Y, Zhang D, Erdjument-Bromage H, Tempst P et al (2006b) The transcriptional repressor JHDM3A demethylates trimethyl histone H3 lysine 9 and lysine 36. Nature 442(7100):312–316. https://doi.org/10.1038/nature04853
Klose RJ, Yan Q, Tothova Z, Yamane K, Erdjument-Bromage H, Tempst P et al (2007) The retinoblastoma binding protein RBP2 is an H3K4 demethylase. Cell 128(5):889–900. https://doi.org/10.1016/j.cell.2007.02.013
Kouzarides T (2007) Chromatin modifications and their function. Cell 128(4):693–705. https://doi.org/10.1016/j.cell.2007.02.005
Lan F, Bayliss PE, Rinn JL, Whetstine JR, Wang JK, Chen S et al (2007) A histone H3 lysine 27 demethylase regulates animal posterior development. Nature 449(7163):689–694. https://doi.org/10.1038/nature06192
Laumonnier F, Holbert S, Ronce N, Faravelli F, Lenzner S, Schwartz CE et al (2005) Mutations in PHF8 are associated with X linked mental retardation and cleft lip/cleft palate. J Med Genet 42(10):780–786. https://doi.org/10.1136/jmg.2004.029439
Lee J, Thompson JR, Botuyan MV, Mer G (2008) Distinct binding modes specify the recognition of methylated histones H3K4 and H4K20 by JMJD2A-tudor. Nat Struct Mol Biol 15(1):109–111. https://doi.org/10.1038/nsmb1326
Lee MG, Norman J, Shilatifard A, Shiekhattar R (2007) Physical and functional association of a trimethyl H3K4 demethylase and Ring6a/MBLR, a polycomb-like protein. Cell 128(5):877–887. https://doi.org/10.1016/j.cell.2007.02.004
Lee MG, Villa R, Trojer P, Norman J, Yan KP, Reinberg D et al (2007) Demethylation of H3K27 regulates polycomb recruitment and H2A ubiquitination. Science 318(5849):447–450. https://doi.org/10.1126/science.1149042
Loenarz C, Ge W, Coleman ML, Rose NR, Cooper CD, Klose RJ et al (2010) PHF8, a gene associated with cleft lip/palate and mental retardation, encodes for an Nepsilon-dimethyl lysine demethylase. Hum Mol Genet 19(2):217–222. https://doi.org/10.1093/hmg/ddp480
Lu Y, Chang Q, Zhang Y, Beezhold K, Rojanasakul Y, Zhao H et al (2009) Lung cancer-associated JmjC domain protein mdig suppresses formation of tri-methyl lysine 9 of histone H3. Cell Cycle 8(13):2101–2109. https://doi.org/10.4161/cc.8.13.8927
Luger K, Mader AW, Richmond RK, Sargent DF, Richmond TJ (1997) Crystal structure of the nucleosome core particle at 2.8 A resolution. Nature 389(6648):251–60. https://doi.org/10.1038/38444
Makalowska I, Ferlanti ES, Baxevanis AD, Landsman D (1999) Histone sequence database: sequences, structures, post-translational modifications and genetic loci. Nucleic Acids Res 27(1):323–324
Morera L, Lubbert M, Jung M (2016) Targeting histone methyltransferases and demethylases in clinical trials for cancer therapy. Clin Epigenetics 8:57. https://doi.org/10.1186/s13148-016-0223-4
Nowak RP, Tumber A, Johansson C, Che KH, Brennan P, Owen D et al (2016) Advances and challenges in understanding histone demethylase biology. Curr Opin Chem Biol 33:151–159. https://doi.org/10.1016/j.cbpa.2016.06.021
Okada Y, Scott G, Ray MK, Mishina Y, Zhang Y (2007) Histone demethylase JHDM2A is critical for Tnp1 and Prm1 transcription and spermatogenesis. Nature 450(7166):119–123. https://doi.org/10.1038/nature06236
Paik WK, Paik DC, Kim S (2007) Historical review: the field of protein methylation. Trends Biochem Sci 32(3):146–152. https://doi.org/10.1016/j.tibs.2007.01.006
Probst AV, Dunleavy E, Almouzni G (2009) Epigenetic inheritance during the cell cycle. Nat Rev Mol Cell Biol 10(3):192–206. https://doi.org/10.1038/nrm2640
Sakurai M, Rose NR, Schultz L, Quinn AM, Jadhav A, Ng SS et al (2010) A miniaturized screen for inhibitors of Jumonji histone demethylases. Mol Biosyst 6(2):357–364. https://doi.org/10.1039/b912993f
Sankar A, Kooistra SM, Gonzalez JM (2017) Maternal expression of the histone demethylase Kdm4a is crucial for pre-implantation development. 144(18):3264–3277. https://doi.org/10.1242/dev.155473
Schneider R, Bannister AJ, Myers FA, Thorne AW, Crane-Robinson C, Kouzarides T (2004) Histone H3 lysine 4 methylation patterns in higher eukaryotic genes. Nat Cell Biol 6(1):73–77. https://doi.org/10.1038/ncb1076
Seward DJ, Cubberley G, Kim S, Schonewald M, Zhang L, Tripet B et al (2007) Demethylation of trimethylated histone H3 Lys4 in vivo by JARID1 JmjC proteins. Nat Struct Mol Biol 14(3):240–242. https://doi.org/10.1038/nsmb1200
Shi Y, Lan F, Matson C, Mulligan P, Whetstine JR, Cole PA et al (2004) Histone demethylation mediated by the nuclear amine oxidase homolog LSD1. Cell 119(7):941–953. https://doi.org/10.1016/j.cell.2004.12.012
Siderius LE, Hamel BC, van Bokhoven H, de Jager F, van den Helm B, Kremer H et al (1999) X-linked mental retardation associated with cleft lip/palate maps to Xp11.3-q21.3. Am J Med Genet 85(3):216–220
Sinha KM, Yasuda H, Coombes MM, Dent SY, de Crombrugghe B (2010) Regulation of the osteoblast-specific transcription factor Osterix by NO66,

a Jumonji family histone demethylase. EMBO J 29(1):68–79. https://doi.org/10.1038/emboj.2009.332

Suzuki T, Minehata K, Akagi K, Jenkins NA, Copeland NG (2006) Tumor suppressor gene identification using retroviral insertional mutagenesis in Blm-deficient mice. Embo J 25(14):3422–3431. https://doi.org/10.1038/sj.emboj.7601215

Tahiliani M, Mei P, Fang R, Leonor T, Rutenberg M, Shimizu F et al (2007) The histone H3K4 demethylase SMCX links REST target genes to X-linked mental retardation. Nature 447(7144):601–605. https://doi.org/10.1038/nature05823

Tan M, Luo H, Lee S, Jin F, Yang JS, Montellier E et al (2011) Identification of 67 histone marks and histone lysine crotonylation as a new type of histone modification. Cell 146(6):1016–1028. https://doi.org/10.1016/j.cell.2011.08.008

Tateishi K, Okada Y, Kallin EM, Zhang Y (2009) Role of Jhdm2a in regulating metabolic gene expression and obesity resistance. Nature 458(7239):757–761. https://doi.org/10.1038/nature07777

Trewick SC, McLaughlin PJ, Allshire RC (2005) Methylation: lost in hydroxylation? EMBO Rep 6(4):315–320. https://doi.org/10.1038/sj.embor.7400379

Tsukada Y, Fang J, Erdjument-Bromage H, Warren ME, Borchers CH, Tempst P et al (2006) Histone demethylation by a family of JmjC domain-containing proteins. Nature 439(7078):811–816. https://doi.org/10.1038/nature04433

Tzschach A, Lenzner S, Moser B, Reinhardt R, Chelly J, Fryns JP et al (2006) Novel JARID1C/SMCX mutations in patients with X-linked mental retardation. Hum Mutat 27(4):389. https://doi.org/10.1002/humu.9420

Walport LJ, Hopkinson RJ, Vollmar M, Madden SK, Gileadi C, Oppermann U et al (2014) Human UTY(KDM6C) is a male-specific N-methyl lysyl demethylase. J Biol Chem 289(26):18302–18313. https://doi.org/10.1074/jbc.M114.555052

Wang J, Scully K, Zhu X, Cai L, Zhang J, Prefontaine GG et al (2007) Opposing LSD1 complexes function in developmental gene activation and repression programmes. Nature 446(7138):882–887. https://doi.org/10.1038/nature05671

Wen H, Li J, Song T, Lu M, Kan PY, Lee MG et al (2010) Recognition of histone H3K4 trimethylation by the plant homeodomain of PHF2 modulates histone demethylation. J Biol Chem 285(13):9322–9326. https://doi.org/10.1074/jbc.C109.097667

Whetstine JR, Nottke A, Lan F, Huarte M, Smolikov S, Chen Z et al (2006) Reversal of histone lysine trimethylation by the JMJD2 family of histone demethylases. Cell 125(3):467–481. https://doi.org/10.1016/j.cell.2006.03.028

Williams ST, Walport LJ, Hopkinson RJ, Madden SK, Chowdhury R, Schofield CJ et al (2014) Studies on the catalytic domains of multiple JmjC oxygenases using peptide substrates. Epigenetics 9(12):1596–1603. https://doi.org/10.4161/15592294.2014.983381

Yamane K, Tateishi K, Klose RJ, Fang J, Fabrizio LA, Erdjument-Bromage H et al (2007) PLU-1 is an H3K4 demethylase involved in transcriptional repression and breast cancer cell proliferation. Mol Cell 25(6):801–812. https://doi.org/10.1016/j.molcel.2007.03.001

Yamane K, Toumazou C, Tsukada Y, Erdjument-Bromage H, Tempst P, Wong J et al (2006) JHDM2A, a JmjC-containing H3K9 demethylase, facilitates transcription activation by androgen receptor. Cell 125(3):483–495. https://doi.org/10.1016/j.cell.2006.03.027

You JS, Jones PA (2012) Cancer genetics and epigenetics: two sides of the same coin? Cancer Cell 22(1):9–20. https://doi.org/10.1016/j.ccr.2012.06.008

Zou MR, Cao J, Liu Z, Huh SJ, Polyak K, Yan Q (2014) Histone demethylase jumonji AT-rich interactive domain 1B (JARID1B) controls mammary gland development by regulating key developmental and lineage specification genes. J Biol Chem 289(25):17620–17633. https://doi.org/10.1074/jbc.M114.570853

Targeting the LSD1/KDM1 Family of Lysine Demethylases in Cancer and Other Human Diseases

2

Fei Mao and Yujiang Geno Shi

Abstract

Lysine-specific demethylase 1 (LSD1) was the first histone demethylase discovered and the founding member of the flavin-dependent lysine demethylase family (KDM1). The human KDM1 family includes KDM1A and KDM1B, which primarily catalyze demethylation of histone H3K4me1/2. The KDM1 family is involved in epigenetic gene regulation and plays important roles in various biological and disease pathogenesis processes, including cell differentiation, embryonic development, hormone signaling, and carcinogenesis. Malfunction of many epigenetic regulators results in complex human diseases, including cancers. Regulators such as KDM1 have become potential therapeutic targets because of the reversibility of epigenetic control of genome function. Indeed, several classes of KDM1-selective small molecule inhibitors have been developed, some of which are currently in clinical trials to treat various cancers. In this chapter, we review the discovery, biochemical, and molecular mechanisms, atomic structure, genetics, biology, and pathology of the KDM1 family of lysine demethylases. Focusing on cancer, we also provide a comprehensive summary of recently developed KDM1 inhibitors and related preclinical and clinical studies to provide a better understanding of the mechanisms of action and applications of these KDM1-specific inhibitors in therapeutic treatment.

Keywords

Histone demethylase · LSD1 · Cancer · Inhibitors

F. Mao · Y. G. Shi (✉)
Longevity and Aging Institute (LAI), IBS and Department of Endocrinology and Metabolism, Zhongshan Hospital, Fudan University, Shanghai 200032, P.R. China
e-mail: shiyujiang@fudan.edu.cn

F. Mao · Y. G. Shi
Division of Endocrinology, Diabetes and Hypertension, Department of Medicine, Brigham and Women's Hospital, Harvard Medical School, Boston, MA, USA

2.1 Introduction: Discovery of the First Histone Demethylase, LSD1/KDM1A

Histone methylation at lysine and arginine residues and DNA methylation at the 5-position of cytosine are key components of the eukaryotic epigenome, playing critical roles in epigenetic regulation. Although some histone

Q. Yan (ed.), *Targeting Lysine Demethylases in Cancer and Other Human Diseases*, Advances in Experimental Medicine and Biology 1433, https://doi.org/10.1007/978-3-031-38176-8_2

modifications, such as acetylation and phosphorylation, are known to be reversible when they were found, DNA and histone methylation were long considered to be stable and irreversible epigenetic marks that constituted the hallmark of epigenetic inheritance. The reversibility of histone and DNA methylation was questioned mainly because of failure to identify active enzymes and chemical mechanisms responsible for DNA and histone demethylation. It was not until 2004, with the discovery of histone lysine-specific demethylase 1 (LSD1, now named KDM1A) (Shi et al. 2004), that the debate on whether histone methylation could be reversibly removed and thus dynamically regulated ended, opening new avenues in the field of epigenetics.

The discovery of KDM1A was unexpected and masks many previous unsuccessful attempts. When Yujiang Geno Shi was a post-doc in Yang Shi's laboratory at Harvard Medical School, he was interested in understanding how metabolic enzymes and their homologs and cofactors were involved in epigenetic gene regulation. In particular, Geno was very curious about a protein isolated from the C-terminal-binding protein (CtBP) complex, then named nuclear polyamine oxidase (nPAO, also called KIAA0601/BHC110 at the time). Based on nPAO's homology with known polyamine oxidases, and given that polyamines such as spermine and spermidine also were minor components of chromatin, nPAO was hypothesized to regulate chromatin structure through a polyamine oxidation mechanism. However, despite months of attempts exhausting all possible biochemical experiments, Geno was unable to unambiguously prove that nPAO was a true polyamine oxidase.

Looking for a turning point, Geno explored alternate angles for new substrates and activities of nPAO. Theoretically, it is chemically possible that oxidation of methylated lysine could lead to demethylation through an amine oxidation reaction. In 2002, Tony Kouzarides nicely proposed a chemical mechanism for potential histone demethylation (Bannister et al. 2002). However, most investigators in the field believed it was unlikely due to 40 years of failing to identify such an oxidase. One day, enlightened by the chemical demethylation scheme proposed by Kouzarides (Bannister et al. 2002), Geno was staring at a drawing of the methylated lysine molecule, which had always been displayed vertically. He accidentally turned the drawing 90 degrees, laying the methylated lysine molecule horizontally and revealing a new angle for nPAO activity—the core portion of the methyl-C-N-lysine now perfectly matched the oxidative breakage point of spermine!

Geno immediately realized that nPAO could be the long-sought histone lysine demethylase. He quickly diagramed all possible chemical mechanisms for the nPAO-mediated histone demethylation reaction and chose histone 3 methylated lysine 4 (H3K4), a mark for gene activation, as the substrate for the first oxidative reaction assay. Unfortunately, however, good things are usually not found easily—the experiment did not yield the expected results. Switching the substrate to histone H3 momo-, di-, or tri-methylated at lysine 4 (H3K4me1/2/3) still did not reveal detection of nPAO-mediated histone demethylation. Yet Geno continued.

After about a month of troubleshooting, he caught a trivial but fatal error in the demethylation assay—the substrate for the nPAO demethylation assay, the 21 amino acid H3K4me1/2/3 (~ 3 kD), was too small to retain on a 10% SDS-PAGE gel and therefore was consistently lost in the assays. Nevertheless, simply switching to a 15% SDS-PAGE gel solved the problem, allowing detection of the apparent demethylation of H3K4me2! A series of subsequent experiments concluded that nPAO was a bona fide histone lysine demethylase—the first identified histone demethylase. nPAO was then renamed LSD1 (hereafter, KDM1A) (Shi et al. 2003, 2004, 2005).

KDM1A catalyzes amine oxidation by oxidative cleavage of the α-carbon bond of methylated lysine to form an imine intermediate, which is hydrolyzed to form formaldehyde, releasing one molecule of H_2O_2 and the demethylated lysine in the histone H3 peptide. Since formation of an imine intermediate requires a protonated nitrogen, KDM1A can only demethylate mono- and di-methylated lysine residues and not the tri-methylated form. Tri-methylated K4 not only correlates with the dynamic on/off gene state, but also widely exists in baker's yeast to humans. However, it is chemically impossible for KDM1A family enzymes to demethylate this species. Thus, the discovery of KDM1A also predicted the existence of additional demethylases that employ other chemical mechanisms to demethylate tri-methylated H3K4, raising the possibility of other HDM classes yet to be discovered.

In 2005, Tsukada et al. identified the first Jumonji C (JmjC) domain-containing histone demethylase, JHDM1 (Tsukada et al. 2006). The histone demethylation field then exploded—in subsequent years, > 20 histone demethylases that can actively catalyze demethylation of almost all major histone methylation sites and states (except for H3K79 methylation), have since been identified by many groups. Identification of these two distinct classes of oxidative chromatin demethylases—flavin-dependent, lysine-specific demethylases (KDM1/LSD family) and JmjC domain-containing demethylases—have shed light on the reversibility of histone methylation and revealed intricate dynamics of methylation signatures. Many laboratories have made pioneering contributions to define these new classes of histone demethylases.

With growing knowledge of their molecular mechanisms of action and biological functions, the KDM1 family has emerged as a key player in regulation of genomic information processing, as well as cellular, physiological, developmental, and pathological processes (Shao et al. 2010; Chen et al. 2012; Burg et al. 2015; Zheng et al. 2015; Maiques-Diaz and Somervaille 2016; Morera et al. 2016). The versatile functions of the KDM1 family are, in part, due to differential expression in distinctive tissue types, developmental stages, or disease processes. Moreover, complexity of their biological functions is also achieved by differential association with a variety of biomolecules that are closely involved in chromatin regulation, control of transcriptional repression, and activation of target genes. Because both genetic as well as epigenetic alterations can cause cancer, and given the unique biochemical properties and broad biological functions of KDM1, it has become increasingly evident that dysregulation of the KDM1 family of histone demethylases is likely an important epigenetic mechanism for tumor onset and progression.

The reversible nature of histone methylation and demethylation catalyzed by the KDM1 family, along with their dysregulation in cancer, makes these histone demethylases attractive and promising drug targets for pharmacological interventions (Lynch et al. 2012; Burg et al. 2015; Nowak et al. 2016; Zhou et al. 2017). A wide range of small molecule KDM1 inhibitors, including monoamine derivatives and polyamine- and peptide-based compounds, have been developed for anticancer therapy and have shown promise in several preclinical and clinical studies. While many clinical trials have been underway in recent years, development of novel KDM1 inhibitors for cancer treatment or other human diseases remains a hot topic in the pharmaceutical industry.

In the following sections, we first briefly overview current knowledge of the biochemical and molecular characterization of KDM1 family members, including their unique structural features, mechanisms of action, and interactions with various protein complexes. We also discuss the biological function and significance of these histone demethylases, with a focus on their role in normal cellular processes and cancer development. We then review the currently available KDM1 inhibitors and discuss their clinical applications to offer future directions for the rapidly growing field of epigenetic mechanism-based therapeutic strategies for cancer.

2.2 Structure, Mechanism, and Biological Function of the KDM1 Family

The highly conserved KDM1 family consists of two lysine-specific demethylases, KDM1A (also known as LSD1/AOF2/BHC110) and KDM1B (also known as LSD2/AOF1). Both use flavin adenine dinucleotide (FAD) as a coenzyme to remove one or two methyl groups from mono- or di-methylated H3K4 (Shi et al. 2004; Fang et al. 2010). Although KDM1A and KDM1B share overall amino acid sequence features critical to their catalytic function, differences in molecular structure of each protein give rise to unique cellular complex formation and diversified biological function.

2.2.1 Domain Organization and Structural Features of the KDM1 Family

Primary amino acid sequence comparison and domain prediction analysis suggests that both KDM1 proteins encompass a C-terminal amine oxidase-like (AOL) domain and a SWIRM (Swi3p/Rsc8c/Moira) domain (Fig. 2.1a). The AOL domain contains a FAD-binding subdomain, which is highly conserved with the known subfamily of amine oxidases, including monoamine oxidases (MAOs), spermine oxidase (SMO), and other polyamine oxidases (PAO) (Burg et al. 2015). This similarity in structures and conserved active catalytic sites for KDM1, MAO, and PAO vindicates that the KDM1 family of demethylases evolved from ancient amine oxidases. While essential to the catalytic action of both KDM1 family members, the SWIRM domain, which is located at the N-terminus of the catalytic domain, is important for protein stability and for interactions with histone tails of the nucleosome.

In 2006, both Stavropoulos et al. (2006) and Yang et al. (2006) presented the crystal structure of KDM1A, showing it is a highly asymmetric, closely packed structure from which a long helical "tower" domain protrudes (Fig. 2.1b). The SWIRM domain of KDM1A is intimately bound to the oxidase domain through an extensive hydrophobic interface, and the interaction between these domains forms a highly conserved cleft that serves as an additional histone tail-binding site. Further comparative analysis of the crystal structures of KDM1A, MAOs, and PAOs demonstrates that KDM1A is distinguishable from related amine oxidases by its active site cavity, as MAOs and PAOs have significantly restricted substrate accommodations and active catalytic cavities (Stavropoulos et al. 2006; Anand et al. 2007). The co-crystal structure of the KDM1A-CoREST complex reveals that the tower domain provides a surface for interaction with other proteins to form multiprotein complexes composed of CoREST, histone deacetylase 1/2 (HDAC1/2), CtBP1, and SNAIL, and it is indispensable for KDM1A demethylase activity (Burg et al. 2015).

In 2013, our group solved the crystal structure of KDM1B and the co-crystal structure of KDM1B in ternary complex with its substrate and cofactor, GLYR1 (Fang et al. 2013). Structural analysis of KDM1B uncovered a tightly packed C-terminal oxidase domain, middle SWIRM domain, and two N-terminal zinc finger domains into a boot-shaped structure (Fig. 2.1b) (Zhang et al. 2013). The active cavity in the oxidase domain is large enough to accommodate several residues of the histone H3 tail and cannot discriminate between different states of H3K4 methylation. The N-terminal zinc finger domains are composed of a novel C4H2C2-type zinc finger and a specific CW-type zinc finger, required for demethylase activity and FAD cofactor binding. The atomic structure reveals a relay of extensive interactions through the zinc finger–SWIRM–oxidase domains, explaining why these zinc fingers are required for KDM1B demethylase activity and FAD binding (Yang et al. 2010b; Zhang et al. 2013). The co-crystal structure of KDM1B ternary complex further provides molecular explanation for how GLYR1 recruits the demethylase to the vicinity of the histone H3 substrate and structurally facilitates enzyme and substrate interaction, thereby enhancing KDM1B H3K4 demethylase activity.

While sharing common enzymatic and structural similarities, KDM1A and KDM1B also have unique structural features (Fig. 2.1a, b). Unlike KDM1A's signature structure, KDM1B does not contain a tower domain. On the other hand, the N-terminal region of KDM1B contains a CW-kind zinc finger domain, while the equivalent region in KDM1A is relatively unstructured.

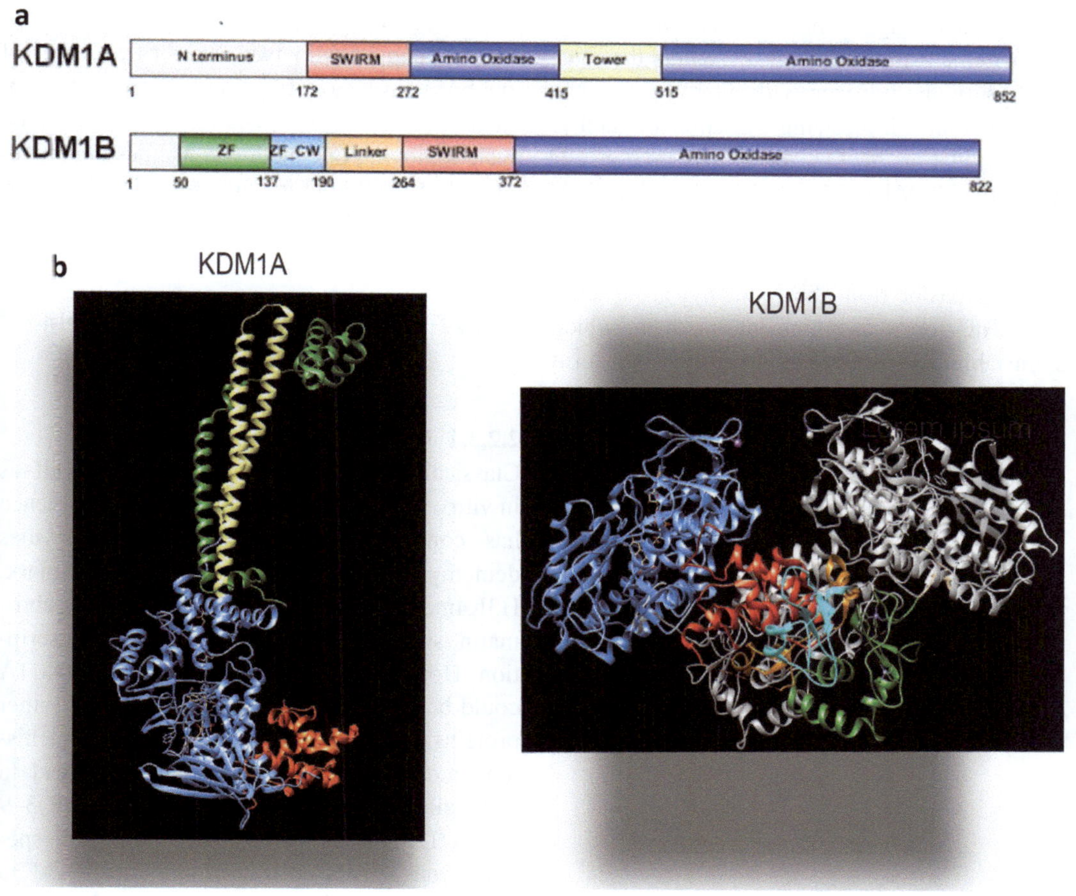

Fig. 2.1 Structural overview of KDM1 family members KDM1A and KDM1B. a Domain structures of KDM1A and KDM1B. SWIRM domains are red, amino oxidase domains are blue, tower domain is yellow, zinc finger domain is green, and linker domain is orange. **b** Ribbon representations show structural features of KDM1A and KDM1B. Left panel shows ribbon representation of KDM1A interaction with CoREST (PDB: 2IW5). Domains are colored as above, although green ribbon represents CoREST. Right panel shows ribbon representation of KDM1B interaction with GLYR1 (PDB: 4GU1). Domains are colored as above, although green ribbon represents GLYR1

Through mutational, deletional, and structural analyses, researchers have confirmed that the tower domain of KDM1A is critical for its enzymatic activity, while the N-terminal zinc finger domain is vital for demethylase activity of KDM1B.

Taken together, these detailed molecular and structural analyses provide valuable insight into protein structure, mechanism of catalysis, and regulation of enzymatic activity of the KDM1 family, laying a foundation to understand their biochemical mechanisms of action and to inform strategies to design future KDM1A- or KDM1B-specific inhibitors (Stavropoulos et al. 2006; Yang et al. 2006; Anand and Marmorstein 2007; Hou and Yu 2010; Chen et al. 2013). This is of paramount importance to develop drugs specifically targeting this family of demethylases (Lee et al. 2006).

2.2.2 Enzymatic Mechanism of Action of the KDM1 Family

Both KDM1 family members require the FAD^+ cofactor and share a similar demethylation mechanism, as they have a conserved catalytic core structure around the FAD^+ binding site.

FAD^+ cofactor tightly binds to the KDM1 protein. After substrate H3K4me1/2 enters the catalytic cavity, the nitrogen with methyl group has to be protonated, allowing initiation of methyl group oxidation by O_2. As shown in Fig. 2.2, during the KDM1-catalyzed demethylation reaction, molecular oxygen is the electron acceptor, and methyl group oxidation then proceeds via hydride transfer from the N-methyl group onto FAD. This forms an imine intermediate, which is unstable and undergoes hydrolysis to form formaldehyde (Forneris et al. 2009). The reaction is coupled with two-electron reduction of the FAD^+ cofactor, resulting in production of one molecule of H_2O_2. As a result, each catalytic cycle removing one methyl consumes one molecule of O_2 while producing one molecule of formaldehyde and H_2O_2 (Shi and Tsukada 2013).

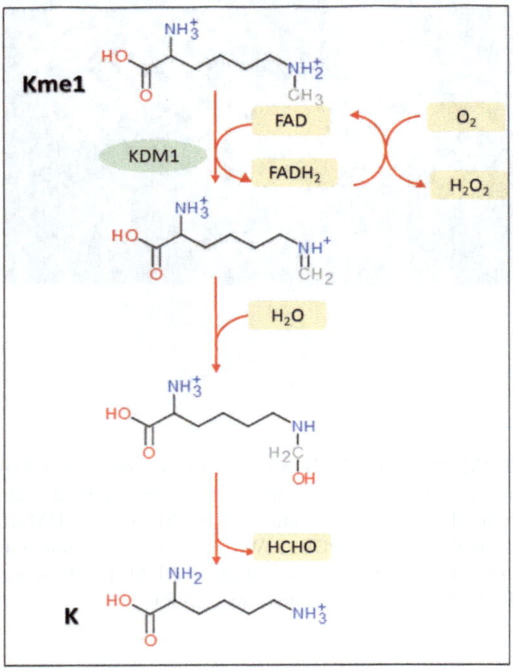

Fig. 2.2 Proposed demethylation reaction mechanism catalyzed by KDM1 (from Yujiang Geno Shi, 2013). Histone demethylation (Kme1 to K) mediated by KDM1 family demethylases through a FAD-dependent amine oxidase reaction requires cofactor FAD^+ and shares a similar demethylation mechanism. KDM1 can demethylate mono- and di-methylated states of histone lysine residues. After substrate H3K4me1 enters the catalytic cavity, KDM1 uses oxygen as the electron acceptor in demethylation reaction, and methyl group oxidation then proceeds via hydride transfer from the N-methyl group onto FAD. This forms an imine intermediate, which is unstable and will undergo hydrolysis to form formaldehyde. The reaction is coupled with two-electron reduction of the cofactor FAD^+, resulting in production of one molecule of H_2O_2

2.2.3 KDM1 Substrates and Protein Interactions

2.2.3.1 Histone Substrates

Classically, a myriad of structural as well as in vitro and in vivo biochemical evidence has concluded that KDM1 family enzymes demethylate a poised or active histone mark, H3K4me1/2, resulting in a more closed chromatin structure that represses gene transcription. However, substrate specificity of KDM1A could be modulated by its interaction with other proteins or the presence of other adjacent histone modifications, e.g., KDM1 could lead to gene silencing by forming HP1/SU(VAR)3–9 or HOTAIR/PRC2 complexes, inhibited specific genes expressed by forming core-BRAF35 or CoREST complexes, or performed nucleosome remodeling by forming NuRD complex, etc. Meanwhile, KDM1 could also act as a transcription co-activator through its ability to demethylate H3K9me1/2. Metzger et al. (2005) reported that when KDM1A is associated with the androgen receptor (AR), enzymatic specificity of KDM1A switches to demethylating the repressive histone mark, H3K9me1/2, thereby stimulating transcription of target genes. Further, Laurent et al. (2015) recently showed that in collaboration with supervillain (SVIL), KDM1A+8a—a neuronal isoform of KDM1A that has eight additional amino acids within the amino oxidase domain—also demethylates H3K9me2 in neuronal cells. This indicates that KDM1A+8a demethylation of H3K9me2 is likely due to insertion of the eight amino acids near the catalytic cavity, thereby switching demethylase activity of H3K4me1/2 to H3K9me2. These findings suggest that alternative splicing may be another underlying molecular mechanism by which KDM1A gains selective substrate specificities (H3K9 vs. H3K4) to differentially manage specific gene expression programs in neurons. Notably, a couple of studies have reported KDM1A can act as a H3K9 histone demethylase in specific cellular contexts, although the molecular mechanism for the switch from H3K4me1/2 to H3K9me1/2 substrates remains unknown (Laurent et al. 2015; Fiszbein and Kornblihtt 2016).

Despite growing evidence supporting the dual enzymatic activity of KDM1 family demethylases (H3K4 and H3K9 demethylation), there is no prevailing and unambiguous structural evidence or biochemical data from in vitro demethylase assays to support H3K9 demethylase activity of the KDM1 family. Thus, the underlying mechanism for demethylation of H3K9 by KDM1 remains elusive. This fundamental issue warrants future investigation, which may give ultimate vindication of the KDM1 family as bona fide H3K9 demethylases.

2.2.3.2 Non-histone Substrates

In addition to the most common substrate H3, non-histone proteins also are substrates for KDM1A. KDM1A can demethylate TP53 (Huang et al. 2007a), DNMT1 (Wang et al. 2008), E2F1 (Kontaki and Talianidis 2010), MYPT1 (Cho et al. 2011), STAT3 (Yang et al. 2010a), HSP90 (Abu-Farha et al. 2011), and MTA1 (Nair et al. 2013), ER α (Perillo et al. 2020), AGO2 (Sheng et al. 2018). The existence of numerous non-histone substrates for KDM1A has not only broadened the spectrum of KDM1A substrates, but also provided new molecular mechanisms of action for KDM1A in gene activation or repression, which are important for executing its diversified and complex biological functions. While both KDM1A and KDM1B have significant structural similarity at their catalytic cavity and share the common substrate H3K4me1/2 (Fang et al. 2010; Yang et al. 2010b), no non-histone substrate has been identified yet for KDM1B. However, future investigations searching for non-histone substrates of KDM1B are expected to inform new mechanisms of action of KDM1B to regulate biological or pathogenic processes.

2.2.4 Functional Interactions of KDM1 Demethylases with Other Biomolecules in Different Cellular Complexes

KDM1 family demethylases often act as catalytic subunits within specific protein complexes that play critical functional roles in a variety of biological or disease processes. KDM1A was initially identified as an unnamed and uncharacterized polypeptide and integral common subunit of the chromatin remodeling NURF complex (Lee et al. 2007; Nair et al. 2013). It was later found that KDM1A interacts with various proteins that coordinate its function in gene regulation by targeting or modulating its enzymatic activity and/or substrate specificity (for both histone and non-histone substrates) (Lee et al. 2005; Shi et al. 2005; Nicholson and Chen 2014).

KDM1A participates in several multi-protein cellular complexes, including CoREST (Lee et al. 2005; Shi et al. 2005; Foster et al. 2010), REST (Ballas et al. 2005), TLX orphan nuclear receptor (Yokoyama et al. 2008; Sun et al. 2010, 2011), CtBP (Chinnadurai 2007; Wang et al. 2007; Ray et al. 2014), NuRD (Wang et al. 2009b; Basta and Rauchman 2015), and TAL1 (Hu et al. 2009; Li et al. 2012). Proteomic analysis and biochemical characterization have revealed that KDM1A along with CoREST and HDAC1 form a core complex, known as the CoREST/KDM1A/HDAC1 complex, that interacts with other cellular factors, such as CtBP, REST, TAL1, and TLX, in different biological, physiological, or pathological processes.

Interactions within different complexes target the activity of KDM1A to distinctive biological processes and cellular activities. Moreover, other subunits associated with the core complexes likely also selectively regulate catalytic activity, substrate specificity, and localization of KDM1A at chromatin and coordinately and/or distinctively control downstream gene transcription programs (Hu et al. 2009; Ouyang et al. 2009; Sun et al. 2011; Baron and Vellore 2012; Fuentes et al. 2012; Li et al. 2012; Zhou et al. 2013; Ray et al. 2014; Burg et al. 2015; Saez et al. 2015; Lopez et al. 2016), e.g., the orphan nuclear hormone receptor TLX interacts directly with AOD and SWIRM domains of KDM1A, thereby recruiting the core complex (Sun et al. 2010) to regulate a gene program during neuronal differentiation. In addition, in breast cancer, the tower domain of KDM1A interacts with the MTA subunit of the NuRD complex to repress target gene expression that is important for control of the epithelial-to-mesenchymal transition (EMT) (Wang et al. 2009b). In both normal hematopoiesis and leukemogenesis, transcription factor TAL1 recruits KDM1A along with the core CoREST/HDAC complex to repress erythroid-specific genes in progenitor cells prior to differentiation (Li et al. 2012). These studies together provide unique insight into the molecular mechanisms of KDM1A in cellular contexts and its subsequent roles in biological processes.

In contrast to KDM1A, KDM1B does not possess a coiled-coil tower domain and hence does not interact with CoREST or cooperate with HDAC. Nevertheless, KDM1B functions as a positive regulator of gene transcription by binding to chromatin in the highly transcribed, H3K36me3-enriched coding regions downstream of gene promoters (Stewart et al. 2015). Biochemical purification and proteomic analysis indicate that KDM1B forms different multiprotein functional complexes from KDM1A. The KDM1B complex is associated with RNA polymerase II and other elongation factors, and it contains the core components GLYR1, which specifically recognizes the histone H3K36me3 mark, and interacts with the SET family histone methyltransferases (HMTs) NSD3 and G9a, which methylate histone H3K36 and H3K9 sites, respectively. Co-crystal structure and biochemical studies demonstrate that GLYR1 acts as a demethylase KDM1B cofactor, specifically enhancing KDM1B demethylation of H3K4me1/2 by binding at its AOD/SWIRM interface (Fang et al. 2013). These findings suggest that, in association with a larger transcription elongation complex, the KDM1B core complex maintains the balance of H3K4, H3K9, and H3K36 methylation at gene coding regions for active gene transcription.

In summary, despite similar catalytic activity of KDM1 family demethylases, it is clear that their association with specific cellular complexes largely determines their function in various cellular, biological, and pathological processes.

2.3 Involvement of the KDM1 Family in Different Biological Processes

Genetic studies in numerous animal models have suggested that both KDM1A and KDM1B play a significant role in cellular, physiological, and developmental processes. While the detailed biological role of KDM1B is beginning to emerge, extensive studies have already shown that KDM1A has distinct roles in stem cell differentiation, adipogenesis, neurogenesis, and skeletal muscle differentiation (Fig. 2.3) (Musri et al. 2010; Sun et al. 2010, 2011; Adamo et al. 2011; Fuentes et al. 2012; Whyte et al. 2012; Zhu et al. 2014; Laurent et al. 2015). In the following section, we review KDM1A in different biological processes.

2.3.1 Role of KDM1A in Stem Cells

The role of KDM1A in stem cell development has been well-studied since Taiping Chen and En Li' group (Wang et al. 2009a) first reported in 2009 its necessity for gastrulation during mouse embryogenesis. They found early embryo lethality in KDM1A-deficient mice at about day E6.5, which may be due to a complex abnormality of the developmental program of the

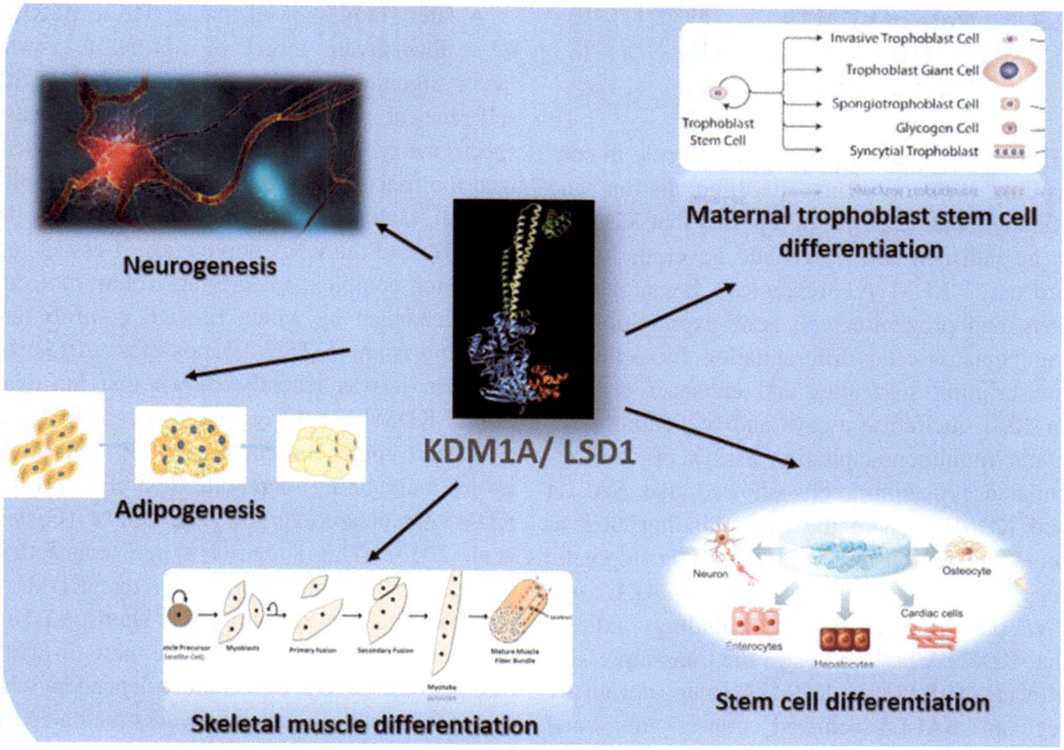

Fig. 2.3 **Summary of KDM1A's functions in physiological processes.** KDM1A has distinct roles in stem cell differentiation, adipogenesis, neurogenesis, and skeletal muscle differentiation, among other functions

KDM1A knockout mouse. Foster et al. (Foster et al. 2010) reported that KDM1A conditional knockout mouse embryonic stem cells (ESCs) were associated with neither abnormal proliferation nor alteration of their stem cell status, but rather a required role to coordinate gene expression as a key catalytic and structural component of the KDM1A/CoREST/HDAC complex required for early embryonic development.

Later chromatin immunoprecipitation-sequencing analysis by Whyte et al. (Whyte et al. 2012) revealed that KDM1A occupies enhancers and core promoters of a substantial population of actively transcribed and bivalent genes that are critical for proper control of ESCs. KDM1A is essential in decommissioning enhancers during differentiation of mouse ESCs, which is partly mediated by the NuRD complex (Whyte et al. 2012). By demethylating H3K4me1 at the enhancer of ESC-specific genes, KDM1A controls suppression of *Oct4/Sox/Nanog*-related target genes upon differentiation. In ESCs, KDM1A–NuRD complex is also proposed to bind to *Oct4*-active enhancers, although it cannot demethylate H3K4 because KDM1A activity is repressed by acetylated histones. Therefore, coordinated regulation of both histone acetyltransferases and NuRD-related HDACs controls histone acetylation at enhancers, fine-tuning KDM1A demethylation to set the on/off switch for activation of an array of enhancers of key pluripotent ESC genes. These studies provide a mechanistic model for how KDM1A is involved in embryonic development, suggesting that KDM1A likely regulates ESC differentiation by silencing active enhancers of key pluripotent ESC genes instead of preserving the ESC state (Whyte et al. 2012).

2.3.2 Role of KDM1A in Hematopoietic Cell Differentiation

Histone methylation plays a central role in controlling hematopoietic cell differentiation, and Kerenyi et al. (2013) first reported that KDM1A is an indispensable epigenetic governor in this process. KDM1A represses hematopoietic stem and progenitor cell gene expression during hematopoietic differentiation by acting at transcription start sites and enhancer regions. In 2013, luciferase assays and sequential chromatin immunoprecipitation assays of undifferentiated progenitor cells showed that SALL4 and KDM1A share the same binding sites at promoter regions of important hematopoietic regulatory genes, including *EBF1*, *GATA1*, and *TNF* (Liu et al. 2013). These findings indicate that KDM1A participates in the trans-repressive effects of SALL4. KDM1A may negatively regulate SALL4-mediated transcription, and the dynamic regulation of SALL4-associated epigenetic events by KDM1A may cooperatively modulate early hematopoietic precursor proliferation.

2.3.3 Role of KDM1A in Maternal Trophoblast Stem Cell Differentiation

Zhu et al. (2014) first demonstrated that KDM1A controls the onset of maternal trophoblast stem cell (TSC) differentiation and that deletion of KDM1A in mice resulted in decreased TSCs, diminished formation of trophectoderm tissues, and early embryonic lethality. KDM1A-deficient TSCs display features of differentiation initiation, including abnormal changes in cell morphology and increased migration and invasion, which are related to early expression of OVOL2, a transcription factor directly suppressed by KDM1A in undifferentiated cells. These findings indicate the role of KDM1A as a gatekeeper for initiation of TSC differentiation and migration (Zhu et al. 2014).

A later study showed that in TSCs, ESRRB is a downstream target of fibroblast growth factor signaling and is critical to drive TSC self-renewal (Latos et al. 2015). Using mass spectrometry, the authors further characterized the functional role of ESRRB in TSC self-renewal. Unlike in ESCs, ESRRB interacts with KDM1A and the RNA polymerase II-associated integrator complex, underlying a new molecular mechanism by which ESRRB controls target expression in TSCs (Latos et al. 2015). In addition, it was recently shown that inactivation of KDM1A can trigger senescence in TSCs and direct epigenetic control of TSC immortality by maintaining metabolic flexibility via the KDM1A-repressed target gene *SIRT4* (Castex et al. 2017). This suggests a new connection between cell metabolic pathways and KDM1A regulation in maternal TSC status. Taken together, these findings provide new insights into both the general and context-dependent wiring of transcription factor networks mediated by KDM1A in TSCs.

2.3.4 Role of KDM1A in Adipose Differentiation and Metabolism

Crosstalk between epigenetic modifications and cell metabolism via different chromatin modifiers has led to new understanding of cellular pathways and molecular mechanisms underlying metabolic disorders. With a growing number of studies on the functional role and molecular mechanism of KDM1A in different fat tissues, mounting evidence has started to shed light on the role of KDM1A as a metabolic environment sensor and on its function in adipogenesis as well as thermogenesis (Hino et al. 2012; Chen et al. 2016; Sambeat et al. 2016; Zeng et al. 2016; Duteil et al. 2017).

KDM1A was first discovered in 2010 to play a role in adipocyte development by maintaining H3K4 di-methylation and decreasing H3K9 di-methylation at the promoter of C/EBP, a key transcription factor for adipogenesis (Musri et al. 2010). KDM1A was later discovered to be a key epigenetic regulator promoting brown adipogenesis by demethylation of H3K4 at promoter regions of Wnt signaling components, which represses transcription and suppresses Wnt signaling—critical for anti-differentiation of brown adipocytes (Chen et al. 2016).

Apart from adipocyte differentiation, KDM1A also plays an important part in adipocyte energy expenditure, the key function of brown adipose tissue (Sambeat et al. 2016; Zeng et al. 2016; Straub and Wolfrum 2017). In mature adipocytes, KDM1A responds to different environmental stimuli to alter metabolic function and enable proper thermogenic and oxidative responses (Hino et al. 2012; Duteil et al. 2014; Zeng et al. 2016). As a pivotal regulator of body energy expenditure, KDM1A interacts with PRDM16 to repress selective white adipose tissue genes (Duteil et al. 2014). Further, KDM1A also represses hydroxysteroid 11-β-dehydrogenase 1 (HSD11B1) to prevent production of glucocorticoids that impair brown adipose tissue functions (Zeng et al. 2016). In recent years, studies have also shown a critical role of KDM1A in programed beige cell loss with aging (Duteil et al. 2017). Taken together, these studies identify KDM1A as a key epigenetic regulator of beige fat cell maintenance and provide new insights into the mechanisms of controlling the age-related beige-to-white adipocyte transition.

2.3.5 Role of KDM1A in Skeletal Muscle Differentiation

Skeletal muscle differentiation is another well-orchestrated biological process and is under tight control of master transcription factors MyoD and Mef2 (Buckingham 1994; Molkentin and Olson 1996; Mal and Harter 2003; Taylor and Hughes 2017). HMTs and HDACs regulate MyoD and Mef2 to switch on and off specific programs of target genes (Lu et al. 2000; Steinbac et al. 2000; Dressel et al. 2001; Chan et al. 2003; Zhang et al. 2016). KDM1A physically interacts with MyoD and MEF2 on promoters of target genes to regulate C2C12 mouse myoblast differentiation (Choi et al. 2010). Interruption of KDM1A by shRNAs or chemical inhibitors leads to aberrant histone modifications on myogenic promoters and results in impaired skeletal muscle differentiation. Further, both G9a and KDM1A regulate MEF2D activity in skeletal muscle differentiation (Choi et al. 2014). Scionti et al. (2017) demonstrated that KDM1A is required for timely expression of MyoD in limb buds by activating RNA polymerase II-dependent transcription of enhancers. They also showed that depletion of KDM1A in myoblasts precludes removal of H3K9 methylation and RNA polymerase II recruitment to the core enhancer, thereby preventing transcription of the non-coding enhancer RNA required for MyoD expression. These studies together provide new perspectives on how KDM1A regulates muscle differentiation together with other key transcription factors.

2.3.6 Role of KDM1A in Neurogenesis

Neuronal differentiation is a highly complex process involving strict regulation of proliferation as well as acquisition of distinct neural morphology and functionality (Kalyani and Rao 1998; Urban and Guillemot 2014). KDM1A regulation of gene expression occurs in the brain and nervous system, regulating neuronal differentiation, proliferation, and memory in neuronal physiology processes (Fuentes et al. 2012). In mouse neural stem cells (NSC), KDM1A is required to maintain proliferative capacity through its interaction with an NSC maintenance factor, TLX (Sun et al. 2010). On the other hand, KDM1A in human NSCs mediates neuronal differentiation by repressing a Notch-target gene, *HEYL*. KDM1A directly associates with the promoter of *HEYL* and controls demethylation of H3K4me2, resulting in repressed *HEYL* expression during NSC differentiation (Hirano and Namihira 2016). As previously described, KDM1A can also mediate H3K9me demethylation via a specific isoform in collaboration with other transcription factors (Laurent et al. 2015). These data suggest that KDM1A differentially controls specific gene expression programs during neuronal differentiation (Laurent et al. 2015). Loss of KDM1A gene expression causes a variety of neurodegenerative diseases, such as Alzheimer's disease (AD), frontotemporal dementia (FTD) (Kim et al. 2021).

2.3.7 Emerging Biological Roles for KDM1B

Compared with the well-studied KDM1A, much less is known about the biological roles of KDM1B. Genetic studies in animal models have suggested that KDM1B also plays a significant yet distinctive role in cellular, physiological, and developmental processes. Some reports have described it as an effector of genomic imprinting (Holmes et al. 2012) and a regulator of cellular metabolism in liver (Nagaoka et al. 2015). However, studies are now emerging concerning the biological function and pathogenic roles of KDM1B. It was recently demonstrated to possess E3 ubiquitin ligase activity and inhibit lung cancer cell growth by promoting ubiquitination and degradation of OGT (Yang et al. 2015). In addition, KDM1B has been implicated in regulating breast cancer proliferation (Huang et al. 2012; Katz et al. 2014; Chen et al. 2017). In recent years, it was also reported that KDM1B could be triggered by type I interferons (IFNs-I), which can function as molecular hubs of resistance during immunogenic chemotherapy, resulting an adaptive yet reversible, transcriptional rewiring of cancer cells toward stemness and immune escape (Musella et al. 2022). While the detailed biological role of KDM1B is just beginning to emerge, new discoveries regarding the biological functions and pathological effects of KDM1B dysfunction on human diseases will continue to add new layers to the understanding of its biology.

2.4 KDM1A and Cancer Development

In the past decade, mounting evidence has indicated that both expression and activity of KDM1A directly relate to cancer development, especially in hematopoietic neoplasms such as acute myeloid leukemia (AML) (Schenk et al. 2012; Sprussel et al. 2012). KDM1A is also overexpressed in numerous solid tumors, including gastric (Zheng et al. 2013), esophageal (Yu et al. 2013; Chen et al. 2014), breast (Lim et al. 2010), lung (Stewart and Byers 2015; Mohammad et al. 2016), colon (Ding et al. 2013; Jie et al. 2013), prostate (Kahl et al. 2006; Willmann et al. 2012), and bladder (Hayami et al. 2011) cancers (Fig. 2.4). Downregulation of KDM1A expression may have anti-proliferative as well as inhibitory effects on cell migration and invasion in cancer cells. The molecular mechanism of action of KDM1A in carcinogenesis remains largely elusive and is still under intensive investigation by many cancer researchers as a therapeutic target.

KDM1A may involve several key aspects of cancer development. (1) KDM1A is involved regulating several cell pathways related to proliferation and cell cycle control (Stazi et al. 2016). For instance, KDM1A knockdown or pharmacological inhibition can reactivate expression of tumor suppressor genes in cancer cells (Huang et al. 2009b; Hayami et al. 2011). In addition, KDM1A deficiency can induce partial cell cycle arrest in G2/M stage as well as DNA damage, which delays p53 stabilization and suppresses cell growth (Huang et al. 2007a; Scoumanne et al. 2007). Further, KDM1A has a pro-oncogenic function by modulating pro-survival gene expression and p53 transcriptional activity (Scoumanne and Chen 2007). (2) KDM1A is intimately linked to regulation of EMT, the process by which an adhesive epithelial cell transforms into an invasive mesenchymal phenotype, representing a hallmark of aggressive cancers with high risk of metastasis (Sun et al. 2016). Several reports have shown

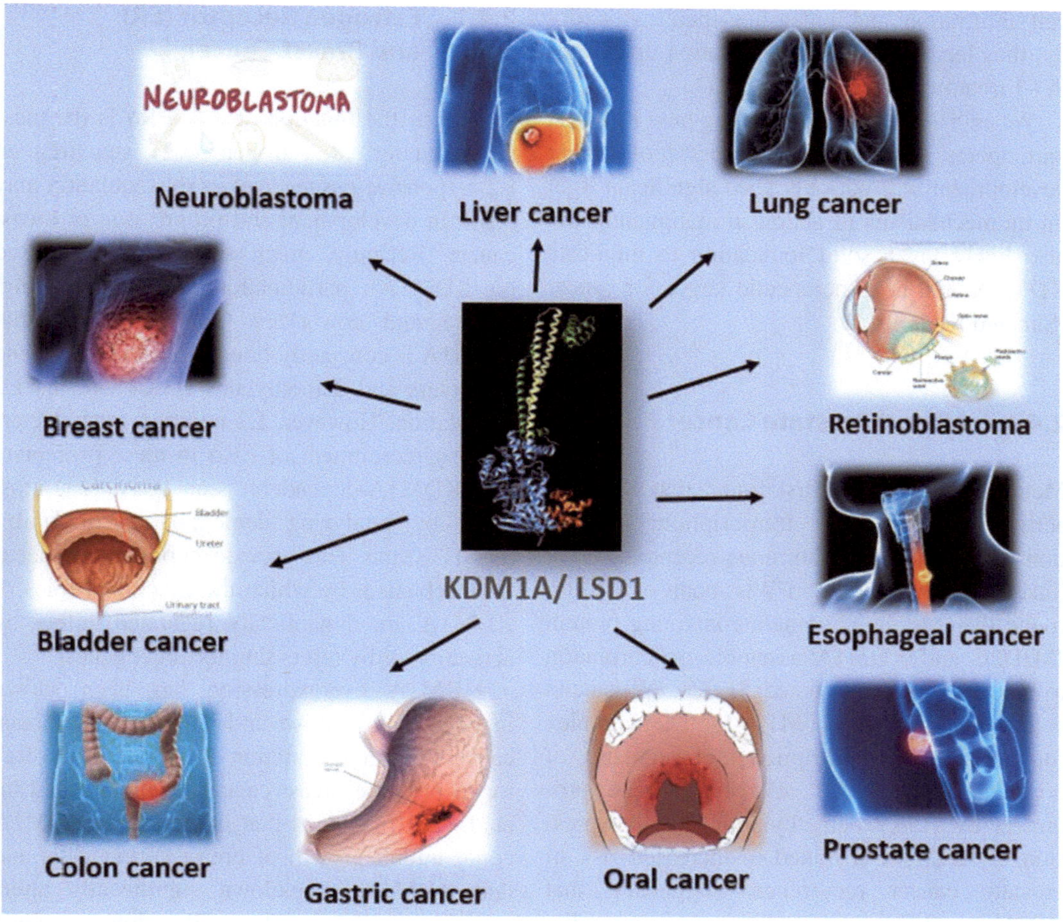

Fig. 2.4 **Summary of KDM1A's involvement in cancer development**. KDM1A is involved in many different types of solid tumors, including gastric, esophageal, breast, lung, colon, prostate, and bladder cancers

that KDM1A, as an established functional partner of the EMT master regulator SNAI1, cooperates to silence epithelial genes (Lin et al. 2010a, b). It also regulates upstream inducers of EMT, including TGFβ (Wang et al. 2009b), WNT (Huang et al. 2009b, 2013, 2017), and NOTCH (Mulligan et al. 2011; Lopez et al. 2016). (3) KDM1A is an integrative regulator of the glycolytic shift in cancer cells and has an essential role in maintaining cancer cells' metabolism. Inhibition of KDM1A reduces glucose uptake and glycolytic activity with concurrent activation of mitochondrial respiration, inducing cancer cell apoptosis (Hino et al. 2016). (4) Several recent studies have also shown that KDM1A plays an important role in disabling cancer immune checkpoints, thereby promoting cancer evasion of immune surveillance (Sheng et al. 2018; Wei et al. 2018). Liu et al. showed that both genetic perturbation or small molecules targeting KDM1A could increase the persistence of the progenitor exhausted CD8+T cells, providing conversion to more terminally exhausted T cells with tumor-killing cytotoxicity, resulting effective and durable responses to anti-PD1 therapy (Liu et al. 2021). A recent study also suggested that co-targeting KDM1A and TGFβ cooperatively could elevate intratumoral CD8+T cell infiltration and unleashes their cytotoxicity, thus leading to tumor eradication upon anti-PD-1 treatment (Sheng et al. 2021).

We envision that understanding how KDM1A participates in these varied aspects of cancer development will not only shed significant light on its mechanisms of action in malignancy, but also likely lay a solid foundation to implicate KDM1A as a new therapeutic target for cancer (Sun and Fang 2016).

2.4.1 AR and Prostate Cancer

Metzger et al. (2005) first found that KDM1A activity is critical for transcriptional regulation by AR, a nuclear hormone receptor closely linked to prostate cancer. Wissmann et al. later found that AR, JmjC domain-containing protein JMJD2C and KDM1A assemble on chromatin to demethylate methylated H3K9 (Wissmann et al. 2007). The KDM1A–JMJD2 complex functions as a transcriptional co-regulator of hormone-activated AR at specific gene promoters by H3K9 demethylation. High expression of KDM1A is linked to increased risk of prostate cancer recurrence, suggesting that KDM1A may be a novel biomarker to predict prostate cancers with aggressive biology (Kahl et al. 2006). Further, KDM1A inhibition silences AR-regulated gene expression and severely impairs androgen-dependent proliferation of cancer cells in vitro and in vivo (Wang et al. 2015). A recent study showed that KDM1A-mediated epigenetic reprogramming in castration-resistant prostate cancer activates cell cycle genes, including *CENPE*, and drives prostate cancer progression (Liang et al. 2017). These studies, together with many others, suggest a possible molecular and epigenetic mechanism of action of KDM1A in prostate cancer. More importantly, they also provide new perspective for drugs targeting KDM1A to treat prostate cancer, particularly castration-resistant prostate cancer (Liang et al. 2017).

2.4.2 Estrogen Receptor (ER) and Breast Cancer

Similar to the function of AR, ERα is the master regulator of estrogen (E2) signaling in E2-responsive tissues, and its dysregulation may result in development and progression of breast cancer. Recently, much attention has focused on KDM1A's participation in ERα signaling. Ombra and coworkers (2013) reported that KDM1A is constantly bound to ERα target gene promoters and demethylates H3K4 with no E2 stimulation. However, E2 addition is characterized by recruitment of ERα to these promoters and KDM1A-dependent gene activation, most likely by catalyzing demethylation of inhibitory H3K9me. This provides a possible molecular mechanism by which the functional roles of KDM1A are dynamically regulated, either by activating or by repressing its target genes.

KDM1A overexpression has been shown in both ERα-positive and ERα-negative breast cancers and may function as an oncogenic factor to promote breast cancer development. Lim et al. (2010) showed that inhibition of KDM1A could inhibit growth of breast cancer cells and that KDM1A knockdown significantly alters expression of several proliferation-associated genes, such as *p21*, *ERBB2*, and *CCNA2*. Other studies also show that the KDM1A/CoREST/HDAC and ZNF217 complex in collaboration with TGFβ signaling controls expression of a key gene program critical to cancer cell invasion and metastasis (Banck et al. 2009; Wang et al. 2009b; Sehrawat et al. 2018).

Recently, several studies have demonstrated that KDM1A-specific inhibitors have synergistic therapeutic effects when used in conjunction with anti-E2 treatment tamoxifen (Bennani-Baiti 2012; Bennesch et al. 2016) and HDAC inhibitors (Vasilatos et al. 2013). In line with these results, Ota et al. (2016) designed PCPA-tamoxifen conjugates that released 4-hydroxy-tamoxifen in the presence of KDM1A in vitro. These conjugates effectively inhibited growth of breast cancer cells and simultaneously inhibited KDM1A and ER without cytotoxicity toward non-cancer cells, paving the way for new drug designs that more effectively treat breast cancer based on the mechanism of action of KDM1A.

2.4.3 Acute Myeloid Leukemia (AML)

AML, a common hematological cancer of myeloid lineage cells, generally has a poor clinical prognosis and thus demands new therapy strategies. With the advancement of next-generation sequencing, mutations or genetic alterations in many epigenetic modifiers, including DNMT3A (Yan et al. 2011; Ribeiro et al. 2012; Russler-Germain et al. 2014), TET2 (He et al. 2011; Pastor et al. 2013; Cimmino et al. 2017), IDH1/2 (Figueroa et al. 2010; Reitman et al. 2011), EZH2 (Ernst et al. 2010, 2012; Nikoloski et al. 2010), and KDM1A (Lokken and Zeleznik-Le 2012; Schenk et al. 2012), have been implied in the initiation and progression of AML. In 2012, Schenk et al. (2012) demonstrated that KDM1A inhibitors unlock the resistance of all-trans retinoic acid (ATRA; the carboxylic acid form of vitamin A)-driven therapeutic response in non-acute promyelocytic leukemia (APL) AML by increasing H3K4me2 and inducing expression of myeloid differentiation-associated genes (Fig. 2.5). This study revealed the mechanism by which KDM1A inhibits the normal pro-differentiated function of ATRA and showed a more potent anti-leukemic effect of ATRA in combination with tranylcypromine (TCP) than ATRA alone. Further, Harris et al. (2012) showed that KDM1A cooperates with the mixed lineage leukemia MTase fusion protein to maintain an oncogenic transcription program in a mouse model of mixed lineage leukemia cells. Importantly, the authors

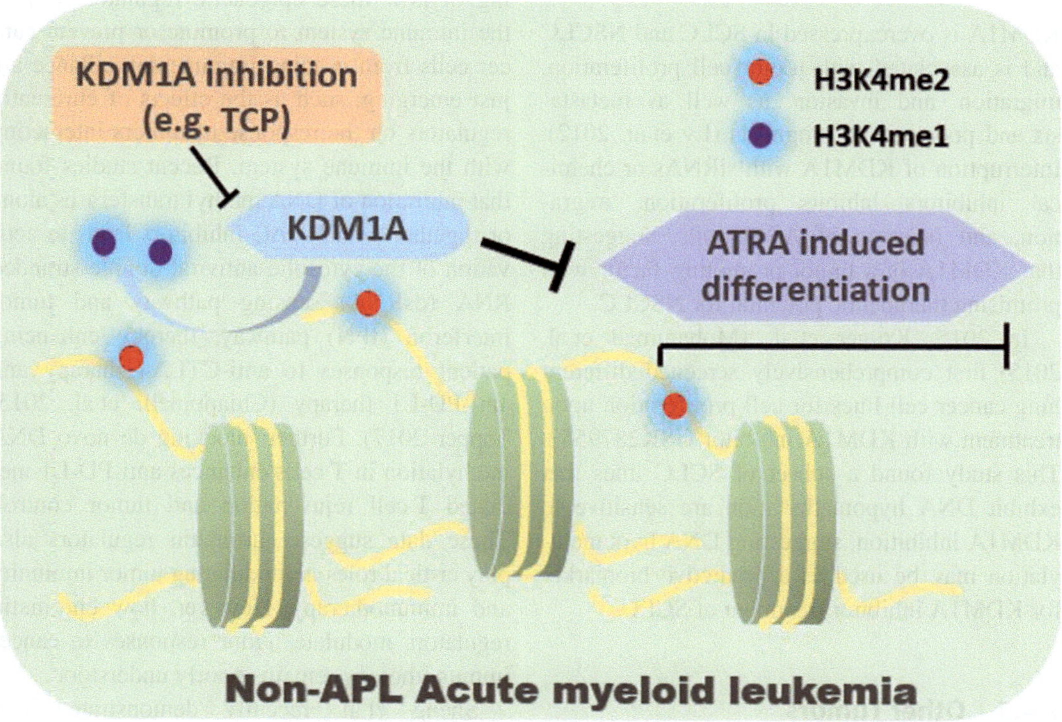

Fig. 2.5 Pharmacological inhibition of KDM1A with ATRA to regulate chromatin modification and gene expression in AML. KDM1A inhibitor TCP can reactivate ATRA-induced differentiation in non-APL AML

also showed that KDM1A inhibitors preferentially reduce the repopulation potential of these leukemia cells over normal hematopoietic cells. In addition, treatment of cultured and primary AML blasts with reversible KDM1A antagonist SP2509 and pan-HDAC inhibitor panobinostat is synergistically lethal (Fiskus et al. 2014).

Due to the growth inhibitory effects of KDM1A inhibitors on AML cells in vitro, KDM1A has emerged as a potential novel target with both preclinical and clinical efficacy in AML. Currently, several different classes of KDM1A inhibitors are being combined with ATRA in clinical trials for AML. In addition, a phase I/II trial of ATRA in conjunction with TCP commenced in 2014 for AML patients who cannot tolerate intensive chemotherapy.

2.4.4 Small Cell Lung Cancer (SCLC) and Non-small Cell Lung Cancer (NSCLC)

KDM1A is overexpressed in SCLC and NSCLC and is associated with tumor cell proliferation, migration, and invasion, as well as metastasis and poor patient prognosis (Lv et al. 2012). Interruption of KDM1A with siRNAs or chemical inhibitors inhibits proliferation, migration, and invasion of A549 cells, suggesting that KDM1A is a tumor-promoting factor with promising therapeutic potential for NSCLC.

In 2015, Kruger et al. (Mohammad et al. 2015) first comprehensively screened different lung cancer cell lines for cell proliferation upon treatment with KDM1A inhibitor GSK2879552. This study found a subset of SCLC lines that exhibit DNA hypomethylation are sensitive to KDM1A inhibition, suggesting DNA hypomethylation may be used as a predictive biomarker for KDM1A inhibitor treatment of SCLC.

2.4.5 Other Tumors

Apart from the most common tumors, KDM1A is also indicated in other tumor types, including colorectal cancer (Ding et al. 2013; Huang et al. 2013), gastrointestinal cancer (Zheng et al. 2013; Ray et al. 2014; Li et al. 2016), neuroblastoma (Schulte et al. 2009), melanoma (Schulte et al. 2009; Xu et al. 2013), and thyroid cancer (Zhang et al. 2022a). Studies show that KDM1A inhibition decreases cell proliferation of these cancers in vitro and reduces tumor growth in xenograft models. However, little research has been done on these cancers, so KDM1A's functional role and mechanism of action are much less understood. Therefore, additional investigation is needed to delineate KDM1A's role in other cancers.

2.4.6 Emerging Role of KDM1 in Cancer Cell Evasion of Immune Surveillance

The functional roles of epigenetic regulators in cancer cells have been broadly and intensively investigated. However, our understanding of how these epigenetic regulators impact the immune system to promote or prevent cancer cells from evading immune surveillance are just emerging, such as the effects of chromatin regulators on the response of tumors interacting with the immune system. Recent studies found that inhibition of DNA methyl transferases alone or together with HDAC inhibitors leads to activation of the cytosolic antiviral double-stranded RNA (dsRNA) sensing pathway and tumor interferon (IFN) pathway, thereby enhancing patient responses to anti-CTLA4 therapy and anti-PD-L1 therapy (Chiappinelli et al. 2015; Topper 2017). Further, blocking de novo DNA methylation in T cells enhances anti-PD-L1-mediated T cell rejuvenation and tumor control. These data suggest chromatin regulators also play critical roles in modulating tumor immunity and immunotherapy. However, how chromatin regulators modulate tumor responses to cancer immunotherapy remains poorly understood.

Sheng et al. recently demonstrated that KDM1A, which is often overexpressed in tumors, plays a critical role in suppressing endogenous dsRNA levels and IFN responses in tumor cells (Sheng et al. 2018). Importantly,

KDM1A inhibition by genetic knockout or chemical inhibitors promotes upregulation of endogenous retroviral elements and activates type I IFN, reactivating potent antitumor T cell immunity and significantly increasing tumor cell responsiveness to anti-PD-1 therapy (Sheng et al. 2018). Mechanistically, on one hand, these results identify TLR3 and MDA5 as critical players responsible for KDM1A loss-induced IFN signaling. On the other hand, KDM1A knockdown downregulates DICER, AGO2, and TRBP2, key components of the RNA-induced silencing complex (Chendrimada et al. 2005; Daniels et al. 2009). Further, AGO2, DICER, or TRBP2 knockdown expectedly results in dsRNA accumulation and activation of IFN signaling. Importantly, these results also reveal that AGO2 is a bona fide KDM1A substrate—KDM1A demethylates AGO2 and promotes AGO2 stabilization, while KDM1A inhibition increases AGO2 methylation and destabilizes the protein. Functionally, KDM1A-depleted tumors have increased CD8+ tumor-infiltrating lymphocytes, MHC class I antigen expression, and immune checkpoint PD-L1. Moreover, KDM1A depletion overcomes resistance to anti-PD-1 antibody in a melanoma model.

In a recent work by Chen et al., it was reported that KDM1A deletion decreases exosomal PD-L1 and restores T cell response in gastric cancer, indicating a new mechanism with which KDM1A may regulate cancer immunity in gastric cancer (Chen et al. 2016). Nguyen et al. also reported a previously uncharacterized role for KDM1A as a regulator of MHC-I antigen presentation in SCLC, as KDM1A inhibition enables MHC-I-restricted T cell cytolysis, induces immune activation, and augments the antitumor immune response to immune checkpoint blockade in SCLC (Nguyen et al. 2022).

Thus, KDM1A is likely a negative regulator of antitumor immunity and overexpression of KDM1A in tumors may be partly responsible for the resistance of tumor cells to immunotherapy—suggesting a key role of KDM1A in cancer immune surveillance. It is possible that chemical inhibitors of KDM1A could potentially turn "cold" tumors "hot." Large-scale mutational analyses have indicated that epigenetic regulators are frequently mutated groups of genes, and chromatin dysregulation is often observed in cancer (Baylin 2011; Baylin and Jones 2011; Dawson and Kouzarides 2012; Dawson et al. 2012; Flavahan et al. 2017).

We envision that understanding the functional roles of other important epigenetic regulators through future investigations involving cancer immune surveillance will pave new avenues for combinational cancer immunotherapy.

2.5 KDM1 Demethylase as a Target in Cancer Therapy

Our growing understanding of the role of epigenetic dysfunction in cancer initiation and progression has paved the way for development of epigenetic-based therapeutics. As discussed throughout the chapter, reversible histone methylation and its role in cancer has led to the identification of lysine methyltransferases and demethylases as promising targets to develop new anticancer drugs. Further, not only is there a strong link between abnormal KDM1A expression and development of various cancer types, but clinical data analysis also demonstrates that KDM1A expression has a close correlation with tumor-node-metastasis staging, distant metastasis, and poor prognosis. Since KDM1A is elevated in various types of tumors, it is considered an important tumor oncogene. Therefore, many pharmacological inhibitors of KDM1A have been increasingly developed and shown to inhibit tumor cell proliferation, invasion, migration, and tested as candidates for anticancer therapy (Table 2.1).

2.6 Classes of KDM1 Inhibitors

2.6.1 MAO Inhibitors and Derivatives

Because KDM1A is a MAO-A/B homolog, the earliest tested KDM1A inhibitors were irreversible MAO inhibitors (MAOi), which were selected based on similarity between the

Table 2.1 Classes of KDM1A inhibitors from in vitro and in vivo studies

Selectivity	First described	Biochemical activity	In vitro study	In vivo study (xenograft)	Other references
Nonselective	Lee et al. (2006)	IC50 = 27.8 μM	AML/breast cancer cell	AML/oral squamous cell carcinoma	Harris et al. (2012), Ferrari-Amorotti et al. (2014), Wang et al. (2016)
MAO-B	Metzger et al. (2005)	Active at 1 mM	Hela/ NSCLC cell	Breast cancer/glioma	Huang et al. (2012), Sareddy et al. (2013)
Nonselective	Culhane et al. (2010)	Ki = 5.6 μM	hiPSCs		Yan et al. (2016)
KDM1A	Gooden et al. (2008)	IC_{50} = 1.9 μM			
KDM1A	Benelkebir et al. (2011)	IC_{50} = 111 μM	LNCaP		
KDM1A	Mimasu et al. (2010)	IC_{50} = 0.99 μM	HEK293		Benner et al. (2013)
Nonselective	Schmitt et al. (2013)	IC50 = 44.0 μM	Breast cancer cell		
KDM1A	Pollock et al. (2012)	Ki = 352 ± 76 μM	Breast cancer cell		
KDM1A	Vianello et al. (2016)	IC50 = 0.084 μM	THP-1 cell	Genetic APL mouse model	
KDM1A	Prusevich et al. (2014)	IC50 = 14 μM	LNCaP/H460		
KDM1A	Ueda et al. (2009)	IC50 = 2.5 μM	HEK293	Prostate cancer xenograft	Ueda et al. (2009), Cortez et al. (2012), Sareddy et al. (2013), Etani et al. (2015), Hoshino et al. (2016)
KDM1A, MAO-A	Neelamegam et al. (2012)	IC_{50} = 0.07 μM		Behaving animals	Benner et al. (2013)
KDM1A	Liang et al. (2013)	IC_{50} = 0.02 μM	HeLa/HFF cell	Mouse ganglion explant model	
KDM1A	Wang et al. (2011)	IC50 = 5.27 μM	Ovarian cancer cell		
KDM1A	Wang et al. (2011)	IC50 = 10.54 μM	Colorectal cancer		Hsu et al. (2015)
KDM1A	Kakizawa et al. (2015)	IC_{50} = 0.148 μM			
KDM1A	Culhane et al. (2010)	Ki = 17.6 μM			
KDM1A	Tortorici et al. (2013)				

(continued)

Table 2.1 (continued)

Selectivity	First described	Biochemical activity	In vitro study	In vivo study (xenograft)	Other references
KDM1A	Huang et al. (2007b)	$IC_{50} = 13\ \mu M$	Breast/lung cancer cell	AML and colon cancer xenograft	Huang et al. (2009a, b), Schenk et al. (2012)
KDM1A	Huang et al. (2009a, b)	$IC_{50} = 5\ \mu M$	Colorectal cancer cell	Colon cancer xenograft	
KDM1A					
KDM1A	Nowotarski et al. (2015)	$IC_{50} = 6\ \mu M$	Breast/lung cancer cell		
KDM1A	Abdulla et al. (2013)				
KDM1A					
KDM1A					
KDM1A	Rotili et al. (2014)	$IC_{50} < 1\ \mu M$			
KDM1A	Han et al. (2015)	$IC_{50} = 0.93\ \mu M$	Colon cancer cell		
KDM1A	Zhou et al. (2015)	$IC_{50} = 1.7$ nM	Different cancer cells		
KDM1A	Willmann et al. (2012)	$IC_{50} = 51\ \mu M$	LNCaP	Prostate cancer	
KDM1A	Wu et al. (2012)		LNCaP/PC3		
KDM1A	(Sorna et al. 2013)	IC50 = 13 nM	Multiple cancer cells	Ewing's sarcoma	Sankar et al. (2013), Fiskus et al. (2014), Zhou et al. (2015)

Abbreviation: *AML* acute myeloid leukemia; *TCP* tranylcypromine; *hiPSC* human induced pluripotent stem cell

catalytic domain of MAO and KDM1A. TCP (brand name: Parnate), a MAOi previously used to treat depression, was one of the first applied KDM1A inhibitors. Lee et al. (2006) assessed inhibition of KDM1A via kinetic analysis and determined that TCP was a mechanistic inactivator that formed a covalent adduct with the FAD cofactor. Pargyline and phenelzine are the other irreversible MAOIs that have also been shown to be weaker KDM1A inhibitors than TCP. Pargyline forms a covalent adduct with FAD and effectively blocks KDM1A-dependent demethylation of H3K9 and, consequently, AR-dependent transcription in LNCaP cell culture (Metzger et al. 2005). Pargyline shows low potency for KDM1A inhibition in vitro and in tumor xenograft models (Schmidt and McCafferty 2007; Kauffman et al. 2011). However, these MAOIs have higher specificity and selectivity for MAOs than KDM1A. Hence, many research groups have tried to develop compounds with higher specificity toward KDM1A, using TCP as the principal skeleton.

In 2009, the Miyata group (Ueda et al. 2009) first designed and synthesized TCP-lysine hybrid compounds 1 and 2 based on the reported X-ray crystal structure of KDM1A. The study identified and characterized these compounds as cell-active and selective-KDM1A inhibitors, both 400–11,000 times more robust than TCP. Guided by predictions of docking of TCP derivatives into the active site of KDM1A, Yokoyama et al. (Mimasu et al. 2010) designed and synthesized candidate KDM1A inhibitor S2101 based on the structures of KDM1A and MAOs in complex with TCP derivative. Compared with TCP, S2101 exhibits stronger and more selective KDM1A inhibition and has weaker inhibition of MAOs. In the same year, Binda et al. (2010) designed compound 14e and evaluated its biological activity in a cellular model of APL. They observed unprecedented synergistic activity of compound 14e with anti-leukemia drugs, suggesting the role of KDM1A inhibitor as an epigenetic tool to alter chromatin state and block tumor progression. In 2011, Benelkebir et al. (2011) synthesized the first enantio-selective TCP analogs as KDM1A inhibitors. They found the *para*-bromo analog compound 4c inhibited growth of prostate cancer cell line LNCaP with an IC_{50} of 111 μM. Ogasawara et al. (2011) reported NCL-1 as the first cell-active, KDM1A-selective inhibitor and showed its preferential inhibition of KDM1A over MAOs. Later, Vianello et al. (2014) designed carbon 1-substituted cyclopropylamine derivatives from the TCP scaffold and proved their selectivity over MAO enzymes.

Except for TCP-based MAO derivatives, irreversible MAOi phenelzine has also been targeted as a feasible skeleton. In 2014, Cole et al. (Prusevich et al. 2014) determined the phenelzine analog bizine is a KDM1A inhibitor that can reduce cell proliferation rate in two cancer cell lines, LNCaP and H460. This inhibitor also has a synergistic effect on cell growth when used in combination with HDAC inhibitors.

Several research groups have further optimized potency and selectivity of the new class of KDM1 inhibitors. More compounds and TCP derivatives have been designed, synthesized, and evaluated both in vitro and in vivo. Among them, several members of an arylcyclopropylamine inhibitor class have reached clinical development, including ORY-1001 (Oryzon Genomics in Spain, also known as RG6016) and GSK2879552 (GlaxoSmithKline in USA). In 2013, Oryzon reported ORY-1001 is a potent and selective KDM1A inhibitor ($IC_{50} = 18$ nM; >1000-fold selectivity over MAOs and KDM1B) that possesses good oral bioavailability. Preclinical studies show that treatment with ORY-1001 results in time- and dose-dependent H3K4me2 accumulation at KDM1A target genes and induction of differentiation markers in THP-1 cells with a mixed lineage leukemia translocation (MLL-AF9). In addition, daily oral administration of doses < 0.020 mg/kg significantly reduces tumor growth in rodent xenografts. Based on these results, ORY-1001 has been in a phase I/II clinical study to establish human pharmacokinetics and safety in blood, bone marrow, and bone cancers after standard treatment or remission.

GSK2879552, as another potent and selective KDM1A inhibitor, shows promising anti-proliferative growth inhibitory effects on differentiation in AML cells and SCLC cells. Further, mouse models of AML and SCLC treated with GSK2879552 show prolonged survival rates. A phase I clinical study commenced in 2014 to investigate the safety, pharmacokinetics, pharmacodynamics, and clinical activity of GSK2879552 in human subjects with SCLC, although the trial was terminated in 2017 since the risk benefits did not favor continuation of the study.

These MAO-derivative molecules have demonstrated specificity for KDM1A in vitro, supporting development of additional structurally similar KDM1A inhibitors. As these studies have compared the activity of TCP or its derivatives with KDM1A and MAOs in vitro, further studies are warranted to investigate whether the in vivo effects of KDM1A inhibitors on tumor suppression could further benefit from combination with inactivation of other enzymes (Jambhekar et al. 2017).

2.6.2 Peptide-Based KDM1A Inhibitors

Peptide-based KDM1A inhibitors have been designed to exploit the highly specific binding of KDM1A to its substrates (Culhane 2006; Schmitt et al. 2013; Tortorici et al. 2013; Kakizawa et al. 2015; Itoh et al. 2016). Because KDM1A can specifically recognize 21 amino acids from the N-terminal tail of histone H3, Culhane et al. (2006) first designed and synthesized propargyl-Lys-derivatized peptide 1 (compound 1), which mimics the 21-amino acid sequence. However, a modification on the fourth lysine of the fourth amino acid site allows the peptide to function as a potent and selective time-dependent inactivator of KDM1A (Culhane 2006). Later in 2010, Culhane et al. (2010) further advanced their study by adding "warheads" in peptide scaffolds to include chlorovinyl, endo-cyclopropylamine, and hydrazine functionalities as KDM1A inactivators. This revealed that the hydrazine analog (compound 18) is a potent time-dependent inhibitor of KDM1A. Two other molecules, CBB1003 and its methyl ester CBB1007, also mimic the H3 substrate and can reduce proliferation of multiple cancers types (Wang et al. 2011).

Because the KDM1A-CoREST complex binds to the SNAI1transcription factor, the co-crystal structure of the triple complex provides further insight into KDM1A's binding specificity to SNAI1. Similar to the conformation of the H3 tail, the N-terminal residues of SNAI1 bind to the enzyme's active site cleft (Baron et al. 2011). This was further confirmed by Tortorici et al. (2013), who then tested the efficacy of a 6-mer peptide derived from SNAI as a competitive inhibitor of KDM1A. Recently, the Suzuki group (Itoh et al. 2016) designed and developed a series of new SNAI1-based KDM1A inhibitors, of which peptide 3 displayed the most potent KDM1A-inhibitory activity in enzyme assays.

2.6.3 Polyamine-Based KDM1A Inhibitors

Polyamines are critical for eukaryotic cell growth and thus the maintenance of appropriate intracellular concentrations via a highly regulated interplay of biosynthesis, catabolism, uptake, and excretion (Huang et al. 2009a). Structural and catalytic similarities between KDM1A and polyamine oxidases facilitate the identification of different polyamine analogs, including biguanide, bisguanidine, and oligoamine, as potent KDM1A inhibitors.

In 2007, Huang et al. (2007b) first reported that bisguanidine and biguanide polyamine analogs are potent inhibitors of KDM1A. These analogs (including compound 2d) inhibit KDM1A in human colon carcinoma cells and affect reexpression of multiple aberrantly silenced genes that are important in the development of colon cancer—including members of the secreted frizzle-related proteins (SFRPs) and the GATA family of transcription factors—concurrent with increased H3K4me2 and decreased H3K9me1 and H3K9me2 markers. Later in 2009, Huang et al. (2009b) reported other novel polyamine analogs (including compounds PG11144 and 11150) also are effective KDM1A inhibitors. Treatment in colon cancer cell lines, including HCT116 and RKO, inhibits growth and leads to reexpression of aberrantly silenced SFRPs and GATA5 genes.

In 2010, Sharma et al. (2010) reported a series of isosteric ureas and thioureas that are also potent KDM1A inhibitors (including compound 6d). These compounds induce methylation at H3K4 and increase cellular levels of secreted SFRPs and GATA4 in Calu-6 lung carcinoma cells. Other studies have also demonstrated that polyamine analogs can effectively inhibit KDM1A and induce reexpression of several aberrantly silenced genes in MDA231 ER-negative breast cancer cells, a human colon cancer cell line, and human AML cell lines (Zhu et al. 2012; Murray-Stewart et al. 2013; Nowotarski et al. 2015).

However, it should be noted that the precise mechanisms of KDM1A inhibition by the polyamine analogs remain unclear. Ongoing crystallographic analysis should facilitate better understanding of the molecular and structural basis of KDM1A inhibition by polyamine analogs and perhaps provide insight to design more effective inhibitors.

2.6.4 Natural Products as KDM1A Inhibitors

Natural products characterized with degree of stereochemistry have been identified as resources for drug discovery (Song et al. 2022). Natural polyphenols, such as resveratrol, have beneficial functions in major human diseases, including cancer, diabetes, and cardiovascular disease. In 2013, Abdulla and coworkers (2013) first studied the effect of natural polyphenols, including resveratrol, curcumin, and quercetin, on KDM1A inhibition with in vitro enzymatic assays. The study surprisingly showed that natural polyphenols display a potent inhibitory effect on KDM1A activity far stronger than known inhibitory effects of TCP on KDM1A. Recently, Duan et al. (2017) designed a novel class of resveratrol derivatives that also are potent KDM1A inhibitors, with compounds 4e and 4m displaying the most potent inhibition in enzyme assays. This finding encourages development of more potent KDM1A inhibitors through further modifications of natural polyphenols. Recently, natural KDM1A inhibitors including coumarin analogs, eupalinilide, spirooxindole derivatives and capsaicin analogs have also been reported, providing further promising skeletons for the synthesis of high selectivity KDM1A inhibitors (Zhang et al. 2022b).

2.6.5 Multifunctional Inhibitors

Different inhibitors may affect different aspects of epigenetic modifier functions, highly implicating the benefits of a combination of epigenetic treatments for cancer therapy, including DNA methyl transferases, histone demethylases, and HDACs. The use of dual HDAC–KDM1A inhibitors provides a good example.

Based on this concept, several groups have already designed inhibitors by fusing two or more features of known KDM1A inhibitors into a single molecule, as multifunctional drugs can improve the efficacy or reduce off-target effects of individual drugs. In 2014, Rotili et al. (2014) first designed and synthesized pan-KDM inhibitors by coupling the skeleton of TCP, a known KDM1A inhibitor, with 4-carboxy-4′-carbomethoxy-2,2′-bipyridine or 5-carboxy-8-hydroxyquinoline, two 2-oxoglutarate competitive templates developed to inhibit JmjC. Both pan-inhibiting compounds increase H3K4 and H3K9 methylation levels and cause cell apoptosis in LNCaP prostate and HCT116 colon cancer cells. Interestingly, these compounds together induce apoptosis more effectively than either inhibitor alone, suggesting combinatory strategies may maximize the potency and specificity of targeting KDM1A.

In 2015, Han et al. coupled the carboxyl group of hydroxylcinnamic acid with TCP (compound 19l) and evaluated its biological activities. They discovered significant selectivity for KDM1A over MAOs and stronger

KDM1A inhibitory and anti-proliferative activities against tumor cells compared with KDM1A inhibitor alone (Han et al. 2015). Although these multifunctional compounds have shown remarkable success, their mechanisms of action remain unresolved. However, combination strategies provide additional possibilities in future cancer therapy.

2.6.6 Other KDM1A Inhibitors

Using a database of commercial compounds and molecular docking tools, several other groups have started to identify candidate KDM1A inhibitors that lack structural similarity to previously identified inhibitor classes. In 2015, based on 2D and 3D structure–activity models followed by computational analyses and biochemical screening, several groups identified novel scaffolds against KDM1A that yielded several anti-KDM1A inhibitor candidates, namely aminothiazoles (compound 16q) and namoline (Zheng et al. 2015). Namoline, a totally reversible KDM1A inhibitor, was identified by screening against MAOs and has an IC_{50} of 51 mM against KDM1A. A previous study reported that namoline impairs KDM1A demethylase activity and reduces cell proliferation and xenograft tumor growth (Willmann et al. 2012).

In the same year, Zhou and coworkers (2015) also garnered success with a pharmacophore-based virtual screening approach to identify novel inhibitors of KDM1A. In vitro tests of these compounds showed IC_{50} values in a low micromolar range against KDM1A. Compound XZ09 showed the highest potency against KDM1A, indicating the compound could serve as another tool to probe KDM1A function.

SP2509 is a novel specific KDM1A antagonist with an IC_{50} of 13 nM. It was previously reported from a structure-based drug discovery approach using solved 3D crystal structures of KDM1A to computationally dock>10 million compounds into the protein's active site. After physically screening a selected group of compounds in KDM1A biochemical assays from the docking experiment and optimization with a structure-based synthetic design strategy, SP2509 was identified as a potent inhibitor of KDM1A enzymatic activity. Treatment with SP2509 attenuates binding of KDM1A with CoREST, increases the permissive H3K4Me3 mark on target gene promoters, and increases p21, p27, and C/EBPα levels in cultured AML cells (Fiskus et al. 2014). Co-treatment with pan-HDAC inhibitor panobinostat and SP2509 significantly improves the survival of mice engrafted with human AML cells, compared with each agent alone, indicating the combination of SP2509 and pan-HDAC inhibitor could be a promising AML therapy (Fiskus et al. 2014). Of note, a possible role of non-covalent SP2509 compounds to blocks non-enzymatic function was recently reported. It was indicated that the molecule's core structure is a pan-assay interference compound and is thus prone to interfering with a wide variety of proteins, suggesting more investigation into the target responsible for the anticancer effects of SP2509. (Sonnemann et al. 2017).

2.6.7 KDM1A Inhibitors in Clinical Trials

A growing list of studies have investigated the effect of KDM1A inhibitors on different tumor cell lines (Table 2.1). These studies reveal that interruption of KDM1A with chemical inhibitors suppresses proliferation, migration, and invasion of different cancer cells that overexpress KDM1A. Further, treatment with KDM1A inhibitors severely blunts xenograft tumor growth in mouse models. When taken together, these in vitro and in vivo studies provide solid evidence for the use of KDM1A inhibitors in cancer treatment and have laid foundations for further clinical studies.

Until now, nine LSD1 inhibitors including tranylcypromine (also known as TCP), ORY-1001, ORY-2001, GSK-2879552, IMG-7289, INCB059872, TAK-418, CC-90011, and SP-2577 have entered the clinical trial stage for disease treatment as either mono- or combinational therapy (Table 2.2). Most KDM1A

Table 2.2 Overview of KDM1A inhibitors in clinical trials

Inhibitors	Diseases	Phases	Year	Trial numbers	Status
TCP	Non-M3 AML	I/II	2016	NCT02717884	Unknown
	AML/MDS	I	2014	NCT02273102	Completed
	AML	I/II	2014	NCT02261779	Unknown
ORY-1001 (RG6016)	AL	I/II	2013	EUDRACT 2013-002447-29	Unknown
	SCLC	I	2016	NCT02913443	Completed
GSK2879552	AML	I	2014	NCT02177812	Terminated
	Relapsed/ refractory SCLC	I	2014	NCT02034123	Terminated
	High risk MDS	II	2016	NCT02929498	Terminated
	MDS	I/II	2017	EudraCT 2016-002294-35	Unknown
CC-90011	Relapsed/refractory solid tumors and Non-Hodgkin lymphomas	I	2016	NCT02875223	Active, not recruiting
	SCLC	I/II	2019	NCT03850067	Active, not recruiting
	Advanced tumors	II	2020	NCT04350463	Active, not recruiting
IMG-7289	MDS/AML	I/II	2016	NCT02842827	Completed
	Myelofibrosis	I	2017	NCT03136185	Completed
	Essential thrombocythemia or polycythemia vera	II	2020	NCT04262141	Recruiting
INCB059872	Advanced malignancies	I/II	2016	NCT02712905	Terminated
	Sickle-cell disease	I	2017	NCT03132324	Terminated
	Relapsed Ewing sarcoma	I	2018	NCT03514407	Terminated
	Solid tumors Advanced malignancies Metastatic cancer	I/II	2016	NCT02959437	Terminated
	MDS/MPN	I/II	2019	NCT04061421	Recruiting
ORY-2001	Mild to moderate Alzheimer's disease	IIa	2019	NCT03867253	Completed
SP2577	Ewing Sarcoma	I	2018	NCT03600649	Recruiting

Abbreviation: *TCP* tranylcypromine; *ATRA* all-trans-retinoic acid; AML, acute myeloid leukemia; *AL* acute leukemia; *SCLC* small cell lung cancer; *MDS* myelodysplastic syndrome; *MPN* myeloproliferative neoplasms. Updated in May 2023

inhibitors tested under clinical trials have targeted different blood cancers, including AML, myelodysplastic syndromes (MDS), and SCLC, with or without combination with other chemotherapeutic agents, e.g., TCP, an FDA-approved drug originally designed to treat depression, is in clinical trials for its repurposed use in cancer treatment. The University of Miami first started a phase I study in 2014 on the safety and tolerability of TCP/ATRA combination therapy in patients with AML and MDS. A phase I study began in 2014 to investigate the safety, pharmacokinetics, pharmacodynamics, and clinical activity of GSK2879552 in human subjects with SCLC.

Three newly developed, orally administered, irreversible KDM1A inhibitors—INCB059872, IMG-7289, and CC-90011—have also started clinical trials to treat different cancers (results from in vitro and in vivo studies not public though). Since 2016, a phase I/II safety and tolerability study of INCB059872 has been ongoing in subjects with advanced malignancies, including AML/MDS, SCLC, myelofibrosis, Ewing's sarcoma, and poorly differentiated neuroendocrine tumors. A phase I clinical study also started in 2016 to assess the safety, pharmacokinetics, and pharmacodynamics of IMG-7289 with and without ATRA in patients with AML or MDS. With the completion of the phase 1 portion in 2017, the phase 2a component of the study is now evaluating safety and antitumor activity of IMG-7289 in combination with ATRA. CC-90011 is also a new orally administered KDM1A inhibitor currently in a phase I dose-finding study to assess the safety, tolerability, pharmacokinetics, and efficacy in subjects with advanced solid tumors and non-Hodgkin lymphoma. In addition, in year 2018, a clinical formulation of SP2509, SP2577, has entered a phase I trial in patients with relapsed or refractory Ewing sarcoma.

Apart from inhibitors addressed above, ORY-2001(Vafidemstat), a dual orally active and blood–brain barrier (BBB)–permeable therapeutic KDM1A/MAO-B inhibitor which shows excellent selectivity to KDM1A and its homology MAO-B over other chromatin modulators, has recently also been approved to enter IIa clinical trial to evaluate the safety, tolerability, and preliminary efficacy in patients with Alzheimer's disease (Fang et al. 2019).

Since KDM1A serves as a promising drug target for disease treatment, KDM1A targeted drug discovery has attracted much attention. As we know, the discovery of KDM1A-targeted drugs has been mainly focusing on the irreversible inhibitors, while the development speed of reversible LSD1 inhibitors is much delayed (Fang et al. 2019). Thereby, further attention could be paid to the natural compounds and in-depth pharmacological investigation is also needed to clarify their effects (Dai et al. 2020). In conclusion, targeting KDM1A for treating diseases is still on the way, and many difficulties need to be overcome to improve the therapeutic outcomes.

2.7 Conclusions and Future Perspectives

Discovery of the first histone demethylase prompted new excitement in the field of chromatin biology. Over the past 19 years, studies have focused on the involvement of the KDM1 family in the epigenetic regulation of chromatin state and resulting biological processes. Of particular interest, KDM1A's activity has been implicated in multiple cancer types and thus has become a crucial target for drug development. KDM1A inhibitors have proven successful in decreasing proliferation in vitro and inducing tumor shrinkage in vivo. However, our understanding of KDM1B has severely lagged behind that of KDM1A, possibly due to the fact that KDM1B is mainly related to the gene bodies of actively transcribed genes and almost completely absent from promoter regions, making it difficult to study. Recent findings demonstrate a critical functional role of KDM1B in immune response, breast cancer biology, and glioblastoma. These findings hold significant new promise to develop KDM1B-specific inhibitors to treat these specific cancers.

With increasing understanding of both the functional role and interactions of KDM1 within multi-protein cellular complexes in cancer biology and the mechanism of action of KDM1 inhibitors, emerging roles of the KDM1 family in immune responsiveness, tissue microenvironment, and antitumor immunity may provide alternative avenues to develop new KDM1 inhibitors. Development of next-generation biochemical probes and screening technologies are providing innovative resources to explore novel drug targeting mechanisms as well as establish novel combinatory regimens for cancer treatment. Although still emerging, results from the preclinical and clinical trials are extremely promising, as KDM1 inhibitors are proving to be highly effective to treat various cancers.

Future research into the roles and functions of the KDM1 family is warranted and will allow expansion of the therapeutic applications of KDM1 inhibitors in the clinic, holding promise to generate more effective cancer therapies. In that sense, the revelation that targeted inactivation of KDM1A increases intracellular dsRNA stress in tumor cells and IFN activation, which in turn promotes antitumor immune responses and sensitizes PD-1 therapy-resistant tumors to PD-1 blockade, reveals several folds of significant clinical and therapeutic implications. This not only provides a way to increase the efficacy of anti-PD-1 cancer therapy and potentially turn "cold" tumors "hot," but also provides a basis for the combinatorial use of KDM1 inhibitors and anti-PD-L1 for cancer therapy. Further works warrant understanding both the functional roles and mechanisms of KDM1A in tumor cells and immune cells. However, it is possible that drugs targeting KDM1A in combination with anti-PD-L1 will prove to be a common new strategy in cancer immunotherapy.

References

Abdulla A, Zhao X, Yang F (2013) Natural polyphenols inhibit lysine-specific demethylase-1 in vitro. J Biochem Pharmacol Res 1:56–63

Abu-Farha M, Lanouette S, Elisma F, Tremblay V, Butson J, Figeys D, Couture JF (2011) Proteomic analyses of the SMYD family interactomes identify HSP90 as a novel target for SMYD2. J Mol Cell Biol 3:301–308

Adamo A, Sese B, Boue S, Castano J, Paramonov I, Barrero MJ, Izpisua Belmonte JC (2011) LSD1 regulates the balance between self-renewal and differentiation in human embryonic stem cells. Nat Cell Biol 13:652–659

Anand R, Marmorstein R (2007) Structure and mechanism of lysine-specific demethylase enzymes. J Biol Chem 282:35425–35429

Ballas N, Grunseich C, Lu DD, Speh JC, Mandel G (2005) REST and its corepressors mediate plasticity of neuronal gene chromatin throughout neurogenesis. Cell 121:645–657

Banck MS, Li S, Nishio H, Wang C, Beutler AS, Walsh MJ (2009) The ZNF217 oncogene is a candidate organizer of repressive histone modifiers. Epigenetics 4:100–106

Bannister AJ, Schneider R, Kouzarides T (2002) Histone methylation: dynamic or static? Cell 109:801–806

Baron R, Binda C, Tortorici M, McCammon JA, Mattevi A (2011) Molecular mimicry and ligand recognition in binding and catalysis by the histone demethylase LSD1-CoREST complex. Structure 19:212–220

Baron R, Vellore NA (2012) LSD1/CoREST reversible opening-closing dynamics: discovery of a nanoscale clamp for chromatin and protein binding. Biochemistry 51:3151–3153

Basta J, Rauchman M (2015) The nucleosome remodeling and deacetylase complex in development and disease. Transl Res J Labor Clin Med 165:36–47

Baylin SB (2011) Resistance, epigenetics and the cancer ecosystem. Nat Med 17:288–289

Baylin SB, Jones PA (2011) A decade of exploring the cancer epigenome—biological and translational implications. Nat Rev Cancer 11:726–734

Benelkebir H, Hodgkinson C, Duriez PJ, Hayden AL, Bulleid RA, Crabb SJ, Packham G, Ganesan A (2011) Enantioselective synthesis of tranylcypromine analogues as lysine demethylase (LSD1) inhibitors. Bioorg Med Chem 19:3709–3716

Bennani-Baiti (2012) Integration of ERα-PELP1-HER2 signaling by LSD1 (KDM1A_AOF2) offers combinatorial therapeutic opportunities to circumventing hormone resistance in breast cancer.pdf. Bennani-Baiti Breast Cancer Res 14:112

Benner C, Konovalov S, Mackintosh C, Hutt KR, Stunnenberg R, Garcia-Bassets I (2013) Decoding a signature-based model of transcription cofactor recruitment dictated by cardinal cis-regulatory elements in proximal promoter regions. PLoS Genet 9:e1003906

Bennesch MA, Segala G, Wider D, Picard D (2016) LSD1 engages a corepressor complex for the activation of the estrogen receptor alpha by estrogen and cAMP. Nucleic Acids Res 44:8655–8670

Binda C, Valente S, Romanenghi M, Pilotto S, Cirilli R, Karytinos A, Ciossani G, Botrugno OA, Forneris F, Tardugno M, Edmondson DE, Minucci S, Mattevi A, Mai A (2010) Biochemical, structural, and biological evaluation of tranylcypromine derivatives as

inhibitors of histone demethylases LSD1 and LSD2. J Am Chem Soc 132:6827–6833
Buckingham M (1994) Molecular biology of muscle development. Cell 78:15–21
Burg JM, Link JE, Morgan BS, Heller FJ, Hargrove AE, McCafferty DG (2015) KDM1 class flavin-dependent protein lysine demethylases. Biopolymers 104:213–246
Castex J, Willmann D, Kanouni T, Arrigoni L, Li Y, Friedrich M, Schleicher M, Wohrle S, Pearson M, Kraut N, Meret M, Manke T, Metzger E, Schule R, Gunther T (2017) Inactivation of Lsd1 triggers senescence in trophoblast stem cells by induction of Sirt4. Cell Death Dis 8:e2631
Chan JK, Sun L, Yang XJ, Zhu G, Wu Z (2003) Functional characterization of an amino-terminal region of HDAC4 that possesses MEF2 binding and transcriptional repressive activity. J Biol Chem 278:23515–23521
Chen F, Yang H, Dong Z, Fang J, Wang P, Zhu T, Gong W, Fang R, Shi YG, Li Z, Xu Y (2013) Structural insight into substrate recognition by histone demethylase LSD2/KDM1b. Cell Res 23:306–309
Chen L, Vasilatos SN, Qin Y, Katz TA, Cao C, Wu H, Tasdemir N, Levine KM, Oesterreich S, Davidson NE, Huang Y (2017) Functional characterization of lysine-specific demethylase 2 (LSD2/KDM1B) in breast cancer progression. Oncotarget 8:81737–81753
Chen L, Xu Y, Xu B, Deng H, Zheng X, Wu C, Jiang J (2014) Over-expression of lysine-specific demethylase 1 predicts tumor progression and poor prognosis in human esophageal cancer. Int J Clin Exp Pathol 7:8929–8934
Chen Y, Jie W, Yan W, Zhou K, Xiao Y (2012) Lysine-specific histone demethylase 1 (LSD1): a potential molecular target for tumor therapy. Crit Rev Eukaryot Gene Expr 22:53–59
Chen Y, Kim J, Zhang R, Yang X, Zhang Y, Fang J, Chen Z, Teng L, Chen X, Ge H, Atadja P, Li E, Chen T, Qi W (2016) Histone demethylase LSD1 promotes adipocyte differentiation through repressing Wnt signaling. Cell Chem Biol 23:1228–1240
Chendrimada TP, Gregory RI, Kumaraswamy E, Norman J, Cooch N, Nishikura K, Shiekhattar R (2005) TRBP recruits the dicer complex to Ago2 for microRNA processing and gene silencing. Nature 436:740–744
Chiappinelli KB, Strissel PL, Desrichard A, Li H, Henke C, Akman B, Hein A, Rote NS, Cope LM, Snyder A, Makarov V, Budhu S, Slamon DJ, Wolchok JD, Pardoll DM, Beckmann MW, Zahnow CA, Merghoub T, Chan TA, Baylin SB, Strick R (2015) Inhibiting DNA methylation causes an interferon response in cancer via dsRNA including endogenous retroviruses. Cell 162:974–986
Chinnadurai G (2007) Transcriptional regulation by C-terminal binding proteins. Int J Biochem Cell Biol 39:1593–1607
Cho HS, Suzuki T, Dohmae N, Hayami S, Unoki M, Yoshimatsu M, Toyokawa G, Takawa M, Chen T, Kurash JK, Field HI, Ponder BA, Nakamura Y, Hamamoto R (2011) Demethylation of RB regulator MYPT1 by histone demethylase LSD1 promotes cell cycle progression in cancer cells. Can Res 71:655–660
Choi J, Jang H, Kim H, Kim ST, Cho EJ, Youn HD (2010) Histone demethylase LSD1 is required to induce skeletal muscle differentiation by regulating myogenic factors. Biochem Biophys Res Commun 401:327–332
Choi J, Jang H, Kim H, Lee JH, Kim ST, Cho EJ, Youn HD (2014) Modulation of lysine methylation in myocyte enhancer factor 2 during skeletal muscle cell differentiation. Nucleic Acids Res 42:224–234
Cimmino L, Dolgalev I, Wang Y, Yoshimi A, Martin GH, Wang J, Ng V, Xia B, Witkowski MT, Mitchell-Flack M, Grillo I, Bakogianni S, Ndiaye-Lobry D, Martin MT, Guillamot M, Banh RS, Xu M, Figueroa ME, Dickins RA, Abdel-Wahab O, Park CY, Tsirigos A, Neel BG, Aifantis I (2017) Restoration of TET2 function blocks aberrant self-renewal and leukemia progression. Cell 170(1079–1095):e1020
Cortez V, Mann M, Tekmal S, Suzuki T, Miyata N, Rodriguez-Aguayo C, Lopez-Berestein G, Sood AK, Vadlamudi RK (2012) Targeting the PELP1-KDM1 axis as a potential therapeutic strategy for breast cancer. Breast Cancer Res BCR 14:R108
Culhane ea (2006) A mechanism-based inactivator for histone demethylase LSD1.pdf. JACS 128:4536–4537
Culhane JC, Szewczuk LM, Liu X, Da G, Marmorstein R, Cole PA (2006) A mechanism-based inactivator for histone demethylase LSD1. J Am Chem Soc 128:4536–4537
Culhane JC, Wang D, Yen PM, Cole PA (2010) Comparative analysis of small molecules and histone substrate analogues as LSD1 lysine demethylase inhibitors. J Am Chem Soc 132:3164–3176
Dai XJ, Liu Y, Xiong XP, Xue LP, Zheng YC, Liu HM (2020) Tranylcypromine based lysine-specific demethylase 1 inhibitor: summary and perspective. J Med Chem 63:14197–14215
Daniels SM, Melendez-Pena CE, Scarborough RJ, Daher A, Christensen HS, El Far M, Purcell DF, Laine S, Gatignol A (2009) Characterization of the TRBP domain required for dicer interaction and function in RNA interference. BMC Mol Biol 10:38
Dawson MA, Kouzarides T (2012) Cancer epigenetics: from mechanism to therapy. Cell 150:12–27
Dawson MA, Kouzarides T, Huntly BJ (2012) Targeting epigenetic readers in cancer. N Engl J Med 367:647–657
Ding J, Zhang ZM, Xia Y, Liao GQ, Pan Y, Liu S, Zhang Y, Yan ZS (2013) LSD1-mediated epigenetic modification contributes to proliferation and metastasis of colon cancer. Br J Cancer 109:994–1003
Dressel U, Bailey PJ, Wang SC, Downes M, Evans RM, Muscat GE (2001) A dynamic role for HDAC7 in MEF2-mediated muscle differentiation. J Biol Chem 276:17007–17013

Duan YC, Guan YY, Zhai XY, Ding LN, Qin WP, Shen DD, Liu XQ, Sun XD, Zheng YC, Liu HM (2017) Discovery of resveratrol derivatives as novel LSD1 inhibitors: design, synthesis and their biological evaluation. Eur J Med Chem 126:246–258

Duteil D, Metzger E, Willmann D, Karagianni P, Friedrichs N, Greschik H, Gunther T, Buettner R, Talianidis I, Metzger D, Schule R (2014) LSD1 promotes oxidative metabolism of white adipose tissue. Nat Commun 5:4093

Duteil D, Tosic M, Willmann D, Georgiadi A, Kanouni T, Schule R (2017) Lsd1 prevents age-programed loss of beige adipocytes. Proc Natl Acad Sci USA 114:5265–5270

Ernst T, Chase AJ, Score J, Hidalgo-Curtis CE, Bryant C, Jones AV, Waghorn K, Zoi K, Ross FM, Reiter A, Hochhaus A, Drexler HG, Duncombe A, Cervantes F, Oscier D, Boultwood J, Grand FH, Cross NC (2010) Inactivating mutations of the histone methyltransferase gene EZH2 in myeloid disorders. Nat Genet 42:722–726

Ernst T, Pflug A, Rinke J, Ernst J, Bierbach U, Beck JF, Hochhaus A, Gruhn B (2012) A somatic EZH2 mutation in childhood acute myeloid leukemia. Leukemia 26:1701–1703

Etani T, Suzuki T, Naiki T, Naiki-Ito A, Ando R, Iida K, Kawai N, Tozawa K, Miyata N, Kohri K, Takahashi S (2015) NCL1, a highly selective lysine-specific demethylase 1 inhibitor, suppresses prostate cancer without adverse effect. Oncotarget 6:2865–2878

Fang R, Barbera AJ, Xu Y, Rutenberg M, Leonor T, Bi Q, Lan F, Mei P, Yuan GC, Lian C, Peng J, Cheng D, Sui G, Kaiser UB, Shi Y, Shi YG (2010) Human LSD2/KDM1b/AOF1 regulates gene transcription by modulating intragenic H3K4me2 methylation. Mol Cell 39:222–233

Fang R, Chen F, Dong Z, Hu D, Barbera AJ, Clark EA, Fang J, Yang Y, Mei P, Rutenberg M, Li Z, Zhang Y, Xu Y, Yang H, Wang P, Simon MD, Zhou Q, Li J, Marynick MP, Li X, Lu H, Kaiser UB, Kingston RE, Xu Y, Shi YG (2013) LSD2/KDM1B and its cofactor NPAC/GLYR1 endow a structural and molecular model for regulation of H3K4 demethylation. Mol Cell 49:558–570

Fang Y, Liao G, Yu B (2019) LSD1/KDM1A inhibitors in clinical trials: advances and prospects. J Hematol Oncol 12:129

Ferrari-Amorotti G, Chiodoni C, Shen F, Cattelani S, Soliera AR, Manzotti G, Grisendi G, Dominici M, Rivasi F, Colombo MP, Fatatis A, Calabretta B (2014) Suppression of invasion and metastasis of triple-negative breast cancer lines by pharmacological or genetic inhibition of slug activity. Neoplasia 16:1047–1058

Figueroa ME, Abdel-Wahab O, Lu C, Ward PS, Patel J, Shih A, Li Y, Bhagwat N, Vasanthakumar A, Fernandez HF, Tallman MS, Sun Z, Wolniak K, Peeters JK, Liu W, Choe SE, Fantin VR, Paietta E, Lowenberg B, Licht JD, Godley LA, Delwel R, Valk PJ, Thompson CB, Levine RL, Melnick A (2010) Leukemic IDH1 and IDH2 mutations result in a hypermethylation phenotype, disrupt TET2 function, and impair hematopoietic differentiation. Cancer Cell 18:553–567

Fiskus W, Sharma S, Shah B, Portier BP, Devaraj SG, Liu K, Iyer SP, Bearss D, Bhalla KN (2014) Highly effective combination of LSD1 (KDM1A) antagonist and pan-histone deacetylase inhibitor against human AML cells. Leukemia 28:2155–2164

Fiszbein A, Kornblihtt AR (2016) Histone methylation, alternative splicing and neuronal differentiation. Neurogenesis (austin) 3:e1204844

Flavahan WA, Gaskell E, Bernstein BE (2017) Epigenetic plasticity and the hallmarks of cancer. Science 357

Forneris F, Battaglioli E, Mattevi A, Binda C (2009) New roles of flavoproteins in molecular cell biology: histone demethylase LSD1 and chromatin. FEBS J 276:4304–4312

Foster CT, Dovey OM, Lezina L, Luo JL, Gant TW, Barlev N, Bradley A, Cowley SM (2010) Lysine-specific demethylase 1 regulates the embryonic transcriptome and CoREST stability. Mol Cell Biol 30:4851–4863

Fuentes P, Canovas J, Berndt FA, Noctor SC, Kukuljan M (2012) CoREST/LSD1 control the development of pyramidal cortical neurons. Cereb Cortex 22:1431–1441

Gooden DM, Schmidt DM, Pollock JA, Kabadi AM, McCafferty DG (2008) Facile synthesis of substituted trans-2-arylcyclopropylamine inhibitors of the human histone demethylase LSD1 and monoamine oxidases A and B. Bioorg Med Chem Lett 18:3047–3051

Han Y, Wu C, Lv H, Liu N, Deng H (2015) Novel tranylcypromine/hydroxylcinnamic acid hybrids as lysine-specific demethylase 1 inhibitors with potent antitumor activity. Chem Pharm Bull (tokyo) 63:882–889

Harris WJ, Huang X, Lynch JT, Spencer GJ, Hitchin JR, Li Y, Ciceri F, Blaser JG, Greystoke BF, Jordan AM, Miller CJ, Ogilvie DJ, Somervaille TC (2012) The histone demethylase KDM1A sustains the oncogenic potential of MLL-AF9 leukemia stem cells. Cancer Cell 21:473–487

Hayami S, Kelly JD, Cho HS, Yoshimatsu M, Unoki M, Tsunoda T, Field HI, Neal DE, Yamaue H, Ponder BA, Nakamura Y, Hamamoto R (2011) Overexpression of LSD1 contributes to human carcinogenesis through chromatin regulation in various cancers. Int J Cancer 128:574–586

He YF, Li BZ, Li Z, Liu P, Wang Y, Tang Q, Ding J, Jia Y, Chen Z, Li L, Sun Y, Li X, Dai Q, Song CX, Zhang K, He C, Xu GL (2011) Tet-mediated formation of 5-carboxylcytosine and its excision by TDG in mammalian DNA. Science 333:1303–1307

Hino S, Kohrogi K, Nakao M (2016) Histone demethylase LSD1 controls the phenotypic plasticity of cancer cells. Cancer Sci 107:1187–1192

Hino S, Sakamoto A, Nagaoka K, Anan K, Wang Y, Mimasu S, Umehara T, Yokoyama S, Kosai K, Nakao M (2012) FAD-dependent lysine-specific demethylase-1 regulates cellular energy expenditure. Nat Commun 3:758

Hirano K, Namihira M (2016) LSD1 mediates neuronal differentiation of human fetal neural stem cells by controlling the expression of a novel target gene, HEYL. Stem Cells 34:1872–1882

Holmes A, Roseaulin L, Schurra C, Waxin H, Lambert S, Zaratiegui M, Martienssen RA, Arcangioli B (2012) Lsd1 and lsd2 control programmed replication fork pauses and imprinting in fission yeast. Cell Rep 2:1513–1520

Hoshino I, Akutsu Y, Murakami K, Akanuma N, Isozaki Y, Maruyama T, Toyozumi T, Matsumoto Y, Suito H, Takahashi M, Sekino N, Komatsu A, Suzuki T, Matsubara H (2016) Histone demethylase LSD1 inhibitors prevent cell growth by regulating gene expression in esophageal squamous cell carcinoma cells. Ann Surg Oncol 23:312–320

Hou H, Yu H (2010) Structural insights into histone lysine demethylation. Curr Opin Struct Biol 20:739–748

Hsu HC, Liu YS, Tseng KC, Yang TS, Yeh CY, You JF, Hung HY, Chen SJ, Chen HC (2015) CBB1003, a lysine-specific demethylase 1 inhibitor, suppresses colorectal cancer cells growth through down-regulation of leucine-rich repeat-containing G-protein-coupled receptor 5 expression. J Cancer Res Clin Oncol 141:11–21

Hu X, Li X, Valverde K, Fu X, Noguchi C, Qiu Y, Huang S (2009) LSD1-mediated epigenetic modification is required for TAL1 function and hematopoiesis. Proc Natl Acad Sci USA 106:10141–10146

Huang J, Sengupta R, Espejo AB, Lee MG, Dorsey JA, Richter M, Opravil S, Shiekhattar R, Bedford MT, Jenuwein T, Berger SL (2007a) p53 is regulated by the lysine demethylase LSD1. Nature 449:105–108

Huang Y, Greene E, Murray Stewart T, Goodwin AC, Baylin SB, Woster PM, Casero RA Jr (2007b) Inhibition of lysine-specific demethylase 1 by polyamine analogues results in reexpression of aberrantly silenced genes. Proc Natl Acad Sci USA 104:8023–8028

Huang M, Chen C, Geng J, Han D, Wang T, Xie T, Wang L, Wang Y, Wang C, Lei Z, Chu X (2017) Targeting KDM1A attenuates Wnt/beta-catenin signaling pathway to eliminate sorafenib-resistant stem-like cells in hepatocellular carcinoma. Cancer Lett 398:12–21

Huang Y, Marton LJ, Woster PM, Casero RA (2009a) Polyamine analogues targeting epigenetic gene regulation. Essays Biochem 46:95–110

Huang Y, Stewart TM, Wu Y, Baylin SB, Marton LJ, Perkins B, Jones RJ, Woster PM, Casero RA Jr (2009b) Novel oligoamine analogues inhibit lysine-specific demethylase 1 and induce reexpression of epigenetically silenced genes. Clin Cancer Res Official J Am Assoc Cancer Res 15:7217–7228

Huang Y, Vasilatos SN, Boric L, Shaw PG, Davidson NE (2012) Inhibitors of histone demethylation and histone deacetylation cooperate in regulating gene expression and inhibiting growth in human breast cancer cells. Breast Cancer Res Treat 131:777–789

Huang Z, Li S, Song W, Li X, Li Q, Zhang Z, Han Y, Zhang X, Miao S, Du R, Wang L (2013) Lysine-specific demethylase 1 (LSD1/KDM1A) contributes to colorectal tumorigenesis via activation of the Wnt/beta-catenin pathway by down-regulating Dickkopf-1 (DKK1) [corrected]. PLoS ONE 8:e70077

Itoh Y, Aihara K, Mellini P, Tojo T, Ota Y, Tsumoto H, Solomon VR, Zhan P, Suzuki M, Ogasawara D, Shigenaga A, Inokuma T, Nakagawa H, Miyata N, Mizukami T, Otaka A, Suzuki T (2016) Identification of SNAIL1 peptide-based irreversible lysine-specific demethylase 1-selective inactivators. J Med Chem 59:1531–1544

Jambhekar A, Anastas JN, Shi Y (2017) Histone lysine demethylase inhibitors. Cold Spring Harbor Perspect Med 7

Jie D, Zhongmin Z, Guoqing L, Sheng L, Yi Z, Jing W, Liang Z (2013) Positive expression of LSD1 and negative expression of E-cadherin correlate with metastasis and poor prognosis of colon cancer. Dig Dis Sci 58:1581–1589

Kahl P, Gullotti L, Heukamp LC, Wolf S, Friedrichs N, Vorreuther R, Solleder G, Bastian PJ, Ellinger J, Metzger E, Schule R, Buettner R (2006) Androgen receptor coactivators lysine-specific histone demethylase 1 and four and a half LIM domain protein 2 predict risk of prostate cancer recurrence. Can Res 66:11341–11347

Kakizawa T, Ota Y, Itoh Y, Tsumoto H, Suzuki T (2015) Histone H3 peptide based LSD1-selective inhibitors. Bioorg Med Chem Lett 25:1925–1928

Kalyani AJ, Rao MS (1998) Cell lineage in the developing neural tube. Biochem Cell Biol 76:1051–1068

Katz TA, Vasilatos SN, Harrington E, Oesterreich S, Davidson NE, Huang Y (2014) Inhibition of histone demethylase, LSD2 (KDM1B), attenuates DNA methylation and increases sensitivity to DNMT inhibitor-induced apoptosis in breast cancer cells. Breast Cancer Res Treat 146:99–108

Kauffman EC, Robinson BD, Downes MJ, Powell LG, Lee MM, Scherr DS, Gudas LJ, Mongan NP (2011) Role of androgen receptor and associated lysine-demethylase coregulators, LSD1 and JMJD2A, in localized and advanced human bladder cancer. Mol Carcinog 50:931–944

Kerenyi MA, Shao Z, Hsu YJ, Guo G, Luc S, O'Brien K, Fujiwara Y, Peng C, Nguyen M, Orkin SH (2013) Histone demethylase Lsd1 represses hematopoietic stem and progenitor cell signatures during blood cell maturation. eLife 2:e00633

Kim D, Kim KI, Baek SH (2021) Roles of lysine-specific demethylase 1 (LSD1) in homeostasis and diseases. J Biomed Sci 28:41

Kontaki H, Talianidis I (2010) Lysine methylation regulates E2F1-induced cell death. Mol Cell 39:152–160

Latos PA, Goncalves A, Oxley D, Mohammed H, Turro E, Hemberger M (2015) Fgf and Esrrb integrate epigenetic and transcriptional networks that regulate self-renewal of trophoblast stem cells. Nat Commun 6:7776

Laurent B, Ruitu L, Murn J, Hempel K, Ferrao R, Xiang Y, Liu S, Garcia BA, Wu H, Wu F, Steen H, Shi Y (2015) A specific LSD1/KDM1A isoform regulates neuronal differentiation through H3K9 demethylation. Mol Cell 57:957–970

Lee MG, Norman J, Shilatifard A, Shiekhattar R (2007) Physical and functional association of a trimethyl H3K4 demethylase and Ring6a/MBLR, a polycomb-like protein. Cell 128:877–887

Lee MG, Wynder C, Cooch N, Shiekhattar R (2005) An essential role for CoREST in nucleosomal histone 3 lysine 4 demethylation. Nature 437:432–435

Lee MG, Wynder C, Schmidt DM, McCafferty DG, Shiekhattar R (2006) Histone H3 lysine 4 demethylation is a target of nonselective antidepressive medications. Chem Biol 13:563–567

Li Y, Deng C, Hu X, Patel B, Fu X, Qiu Y, Brand M, Zhao K, Huang S (2012) Dynamic interaction between TAL1 oncoprotein and LSD1 regulates TAL1 function in hematopoiesis and leukemogenesis. Oncogene 31:5007–5018

Li Y, Tian X, Sui CG, Jiang YH, Liu YP, Meng FD (2016) Interference of lysine-specific demethylase 1 inhibits cellular invasion and proliferation in vivo in gastric cancer MKN-28 cells. Biomed Pharmacother 82:498–508

Liang Y, Ahmed M, Guo H, Soares F, Hua JT, Gao S, Lu C, Poon C, Han W, Langstein J, Ekram MB, Li B, Davicioni E, Takhar M, Erho N, Karnes RJ, Chadwick D, van der Kwast T, Boutros PC, Arrowsmith CH, Feng FY, Joshua AM, Zoubeidi A, Cai C, He HH (2017) LSD1-mediated epigenetic reprogramming drives CENPE expression and prostate cancer progression. Can Res 77:5479–5490

Liang Y, Quenelle D, Vogel JL, Mascaro C, Ortega A, Kristie TM (2013) A novel selective LSD1/KDM1A inhibitor epigenetically blocks herpes simplex virus lytic replication and reactivation from latency. mBio 4:e00558-00512

Lim S, Janzer A, Becker A, Zimmer A, Schule R, Buettner R, Kirfel J (2010) Lysine-specific demethylase 1 (LSD1) is highly expressed in ER-negative breast cancers and a biomarker predicting aggressive biology. Carcinogenesis 31:512–520

Lin T, Ponn A, Hu X, Law BK, Lu J (2010a) Requirement of the histone demethylase LSD1 in Snai1-mediated transcriptional repression during epithelial-mesenchymal transition. Oncogene 29:4896–4904

Lin Y, Wu Y, Li J, Dong C, Ye X, Chi YI, Evers BM, Zhou BP (2010b) The SNAG domain of Snail1 functions as a molecular hook for recruiting lysine-specific demethylase 1. EMBO J 29:1803–1816

Liu L, Souto J, Liao W, Jiang Y, Li Y, Nishinakamura R, Huang S, Rosengart T, Yang VW, Schuster M, Ma Y, Yang J (2013) Histone lysine-specific demethylase 1 (LSD1) protein is involved in Sal-like protein 4 (SALL4)-mediated transcriptional repression in hematopoietic stem cells. J Biol Chem 288:34719–34728

Liu Y, Debo B, Li M, Shi Z, Sheng W, Shi Y (2021) LSD1 inhibition sustains T cell invigoration with a durable response to PD-1 blockade. Nat Commun 12:6831

Lokken AA, Zeleznik-Le NJ (2012) Breaking the LSD1/KDM1A addiction: therapeutic targeting of the epigenetic modifier in AML. Cancer Cell 21:451–453

Lopez CI, Saud KE, Aguilar R, Berndt FA, Canovas J, Montecino M, Kukuljan M (2016) The chromatin modifying complex CoREST/LSD1 negatively regulates notch pathway during cerebral cortex development. Dev Neurobiol 76:1360–1373

Lu J, McKinsey TA, Zhang CL, Olson EN (2000) Regulation of skeletal myogenesis by association of the MEF2 transcription factor with class II histone deacetylases. Mol Cell 6:233–244

Lv T, Yuan D, Miao X, Lv Y, Zhan P, Shen X, Song Y (2012) Over-expression of LSD1 promotes proliferation, migration and invasion in non-small cell lung cancer. PLoS ONE 7:e35065

Lynch JT, Harris WJ, Somervaille TC (2012) LSD1 inhibition: a therapeutic strategy in cancer? Expert Opin Ther Targets 16:1239–1249

Maiques-Diaz A, Somervaille TC (2016) LSD1: biologic roles and therapeutic targeting. Epigenomics 8:1103–1116

Mal A, Harter ML (2003) MyoD is functionally linked to the silencing of a muscle-specific regulatory gene prior to skeletal myogenesis. Proc Natl Acad Sci USA 100:1735–1739

Metzger E, Wissmann M, Yin N, Muller JM, Schneider R, Peters AH, Gunther T, Buettner R, Schule R (2005) LSD1 demethylates repressive histone marks to promote androgen-receptor-dependent transcription. Nature 437:436–439

Mimasu S, Umezawa N, Sato S, Higuchi T, Umehara T, Yokoyama S (2010) Structurally designed trans-2-phenylcyclopropylamine derivatives potently inhibit histone demethylase LSD1/KDM1. Biochemistry 49:6494–6503

Mohammad HP, Kruger RG (2016) Antitumor activity of LSD1 inhibitors in lung cancer. Molecular Cell Oncol 3:e1117700

Mohammad HP, Smitheman KN, Kamat CD, Soong D, Federowicz KE, Van Aller GS, Schneck JL, Carson JD, Liu Y, Butticello M, Bonnette WG, Gorman SA, Degenhardt Y, Bai Y, McCabe MT, Pappalardi MB, Kasparec J, Tian X, McNulty KC, Rouse M, McDevitt P, Ho T, Crouthamel M, Hart TK, Concha NO, McHugh CF, Miller WH, Dhanak D, Tummino

PJ, Carpenter CL, Johnson NW, Hann CL, Kruger RG (2015) A DNA hypomethylation signature predicts antitumor activity of LSD1 inhibitors in SCLC. Cancer Cell 28:57–69

Molkentin JD, Olson EN (1996) Defining the regulatory networks for muscle development. Curr Opin Genet Dev 6:445–453

Morera L, Lubbert M, Jung M (2016) Targeting histone methyltransferases and demethylases in clinical trials for cancer therapy. Clin Epigenetics 8:57

Mulligan P, Yang F, Di Stefano L, Ji JY, Ouyang J, Nishikawa JL, Toiber D, Kulkarni M, Wang Q, Najafi-Shoushtari SH, Mostoslavsky R, Gygi SP, Gill G, Dyson NJ, Naar AM (2011) A SIRT1-LSD1 corepressor complex regulates Notch target gene expression and development. Mol Cell 42:689–699

Murray-Stewart T, Woster PM, Casero RA (2013) The re-expression of the epigenetically silenced e-cadherin gene by a polyamine analogue lysine-specific demethylase-1 (LSD1) inhibitor in human acute myeloid leukemia cell lines. Amino Acids 46:585–594

Musella M, Guarracino A, Manduca N, Galassi C, Ruggiero E, Potenza A, Maccafeo E, Manic G, Mattiello L, Soliman Abdel Rehim S, Signore M, Pietrosanto M, Helmer-Citterich M, Pallocca M, Fanciulli M, Bruno T, De Nicola F, Corleone G, Di Benedetto A, Ercolani C, Pescarmona E, Pizzuti L, Guidi F, Sperati F, Vitale S, Macchia D, Spada M, Schiavoni G, Mattei F, De Ninno A, Businaro L, Lucarini V, Bracci L, Arico E, Ziccheddu G, Facchiano F, Rossi S, Sanchez M, Boe A, Biffoni M, De Maria R, Vitale I, Sistigu A (2022) Type I IFNs promote cancer cell stemness by triggering the epigenetic regulator KDM1B. Nat Immunol 23:1379–1392

Musri MM, Carmona MC, Hanzu FA, Kaliman P, Gomis R, Parrizas M (2010) Histone demethylase LSD1 regulates adipogenesis. J Biol Chem 285:30034–30041

Nagaoka K, Hino S, Sakamoto A, Anan K, Takase R, Umehara T, Yokoyama S, Sasaki Y, Nakao M (2015) Lysine-specific demethylase 2 suppresses lipid influx and metabolism in hepatic cells. Mol Cell Biol 35:1068–1080

Nair SS, Li DQ, Kumar R (2013) A core chromatin remodeling factor instructs global chromatin signaling through multivalent reading of nucleosome codes. Mol Cell 49:704–718

Neelamegam R, Ricq EL, Malvaez M, Patnaik D, Norton S, Carlin SM, Hill IT, Wood MA, Haggarty SJ, Hooker JM (2012) Brain-penetrant LSD1 inhibitors can block memory consolidation. ACS Chem Neurosci 3:120–128

Nguyen EM, Taniguchi H, Chan JM, Zhan YA, Chen X, Qiu J, de Stanchina E, Allaj V, Shah NS, Uddin F, Manoj P, Liu M, Cai SF, Levine R, Quintanal-Villalonga A, Sen T, Chow A, Rudin CM (2022) Targeting lysine-specific demethylase 1 rescues major histocompatibility complex class I antigen presentation and overcomes programmed death-ligand 1 blockade resistance in SCLC. J Thorac Oncol 17:1014–1031

Nicholson TB, Chen T (2014) LSD1 demethylates histone and non-histone proteins. Epigenetics 4:129–132

Nikoloski G, Langemeijer SM, Kuiper RP, Knops R, Massop M, Tonnissen ER, van der Heijden A, Scheele TN, Vandenberghe P, de Witte T, van der Reijden BA, Jansen JH (2010) Somatic mutations of the histone methyltransferase gene EZH2 in myelodysplastic syndromes. Nat Genet 42:665–667

Nowak RP, Tumber A, Johansson C, Che KH, Brennan P, Owen D, Oppermann U (2016) Advances and challenges in understanding histone demethylase biology. Curr Opin Chem Biol 33:151–159

Nowotarski SL, Pachaiyappan B, Holshouser SL, Kutz CJ, Li Y, Huang Y, Sharma SK, Casero RA Jr, Woster PM (2015) Structure-activity study for (bis)ureidopropyl- and (bis)thioureidopropyldiamine LSD1 inhibitors with 3-5-3 and 3-6-3 carbon backbone architectures. Bioorg Med Chem 23:1601–1612

Ogasawara D, Suzuki T, Mino K, Ueda R, Khan MN, Matsubara T, Koseki K, Hasegawa M, Sasaki R, Nakagawa H, Mizukami T, Miyata N (2011) Synthesis and biological activity of optically active NCL-1, a lysine-specific demethylase 1 selective inhibitor. Bioorg Med Chem 19:3702–3708

Ombra MN, Di Santi A, Abbondanza C, Migliaccio A, Avvedimento EV, Perillo B (2013) Retinoic acid impairs estrogen signaling in breast cancer cells by interfering with activation of LSD1 via PKA. Biochem Biophys Acta 1829:480–486

Ota Y, Itoh Y, Kaise A, Ohta K, Endo Y, Masuda M, Sowa Y, Sakai T, Suzuki T (2016) Targeting cancer with PCPA-drug conjugates: LSD1 inhibition-triggered release of 4-hydroxytamoxifen. Angew Chem 55:16115–16118

Ouyang J, Shi Y, Valin A, Xuan Y, Gill G (2009) Direct binding of CoREST1 to SUMO-2/3 contributes to gene-specific repression by the LSD1/CoREST1/HDAC complex. Mol Cell 34:145–154

Pastor WA, Aravind L, Rao A (2013) TETonic shift: biological roles of TET proteins in DNA demethylation and transcription. Nat Rev Mol Cell Biol 14:341–356

Perillo B, Tramontano A, Pezone A, Migliaccio A (2020) LSD1: more than demethylation of histone lysine residues. Exp Mol Med 52:1936–1947

Pollock JA, Larrea MD, Jasper JS, McDonnell DP, McCafferty DG (2012) Lysine-specific histone demethylase 1 inhibitors control breast cancer proliferation in ERalpha-dependent and -independent manners. ACS Chem Biol 7:1221–1231

Prusevich P, Kalin JH, Ming SA, Basso M, Givens J, Li X, Hu J, Taylor MS, Cieniewicz AM, Hsiao PY, Huang R, Roberson H, Adejola N, Avery LB, Casero RA Jr, Taverna SD, Qian J, Tackett AJ, Ratan RR, McDonald OG, Feinberg AP, Cole PA (2014) A selective phenelzine analogue inhibitor of histone demethylase LSD1. ACS Chem Biol 9:1284–1293

Ray SK, Li HJ, Metzger E, Schule R, Leiter AB (2014) CtBP and associated LSD1 are required for transcriptional activation by NeuroD1 in gastrointestinal endocrine cells. Mol Cell Biol 34:2308–2317

Reitman ZJ, Jin G, Karoly ED, Spasojevic I, Yang J, Kinzler KW, He Y, Bigner DD, Vogelstein B, Yan H (2011) Profiling the effects of isocitrate dehydrogenase 1 and 2 mutations on the cellular metabolome. Proc Natl Acad Sci USA 108:3270–3275

Ribeiro AF, Pratcorona M, Erpelinck-Verschueren C, Rockova V, Sanders M, Abbas S, Figueroa ME, Zeilemaker A, Melnick A, Lowenberg B, Valk PJ, Delwel R (2012) Mutant DNMT3A: a marker of poor prognosis in acute myeloid leukemia. Blood 119:5824–5831

Rotili D, Tomassi S, Conte M, Benedetti R, Tortorici M, Ciossani G, Valente S, Marrocco B, Labella D, Novellino E, Mattevi A, Altucci L, Tumber A, Yapp C, King ON, Hopkinson RJ, Kawamura A, Schofield CJ, Mai A (2014) Pan-histone demethylase inhibitors simultaneously targeting Jumonji C and lysine-specific demethylases display high anticancer activities. J Med Chem 57:42–55

Russler-Germain DA, Spencer DH, Young MA, Lamprecht TL, Miller CA, Fulton R, Meyer MR, Erdmann-Gilmore P, Townsend RR, Wilson RK, Ley TJ (2014) The R882H DNMT3A mutation associated with AML dominantly inhibits wild-type DNMT3A by blocking its ability to form active tetramers. Cancer Cell 25:442–454

Saez JE, Gomez AV, Barrios AP, Parada GE, Galdames L, Gonzalez M, Andres ME (2015) Decreased expression of CoREST1 and CoREST2 together with LSD1 and HDAC1/2 during neuronal differentiation. PLoS ONE 10:e0131760

Sambeat A, Gulyaeva O, Dempersmier J, Tharp KM, Stahl A, Paul SM, Sul HS (2016) LSD1 interacts with Zfp516 to promote UCP1 transcription and brown fat program. Cell Rep 15:2536–2549

Sankar S, Bell R, Stephens B, Zhuo R, Sharma S, Bearss DJ, Lessnick SL (2013) Mechanism and relevance of EWS/FLI-mediated transcriptional repression in Ewing sarcoma. Oncogene 32:5089–5100

Sareddy GR, Nair BC, Krishnan SK, Gonugunta VK, Zhang QG, Suzuki T, Miyata N, Brenner AJ, Brann DW, Vadlamudi RK (2013) KDM1 is a novel therapeutic target for the treatment of gliomas. Oncotarget 4:18–28

Schenk T, Chen WC, Gollner S, Howell L, Jin L, Hebestreit K, Klein HU, Popescu AC, Burnett A, Mills K, Casero RA Jr, Marton L, Woster P, Minden MD, Dugas M, Wang JC, Dick JE, Muller-Tidow C, Petrie K, Zelent A (2012) Inhibition of the LSD1 (KDM1A) demethylase reactivates the all-trans-retinoic acid differentiation pathway in acute myeloid leukemia. Nat Med 18:605–611

Schmidt DM, McCafferty DG (2007) Trans-2-phenylcyclopropylamine is a mechanism-based inactivator of the histone demethylase LSD1. Biochemistry 46:4408–4416

Schmitt ML, Hauser AT, Carlino L, Pippel M, Schulz-Fincke J, Metzger E, Willmann D, Yiu T, Barton M, Schule R, Sippl W, Jung M (2013) Nonpeptidic propargylamines as inhibitors of lysine specific demethylase 1 (LSD1) with cellular activity. J Med Chem 56:7334–7342

Schulte JH, Lim S, Schramm A, Friedrichs N, Koster J, Versteeg R, Ora I, Pajtler K, Klein-Hitpass L, Kuhfittig-Kulle S, Metzger E, Schule R, Eggert A, Buettner R, Kirfel J (2009) Lysine-specific demethylase 1 is strongly expressed in poorly differentiated neuroblastoma: implications for therapy. Cancer Res 69:2065–2071

Scionti I, Hayashi S, Mouradian S, Girard E, Esteves de Lima J, Morel V, Simonet T, Wurmser M, Maire P, Ancelin K, Metzger E, Schule R, Goillot E, Relaix F, Schaeffer L (2017) LSD1 controls timely MyoD expression via MyoD core enhancer transcription. Cell Rep 18:1996–2006

Scoumanne A, Chen X (2007) The lysine-specific demethylase 1 is required for cell proliferation in both p53-dependent and -independent manners. J Biol Chem 282:15471–15475

Sehrawat A, Gao L, Wang Y, Bankhead A 3rd, McWeeney SK, King CJ, Schwartzman J, Urrutia J, Bisson WH, Coleman DJ, Joshi SK, Kim DH, Sampson DA, Weinmann S, Kallakury BVS, Berry DL, Haque R, Van Den Eeden SK, Sharma S, Bearss J, Beer TM, Thomas GV, Heiser LM, Alumkal JJ (2018) LSD1 activates a lethal prostate cancer gene network independently of its demethylase function. Proc Natl Acad Sci USA 115:E4179–E4188

Shao GB, Huang XJ, Gong AH, Zhang ZJ, Lu RZ, Sang JR (2010) Histone demethylase LSD1 and its biological functions. Yi Chuan 32:331–338

Sharma SK, Wu Y, Steinbergs N, Crowley ML, Hanson AS, Casero RA, Woster PM (2010) (Bis)urea and (bis)thiourea inhibitors of lysine-specific demethylase 1 as epigenetic modulators. J Med Chem 53:5197–5212

Sheng W, LaFleur MW, Nguyen TH, Chen S, Chakravarthy A, Conway JR, Li Y, Chen H, Yang H, Hsu PH, Van Allen EM, Freeman GJ, De Carvalho DD, He HH, Sharpe AH, Shi Y (2018) LSD1 ablation stimulates anti-tumor immunity and enables checkpoint blockade. Cell 174(549–563):e519

Sheng W, Liu Y, Chakraborty D, Debo B, Shi Y (2021) Simultaneous inhibition of LSD1 and TGFbeta enables eradication of poorly immunogenic tumors with anti-PD-1 treatment. Cancer Discov 11:1970–1981

Shi Y, Lan F, Matson C, Mulligan P, Whetstine JR, Cole PA, Casero RA, Shi Y (2004) Histone demethylation mediated by the nuclear amine oxidase homolog LSD1. Cell 119:941–953

Shi Y, Sawada J, Sui G, el Affar B, Whetstine JR, Lan F, Ogawa H, Luke MP, Nakatani Y, Shi Y (2003)

Coordinated histone modifications mediated by a CtBP co-repressor complex. Nature 422:735–738

Shi YG, Tsukada Y (2013) The discovery of histone demethylases. Cold Spring Harbor Perspect Biol 5

Shi YJ, Matson C, Lan F, Iwase S, Baba T, Shi Y (2005) Regulation of LSD1 histone demethylase activity by its associated factors. Mol Cell 19:857–864

Song Y, Zhang H, Yang X, Shi Y, Yu B (2022) Annual review of lysine-specific demethylase 1 (LSD1/KDM1A) inhibitors in 2021. Euro J Med Chem 228

Sonnemann J, Zimmermann M, Marx C, Ebert F, Becker S, Lauterjung ML, Beck JF (2017) LSD1 (KDM1A)-independent effects of the LSD1 inhibitor SP2509 in cancer cells. Br J Haematol

Sorna V, Theisen ER, Stephens B, Warner SL, Bearss DJ, Vankayalapati H, Sharma S (2013) High-throughput virtual screening identifies novel N'-(1-phenylethylidene)-benzohydrazides as potent, specific, and reversible LSD1 inhibitors. J Med Chem 56 9496–9508

Sprussel A, Schulte JH, Weber S, Necke M, Handschke K, Thor T, Pajtler KW, Schramm A, Konig K, Diehl L, Mestdagh P, Vandesompele J, Speleman F, Jastrow H, Heukamp LC, Schule R, Duhrsen U, Buettner R, Eggert A, Gothert JR (2012) Lysine-specific demethylase 1 restricts hematopoietic progenitor proliferation and is essential for terminal differentiation. Leukemia 26:2039–2051

Stavropoulos P, Blobel G, Hoelz A (2006) Crystal structure and mechanism of human lysine-specific demethylase-1. Nat Struct Mol Biol 13:626–632

Stazi G, Zwergel C, Valente S, Mai A (2016) LSD1 inhibitors: a patent review (2010–2015). Expert Opin Ther Pat 26:565–580

Steinbac OC, Wolffe AP, Rupp RA (2000) Histone deacetylase activity is required for the induction of the MyoD muscle cell lineage in Xenopus. Biol Chem 381:1013–1016

Stewart CA, Byers LA (2015) Altering the course of small cell lung cancer: targeting cancer stem cells via LSD1 inhibition. Cancer Cell 28:4–6

Stewart KR, Veselovska L, Kim J, Huang J, Saadeh H, Tomizawa S, Smallwood SA, Chen T, Kelsey G (2015) Dynamic changes in histone modifications precede de novo DNA methylation in oocytes. Genes Dev 29:2449–2462

Straub LG, Wolfrum C (2017) LSD1 makes fat colorful. Trends Endocrinol Metab 28:1–2

Sun G, Alzayady K, Stewart R, Ye P, Yang S, Li W, Shi Y (2010) Histone demethylase LSD1 regulates neural stem cell proliferation. Mol Cell Biol 30:1997–2005

Sun G, Ye P, Murai K, Lang MF, Li S, Zhang H, Li W, Fu C, Yin J, Wang A, Ma X, Shi Y (2011) miR-137 forms a regulatory loop with nuclear receptor TLX and LSD1 in neural stem cells. Nat Commun 2:529

Sun L, Fang J (2016) Epigenetic regulation of epithelial-mesenchymal transition. Cell Mole Life Sci CMLS 73:4493–4515

Taylor MV, Hughes SM (2017) Mef2 and the skeletal muscle differentiation program. Semin Cell Dev Biol 72:33–44

Topper MJ (2017) Leading the way in veterinary research; acknowledging these passionate professionals. J Am Vet Med Assoc 251:478

Tortorici M, Borrello MT, Tardugno M, Chiarelli LR, Pilotto S, Ciossani G, Vellore NA, Bailey SG, Cowan J, O'Connell M, Crabb SJ, Packham G, Mai A, Baron R, Ganesan A, Mattevi A (2013) Protein recognition by short peptide reversible inhibitors of the chromatin-modifying LSD1/CoREST lysine demethylase. ACS Chem Biol 8:1677–1682

Tsukada Y, Fang J, Erdjument-Bromage H, Warren ME, Borchers CH, Tempst P, Zhang Y (2006) Histone demethylation by a family of JmjC domain-containing proteins. Nature 439:811–816

Ueda R, Suzuki T, Mino K, Tsumoto H, Nakagawa H, Hasegawa M, Sasaki R, Mizukami T, Miyata N (2009) Identification of cell-active lysine specific demethylase 1-selective inhibitors. J Am Chem Soc 131:17536–17537

Urban N, Guillemot F (2014) Neurogenesis in the embryonic and adult brain: same regulators, different roles. Front Cell Neurosci 8:396

Vasilatos SN, Katz TA, Oesterreich S, Wan Y, Davidson NE, Huang Y (2013) Crosstalk between lysine-specific demethylase 1 (LSD1) and histone deacetylases mediates antineoplastic efficacy of HDAC inhibitors in human breast cancer cells. Carcinogenesis 34:1196–1207

Vianello P, Botrugno OA, Cappa A, Ciossani G, Dessanti P, Mai A, Mattevi A, Meroni G, Minucci S, Thaler F, Tortorici M, Trifiro P, Valente S, Villa M, Varasi M, Mercurio C (2014) Synthesis, biological activity and mechanistic insights of 1-substituted cyclopropylamine derivatives: a novel class of irreversible inhibitors of histone demethylase KDM1A. Eur J Med Chem 86:352–363

Vianello P, Botrugno OA, Cappa A, Dal Zuffo R, Dessanti P, Mai A, Marrocco B, Mattevi A, Meroni G, Minucci S, Stazi G, Thaler F, Trifiro P, Valente S, Villa M, Varasi M, Mercurio C (2016) Discovery of a novel inhibitor of histone lysine-specific demethylase 1A (KDM1A/LSD1) as orally active antitumor agent. J Med Chem 59:1501–1517

Wang J, Hevi S, Kurash JK, Lei H, Gay F, Bajko J, Su H, Sun W, Chang H, Xu G, Gaudet F, Li E, Chen T (2008) The lysine demethylase LSD1 (KDM1) is required for maintenance of global DNA methylation. Nat Genet 41:125–129

Wang J, Hevi S, Kurash JK, Lei H, Gay F, Bajko J, Su H, Sun W, Chang H, Xu G, Gaudet F, Li E, Chen T (2009a) The lysine demethylase LSD1 (KDM1) is required for maintenance of global DNA methylation. Nat Genet 41:125–129

Wang J, Lu F, Ren Q, Sun H, Xu Z, Lan R, Liu Y, Ward D, Quan J, Ye T, Zhang H (2011) Novel histone demethylase LSD1 inhibitors selectively target cancer cells with pluripotent stem cell properties. Can Res 71:7238–7249

Wang J, Scully K, Zhu X, Cai L, Zhang J, Prefontaine GG, Krones A, Ohgi KA, Zhu P, Garcia-Bassets I, Liu F, Taylor H, Lozach J, Jayes FL, Korach KS, Glass CK, Fu XD, Rosenfeld MG (2007) Opposing LSD1 complexes function in developmental gene activation and repression programmes. Nature 446:882–887

Wang M, Liu X, Guo J, Weng X, Jiang G, Wang Z, He L (2015) Inhibition of LSD1 by pargyline inhibited process of EMT and delayed progression of prostate cancer in vivo. Biochem Biophys Res Commun 467:310–315

Wang Y, Wu Q, Yang P, Wang C, Liu J, Ding W, Liu W, Bai Y, Yang Y, Wang H, Gao S, Wang X (2016) LSD1 co-repressor Rcor2 orchestrates neurogenesis in the developing mouse brain. Nat Commun 7:10481

Wang Y, Zhang H, Chen Y, Sun Y, Yang F, Yu W, Liang J, Sun L, Yang X, Shi L, Li R, Li Y, Zhang Y, Li Q, Yi X, Shang Y (2009b) LSD1 is a subunit of the NuRD complex and targets the metastasis programs in breast cancer. Cell 138:660–672

Wei X, Calvo-Vidal MN, Chen S, Wu G, Revuelta MV, Sun J, Zhang J, Walsh MF, Nichols KE, Joseph V, Snyder C, Vachon CM, McKay JD, Wang SP, Jayabalan DS, Jacobs LM, Becirovic D, Waller RG, Artomov M, Viale A, Patel J, Phillip J, Chen-Kiang S, Curtin K, Salama M, Atanackovic D, Niesvizky R, Landgren O, Slager SL, Godley LA, Churpek J, Garber JE, Anderson KC, Daly MJ, Roeder RG, Dumontet C, Lynch HT, Mullighan CG, Camp NJ, Offit K, Klein RJ, Yu H, Cerchietti L, Lipkin SM (2018) Germline lysine-specific demethylase 1 (LSD1/KDM1A) mutations confer susceptibility to multiple myeloma. Can Res 78:2747–2759

Whyte WA, Bilodeau S, Orlando DA, Hoke HA, Frampton GM, Foster CT, Cowley SM, Young RA (2012) Enhancer decommissioning by LSD1 during embryonic stem cell differentiation. Nature 482:221–225

Willmann D, Lim S, Wetzel S, Metzger E, Jandausch A, Wilk W, Jung M, Forne I, Imhof A, Janzer A, Kirfel J, Waldmann H, Schule R, Buettner R (2012) Impairment of prostate cancer cell growth by a selective and reversible lysine-specific demethylase 1 inhibitor. Int J Cancer 131:2704–2709

Wissmann M, Yin N, Muller JM, Greschik H, Fodor BD, Jenuwein T, Vogler C, Schneider R, Gunther T, Buettner R, Metzger E, Schule R (2007) Cooperative demethylation by JMJD2C and LSD1 promotes androgen receptor-dependent gene expression. Nat Cell Biol 9:347–353

Wu CY, Hsieh CY, Huang KE, Chang C, Kang HY (2012) Cryptotanshinone down-regulates androgen receptor signaling by modulating lysine-specific demethylase 1 function. Int J Cancer 131:1423–1434

Xu G, Xiao Y, Hu J, Xing L, Zhao O, Wu Y (2013) The combined effect of retinoic acid and LSD1 siRNA inhibition on cell death in the human neuroblastoma cell line SH-SY5Y. Cell Physiol Biochem Int J Exper Cell Physiol Biochem Pharmacol 31:854–862

Yan HJ, Zhou SY, Li Y, Zhang H, Deng CY, Qi H, Li FR (2016) The effects of LSD1 inhibition on self-renewal and differentiation of human induced pluripotent stem cells. Exp Cell Res 340:227–237

Yan XJ, Xu J, Gu ZH, Pan CM, Lu G, Shen Y, Shi JY, Zhu YM, Tang L, Zhang XW, Liang WX, Mi JQ, Song HD, Li KQ, Chen Z, Chen SJ (2011) Exome sequencing identifies somatic mutations of DNA methyltransferase gene DNMT3A in acute monocytic leukemia. Nat Genet 43:309–315

Yang J, Huang J, Dasgupta M, Sears N, Miyagi M, Wang B, Chance MR, Chen X, Du Y, Wang Y, An L, Wang Q, Lu T, Zhang X, Wang Z, Stark GR (2010a) Reversible methylation of promoter-bound STAT3 by histone-modifying enzymes. Proc Natl Acad Sci USA 107:21499–21504

Yang M, Gocke CB, Luo X, Borek D, Tomchick DR, Machius M, Otwinowski Z, Yu H (2006) Structural basis for CoREST-dependent demethylation of nucleosomes by the human LSD1 histone demethylase. Mol Cell 23:377–387

Yang Y, Yin X, Yang H, Xu Y (2015) Histone demethylase LSD2 acts as an E3 ubiquitin ligase and inhibits cancer cell growth through promoting proteasomal degradation of OGT. Mol Cell 58:47–59

Yang Z, Jiang J, Stewart MD, Qi S, Yamane K, Li J, Zhang Y, Wong J (2010b) AOF1 is a histone H3K4 demethylase possessing demethylase activity-independent repression function. Cell Res 20:276–287

Yokoyama A, Takezawa S, Schule R, Kitagawa H, Kato S (2008) Transrepressive function of TLX requires the histone demethylase LSD1. Mol Cell Biol 28:3995–4003

Yu Y, Wang B, Zhang K, Lei Z, Guo Y, Xiao H, Wang J, Fan L, Lan C, Wei Y, Ma Q, Lin L, Mao C, Yang X, Chen X, Li Y, Bai Y, Chen D (2013) High expression of lysine-specific demethylase 1 correlates with poor prognosis of patients with esophageal squamous cell carcinoma. Biochem Biophys Res Commun 437:192–198

Zeng X, Jedrychowski MP, Chen Y, Serag S, Lavery GG, Gygi SP, Spiegelman BM (2016) Lysine-specific demethylase 1 promotes brown adipose tissue thermogenesis via repressing glucocorticoid activation. Genes Dev 30:1822–1836

Zhang Q, Qi S, Xu M, Yu L, Tao Y, Deng Z, Wu W, Li J, Chen Z, Wong J (2013) Structure-function analysis reveals a novel mechanism for regulation of histone demethylase LSD2/AOF1/KDM1b. Cell Res 23:225–241

Zhang RH, Judson RN, Liu DY, Kast J, Rossi FM (2016) The lysine methyltransferase Ehmt2/G9a is dispensable for skeletal muscle development and regeneration. Skelet Muscle 6:22

Zhang W, Ruan X, Li Y, Zhi J, Hu L, Hou X, Shi X, Wang X, Wang J, Ma W, Gu P, Zheng X, Gao M (2022a) KDM1A promotes thyroid cancer progression and maintains stemness through the Wnt/beta-catenin signaling pathway. Theranostics 12:1500–1517

Zhang X, Wang X, Wu T, Yin W, Yan J, Sun Y, Zhao D (2022b) Therapeutic potential of targeting LSD1/KDM1A in cancers. Pharmacol Res 175:105958

Zheng YC, Duan YC, Ma JL, Xu RM, Zi X, Lv WL, Wang MM, Ye XW, Zhu S, Mobley D, Zhu YY, Wang JW, Li JF, Wang ZR, Zhao W, Liu HM (2013) Triazole-dithiocarbamate based selective lysine specific demethylase 1 (LSD1) inactivators inhibit gastric cancer cell growth, invasion, and migration. J Med Chem 56:8543–8560

Zheng YC, Ma J, Wang Z, Li J, Jiang B, Zhou W, Shi X, Wang X, Zhao W, Liu HM (2015) A systematic review of histone lysine-specific demethylase 1 and its inhibitors. Med Res Rev 35:1032–1071

Zhou C, Kang D, Xu Y, Zhang L, Zha X (2015) Identification of novel selective lysine-specific demethylase 1 (LSD1) inhibitors using a pharmacophore-based virtual screening combined with docking. Chem Biol Drug Des 85:659–671

Zhou C, Wu F, Lu L, Wei L, Pai E, Yao Y, Song Y (2017) Structure activity relationship and modeling studies of inhibitors of lysine specific demethylase 1. PLoS ONE 12:e0170301

Zhou G, Du T, Roizman B (2013) The role of the CoREST/REST repressor complex in herpes simplex virus 1 productive infection and in latency. Viruses 5:1208–1218

Zhu D, Holz S, Metzger E, Pavlovic M, Jandausch A, Jilg C, Galgoczy P, Herz C, Moser M, Metzger D, Gunther T, Arnold SJ, Schule R (2014) Lysine-specific demethylase 1 regulates differentiation onset and migration of trophoblast stem cells. Nat Commun 5:3174

Zhu Q, Huang Y, Marton LJ, Woster PM, Davidson NE, Casero RA Jr (2012) Polyamine analogs modulate gene expression by inhibiting lysine-specific demethylase 1 (LSD1) and altering chromatin structure in human breast cancer cells. Amino Acids 42:887–898

Biological Functions of the KDM2 Family of Histone Demethylases

3

Jaclyn Andricovich and Alexandros Tzatsos

Abstract

The histone lysine demethylase 2 (KDM2) family of α-Ketoglutarate-Fe^{++}-dependent dioxygenases were the first Jumonji-domain-containing proteins reported to harbor demethylase activity. This landmark discovery paved the way for the characterization of more than 25 enzymes capable of demethylating lysine residues on histones—an epigenetic modification previously thought to be irreversible. The KDM2 family is comprised of KDM2A and KDM2B which share significant structural similarities and demethylate lysine 36 on histone H3. However, they exert distinct cellular functions and are frequently deregulated in a broad spectrum of human cancers. With the advent of next generation sequencing and development of genetically engineered mouse models, it was shown that KDM2A and KDM2B play critical roles in stem cell biology, somatic cell reprograming, and organismal development by regulating cell fate and lineage commitment decisions. Thus, understanding the biochemistry and elucidating the context-dependent function of these enzymes is an emerging new frontier for the development of small molecule inhibitors to treat cancer and other diseases.

Keywords

KDM2A · KDM2B · Jumonji · Histone demethylase · Cancer · Leukemia · Pancreatic cancer · DNA methylation · Histone modification

3.1 Introduction

Histone N^{ε}-methylated lysine specific demethylases (KDMs) contribute to cellular homeostasis by reversing the degree of methylation on nucleosomes. They are classified into two families based on their sequence homology and catalytic mechanisms (Shi et al. 2004; Tsukada et al. 2006; Kooistra and Helin 2012). The first family encompasses two members, KDM1A and KDM1B (also known as LSD1A and LSD1B), which employ flavin adenine dinucleotide (FAD) as a cofactor. Demethylation occurs through a FAD-dependent oxidative reaction via formation of an imine intermediate, which spontaneously degrades to produce formaldehyde and the demethylated amine, while the reduced FAD is re-oxidized by oxygen (Shi et al. 2004; Kooistra and Helin 2012). However, this mechanism cannot apply to quaternary amines; hence,

J. Andricovich · A. Tzatsos (✉)
Cancer Epigenetics Laboratory, George Washington University Cancer Center, 800 22nd St NW, Suite 8850, Washington DC 20052, USA
e-mail: atzatsos@gwu.edu

Q. Yan (ed.), *Targeting Lysine Demethylases in Cancer and Other Human Diseases*, Advances in Experimental Medicine and Biology 1433, https://doi.org/10.1007/978-3-031-38176-8_3

the KDM1 family does not act on tri-methylated lysine residues (Shi et al. 2004; Kooistra and Helin 2012). The second family encompasses the α-ketoglutarate (α-KG)-dependent Jumonji (JmjC) domain-containing KDMs, which are part of the dioxygenase superfamily that use α-KG and molecular oxygen as cofactors (Tsukada et al. 2006; Kooistra and Helin 2012). The JmjC family of KDMs belongs to the cupin superfamily of metalloenzymes (Clissold and Ponting 2001; Tsukada et al. 2006), consists of approximately thirty members, and is further divided into KDM2, KDM3, KDM4, KDM5, KDM6, KDM7, and KDM8 subfamilies (Tsukada et al. 2006; Kooistra and Helin 2012). JmjC domain KDMs catalyze the removal of methyl groups through an oxidative reaction that requires Fe^{++} and α-KG as cofactors; their interaction with oxygen forms a highly reactive oxo-ferryl intermediate which hydroxylates the methylated lysine substrate with the concomitant conversion of α-KG to succinate and carbon dioxide. The resulting carbinolamine is unstable and degrades into unmethylated lysine and formaldehyde (Tsukada et al. 2006). Unlike KDM1A/B which demethylate mono- and dimethylated lysine 4 at histone H3 (H3K4) (Shi et al. 2004), the JmjC family of KDMs shows broad activity toward methylated lysines on histone H3 and is also capable of demethylating trimethylated lysine residues (Kooistra and Helin 2012).

Mounting evidence indicates that KDMs not only play important roles in homeostasis, but are also deregulated in cancer. Thereby, these enzymes are emerging as attractive candidates for therapeutic targeting by small molecule inhibitors. Here, we discuss the KDM2 family which consists of two members—KDM2A and KDM2B—which were the first JmjC domain proteins shown to reverse lysine methylation on histone tails (Tsukada et al. 2006). Since their discovery, compelling evidence indicates that KDM2A and KDM2B play essential roles in stem cell biology, somatic cell reprogramming, and oncogenesis, while the generation of genetically engineered mice with tissue-specific knockout and overexpression of KDM2A/B highlighted important roles during development, tissue maintenance, and regeneration. At the molecular level, KDM2A and KDM2B regulate pathways linked to cell fate and proliferation; consequently, their deregulation contributes to cell transformation and their pharmacological inhibition holds promise for treating a spectrum of human malignancies.

3.2 Structure and Function of KDM2 Demethylases

Histone methylation impacts chromatin structure and function, contributing to the temporal and spatial aspects of gene expression. Using an activity-based biochemical purification scheme coupled to monitoring radioactive formaldehyde released due to demethylation of radiolabeled nucleosomal substrates methylated on histone H3 lysine 36 (H3K36), it was discovered that KDM2A (also known as FBXL11 and JHDM1A) is capable of demethylating di- and mono-methylated H3K36 (Tsukada et al. 2006). Point mutations of the amino acid residues required for Fe^{++} and α-KG binding inhibited the demethylation reaction, establishing that the JmjC domain harbors the enzymatic activity (Tsukada et al. 2006) (Figs. 3.1 and 3.2). Shortly after, KDM2B (also known as FBXL10 and JHDM1B) and KDM2A were independently cloned as targets of provirus integration from Moloney Murine Leukemia Virus (MoMuLV)-induced T-cell lymphomas in rodents and showed to possess histone H3K36 di-demethylase activity (Pfau et al. 2008; Tzatsos et al. 2009). Structural studies of the JmjC domain of KDM2A revealed that the methylated H3K36 histone tail forms a U-shape that is threaded through the catalytic groove and the side chain of methylated K36 inserts into the catalytic pocket where it is positioned for demethylation in the presence of Fe^{++} and α-KG bound to conserved amino acid residues following the His^1-X-Asp/Glu-X_n-His^2 sequence motif required for chelation of the Fe^{++} atom (Cheng et al. 2014) (Fig. 3.2). Interestingly, although KDM2A is capable of binding to H3K36me3 peptides,

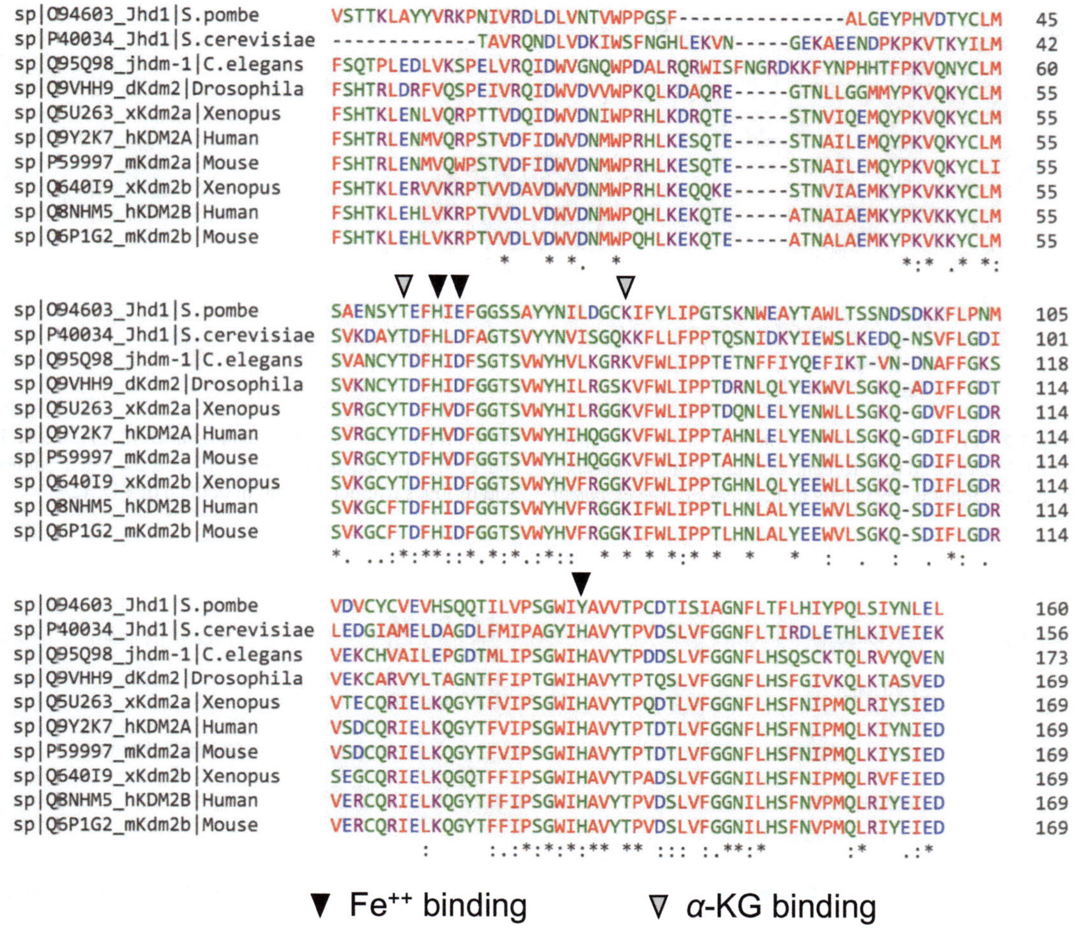

Fig. 3.1 Sequence alignment of the JmjC domain of KDM2 family members across different species using the Clustal Omega software (http://www.ebi.ac.uk/Tools/msa/clustalo/). The amino acids involved in Fe^{++} and α-KG binding are indicated by black and gray triangles, respectively. Epe1 (S. pombe) contains a naturally occurring mutation in the third Fe^{++}-binding residue (histidine to tyrosine) which abolishes the demethylase activity

steric constrains prevent α-KG from undergoing an "off-line" to "in-line" transition necessary for the demethylation reaction (Cheng et al. 2014). Overall, these studies provided the structural basis for understanding H3K36 di-demethylation and will facilitate ongoing efforts for the development of small molecule inhibitors.

The KDM2 family is evolutionary conserved as homologs have been identified in yeast, nematodes, and flies (Fig. 3.3). In *Saccharomyces cerevisiae* (budding yeast), Jhd1 is an active JmjC domain-containing histone H3K36 di-demethylase that also employs Fe^{++} and α-KG as cofactors (Fang et al. 2007; Tu et al. 2007). Although its biological role is poorly defined, Jhd1 has been implicated in the regulation of pre-mRNA splicing (Sorenson et al. 2016). Interestingly, in *Schizosaccharomyces pombe* (fission yeast), Epe1—a negative regulator of heterochromatin spreading (Trewick et al. 2007)—harbors a JmjC domain with sequence similarities to the KDM2 family and was predicted to demethylate H3K36me2. However, it was shown that Epe1 does not exhibit demethylase activity because it lacks a key residue involved in Fe^{++} binding (Tsukada et al. 2006) (Fig. 3.1). The *Drosophila melanogaster* genome encodes a unique histone H3K36

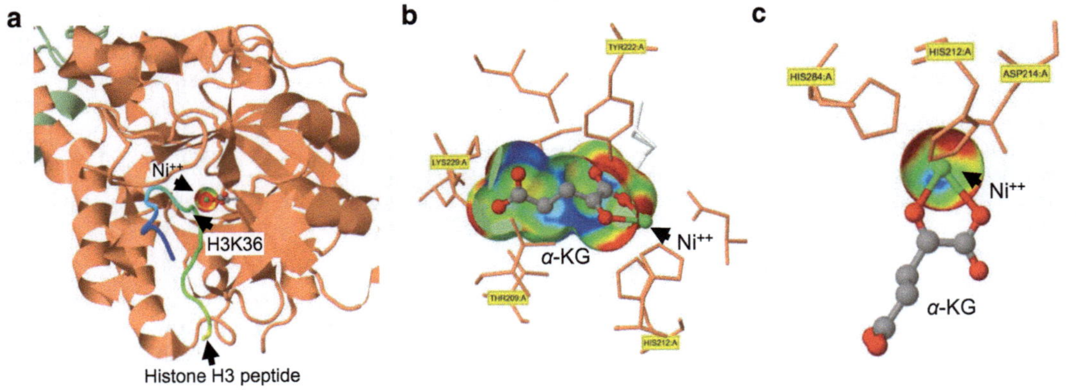

Fig. 3.2 **a** A ribbon representation of the Jumonji domain of KDM2A bound to α-KG and crystalized in the presence of Ni^{++} as reported by Cheng et al. (*Genes & Development* 2014, Protein data bank accession number 4QX7). **b** α-KG and **c** Ni^{++} pocket interactions with the indicated amino acid residues within the Jumonji domain of KDM2A

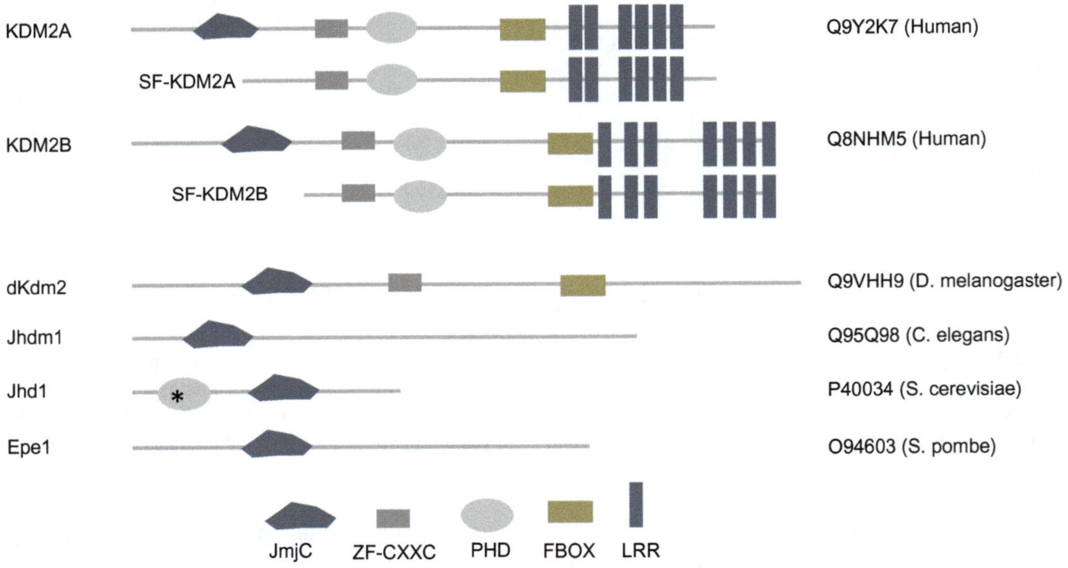

Fig. 3.3 Diagram showing the family of KDM2 demethylases across different species with the corresponding domains. The protein accession number in the UniProt (http://www.uniprot.org/) database is shown on the right. *, atypical PHD domain

di-demethylase, dKdm2, which plays important developmental roles by coupling histone H2A ubiquitination to histone H3 demethylation in gene silencing mediated by Polycomb group (PcG) proteins (Lagarou et al. 2008).

KDM2 homologs in yeast and *Caenorhabditis elegans* contain a JmjC domain, but they lack the zinc-finger CXXC (ZF-CXXC), PHD zinc-finger, F-box, and leucine-rich repeat (LRR) domains that are present in flies and mammals (Fig. 3.3). This suggests that during evolution those proteins acquired additional functions, besides lysine demethylation, to accomplish novel functions through interaction with other proteins or DNA per se. For instance, the ZF-CXXC domains of KDM2A and KDM2B bind unmethylated CpG islands (CGIs) and contribute to genome-wide targeting of those enzymes and associated protein complexes to chromatin (Blackledge et al. 2010; Farcas et al. 2012; He et al. 2013; Wu et al. 2013). On the other hand, the other domains are less characterized in terms of KDM2 function. The PHD domain has been implicated in protein–protein interactions, as well as in recognizing methylated histone tails such as H3K4me3 (Wysocka et al. 2006). The F-Box domain, which is frequently accompanied with a C-terminal LRR, interacts with SKP1 and may serve as a substrate-recognition component of the SCF (SKP-CUL-F-box protein) E3 ubiquitin ligase complex that exhibits phosphorylation-dependent ubiquitination and degradation of target proteins (Skaar et al. 2013). In this regard, it has been reported that KDM2B targets c-FOS for poly-ubiquitination in a phosphorylation-dependent manner to regulate its stability (Han et al. 2016). In addition to the full-length proteins, KDM2A and KDM2B are expressed in several shorter isoforms due to either alternative splicing or use of internal transcription start sites (Pfau et al. 2008). The most prominent and well-characterized isoforms arise from an internal transcription start site encoding short form KDM2A (SF-KDM2A) and KDM2B (SF-KDM2B) which lack the JmjC but retain all other domains (Fig. 3.3). The short isoforms of KDM2A and KDM2B may play important roles in cellular homeostasis independently of histone demethylation.

3.3 KDM2 Demethylases in Polycomb-Mediated Gene Silencing

Polycomb group (PcG) proteins are chromatin-associated factors that form evolutionary conserved complexes to epigenetically silence gene transcription through histone H3K27 tri-methylation and H2AK119 ubiquitination (Entrevan et al. 2016). PcG proteins play critical roles in mediating cellular differentiation and cell identity and are frequently deregulated in cancer. In general, PcG proteins reside in two complexes: Polycomb Repressive Complex 1 (PRC1) and 2 (PRC2). PRC2 consists of SUZ12, EED, JARID2, and EZH2 which methylates H3K27. PRC1 consists of five subunits (PCGF, PHC, CBX, SCM, and RING1), is recruited to H3K27 marked chromatin through CBX proteins, and catalyzes RING1-mediated H2AK119 ubiquitination (Gao et al. 2012; Entrevan et al. 2016). The human genome encodes multiple paralogs of PRC1 subunits: six Polycomb group ring finger proteins (PCGF1-6), three polyhomeotic homologue proteins (PHC1-3), five CBX members (CBX2,4,6-8), three SCM members (SCML1-2 and SCMH1), and two RING1 members (RING1A-B). Mass spectrometry proteomic studies identified at least six PRC1 complexes that exhibit distinct chromatin-binding patterns and are further divided into canonical and non-canonical based on their composition (Gao et al. 2012). Both canonical and non-canonical PRC1 contain the catalytic subunit RING1A or RING1B. Canonical PRC1 contains one CBX member, one PHC member, and PCGF4 (BMI1) or PCGF2 (MEL18). In the hierarchical model, the chromo-domain in CBX proteins recognizes and binds H3K27me3, catalyzed by PRC2, and this is believed to be a mechanism by which PRC2 guides PRC1 recruitment to chromatin (Simon and Kingston 2013). On the other hand, non-canonical PRC1 complexes contain RYBP (Ring and YY1-binding protein) or YAF2 (YY1-associated factor 2), and PCGF1, 3, 5, or 6, but lack CBX, PHC, and SCM subunits. KDM2B, and likely KDM2A, are integral components of a non-canonical PRC1, named PRC1.1, which contains PCGF1, RING1B, RYBP, SKP1, and BCOR (Gearhart et al. 2006; Sanchez et al. 2007; Gao et al. 2012) (Fig. 3.4). Structural studies of PRC1.1 revealed a crucial role of the PCGF1/BCOR heterodimer in creating a docking interface for KDM2B binding, whereas RYBP/YAF2 were shown to enhance the RING1-dependent H2AK119 E3 ligase activity (Rose et al. 2016). These studies highlight PRC1.1 as a highly modular complex and support the idea that KDM2B might simultaneously participate in PRC1.1 and in a SCF ubiquitin ligase complex

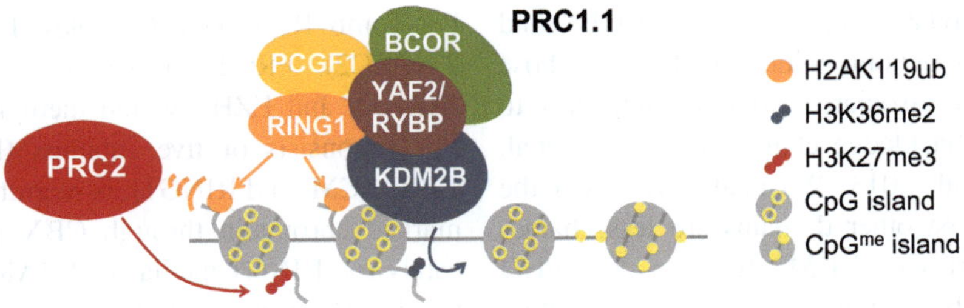

Fig. 3.4 Model of PRC1.1-mediated PRC2 recruitment. PRC1.1 is recruited to unmethylated CGIs via KDM2B, while RING1 ubiquitinates H2AK119 which is recognized by PRC2 that tri-methylates H3K27 to repress gene expression

(Wong et al. 2016), although further studies and identification of downstream targets are needed to confirm its role in SCF-mediated protein ubiquitination.

In *Drosophila melanogaster*, the corresponding dPRC1 contains the CBX homolog Polycomb (Pc), the RING1 homolog Sex combs extra (Sce or dRing), the PCGF homolog Posterior sec combs (Psc), and the PHC homolog Polyhomeotic (Ph) (Entrevan et al. 2016). In an analogous manner to mammalian cells, combinatorial association of those proteins give rise to multiple canonical dPRC1 complexes, whereas a non-canonical dPRC1, known as dRing-associated factors complex (dRAF) (Lagarou et al. 2008), contains dRing, Psc, and dKdm2 as well as dRybp or dYaf2 instead of Pc. Gene expression profiling in flies and mammalian cells revealed that canonical and non-canonical-PRC1 regulate distinct transcriptional programs, and that KDM2B is required not only for H3K36me2 demethylation but also for efficient H2AK119 ubiquitination (Lagarou et al. 2008; Farcas et al. 2012; Blackledge et al. 2014; Cooper et al. 2014; Rose et al. 2016). Surprisingly, PRC1.1 and dRAF, rather canonical-PRC1, are responsible for depositing most H2AK119 ubiquitination both in mammalian cells and in flies, respectively. Genetic studies in flies showed that *dKdm2* mutants increased the frequency of homeotic transformations, including the appearance of ectopic sex combs, transformation of the fourth abdominal segment into the semblance of the fifth, and wing-to-haltere transformations, suggesting that dKdm2 acts as enhancer of Pc silencing. Notably, transgenic mice expressing a Kdm2b mutant lacking a functional ZF-CXXC domain—required to recruit PRC1.1 in non-methylated CGIs—also presented with posterior transformation of the vertebral column and were born with phenotypes mimicking Polycomb mutations (Blackledge et al. 2014). On the other hand, dKdm2 counteracted homeotic transformation driven by *Trithorax1 (trx1)* and *Ash1*, which encode H3K4- and H3K36-methyltransferases, respectively (Lagarou et al. 2008; Gao et al. 2012; Entrevan et al. 2016; Piunti and Shilatifard 2016). In mammalian cells, Trithorax (TrxG) proteins MLL1-4 reside in a complex that includes WDR5, RBBP5, ASH2L, and DPY30 core proteins; MLL1-4 methylate histone H3K4 to activate transcription and antagonize the function of PcG proteins (Schuettengruber et al. 2007; Piunti and Shilatifard 2016). A fine balance between the function of PcG and TrxG proteins is critical during development, and their deregulation has been causatively linked with human cancers and developmental abnormalities. Altogether, KDM2 demethylases play evolutionary conserved roles at the nexus of PcG- and TrxG-orchestrated programs of cell fate decisions, to epigenetically regulate development.

Unlike *Drosophila* where site-specific transcription factors play an important role in recruiting PcG proteins to Polycomb responsive elements (PREs) (Schuettengruber et al. 2007; Entrevan et al. 2016; Piunti and Shilatifard 2016), mammalian cells lack a similar mechanism raising the question on how PcG proteins are recruited to bind specific genomic loci and orchestrate temporal- and spatial-transcriptional responses. Several studies demonstrated that PcG protein complexes are recruited to chromatin through different mechanisms, which involve transcription factors, unmethylated CGIs, and non-coding RNAs (Simon and Kingston 2013; Entrevan et al. 2016). A general mechanism proposed for non-canonical PRC1.1 targeting involves the ability of KDM2 demethylases to bind unmethylated CGIs via the ZF-CXXC domain. Once targeted, PRC1.1 ubiquitinates H2A at K119 to induce gene silencing (Blackledge et al. 2010, 2014; Farcas et al. 2012; Cooper et al. 2014; Rose et al. 2016) (Fig. 3.4). The latter also serves as a signal for the recruitment of PRC2 and H3K27 methylation, likely through direct binding of JARID2 to mono-ubiquitinated H2A (Cooper et al. 2016). In support of this model, studies have shown that deletion of Ring1B in mouse embryonic stem cells (ESCs) resulted in a reduction in PRC2 occupancy and H3K27me3 at target sites (Blackledge et al. 2010, 2014; Farcas et al. 2012; Cooper et al. 2014; Rose et al. 2016). Similarly, knockdown of KDM2B reduced PRC1.1 recruitment and H2A ubiquitination at target loci in a subset of CGIs (Blackledge et al. 2014; Cooper et al. 2014). Moreover, transgenic animals engineered to express KDM2B lacking the ZF-CXXC domain failed to target non-canonical PRC1.1 to CGIs causing severe developmental defects and embryonic lethality (Blackledge et al. 2014). This mode of action for targeting non-canonical PRC1, although it deviates from the hierarchical model (Simon and Kingston 2013), provides an alternative model supporting the idea that PRC1 complexes are not simply downstream readers of PRC2 activity, and instead PRC1 can be actively recruited to target sites and act as central players by driving de novo PRC2 occupancy. It is noteworthy to mention that although both KDM2 members bind CGIs, KDM2B—rather KDM2A—co-binds genes along with PRC1 and PRC2 suggesting additional, currently unknown, features that instill target specificity (Farcas et al. 2012). On the other hand, KDM2A, but not KDM2B, has been shown to integrate DNA and histone modification signals through the ZF-CXXC and PHD domains and direct interaction with HP1 bound to heterochromatin. This interaction enables KDM2A to decode H3K9me3 in addition to CpG methylation signals. Despite the overall similarity of these enzymes, HP1 exclusively interacts with KDM2A (Borgel et al. 2016). Overall, these data highlight the modular function of PcG protein complexes, the reciprocal crosstalk between PRC1 and PRC2 in the formation of Polycomb repressive chromatin domains, and the important roles for both KDM2A and KDM2B in regulating genome-wide gene silencing in a cell specific and context-dependent manner.

3.4 Non-histone Targets of KDM2 Demethylases

JmjC domain KDMs are well characterized biochemically regarding their preference to histone substrates; however, little is known about non-histone substrates of these enzymes. The advent of high-throughput mass spectrometry along with protein labeling and tracing techniques indicated that proteins, including key signaling molecules and transcription factors, are reversibly methylated on lysine residues. Protein methylation may regulate stability, activity, or protein–protein interactions (Biggar and Li 2015). The biological significance of protein methylation is an emerging research topic expected to expand the repertoire of KDMs beyond erasing the histone code. The first hint that a demethylase can erase the methyl mark on a protein came with the discovery that KDM1A interacts with p53 to repress its pro-apoptotic role by removing K370me2, a modification that promotes association with the coactivator 53BP1 (Huang et al. 2007).

In an analogous manner, JmjC domain KDMs have also been implicated in protein demethylation. In this regard, KDM2A was shown to demethylate RelA (p65) which forms a heterodimer with NF-κB (p50) to regulate transcriptional programs linked to the innate and adaptive immune responses (Lu et al. 2009, 2010). Cytokines (such as IL-1β or TNFα) or conditions that activate NF-κB (such as LPS or dsRNA) potently increased the methylation of RelA at K218/221 causing activation of the pathway, and gene expression changes that enhance cell proliferation and oncogenic potential. KDM2A-dependent demethylation of those residues inhibited the activity of the pathway and reversed changes in gene expression in a JmjC domain-dependent manner (Lu et al. 2009, 2010). Although it remains to be elucidated whether K218/221 methylation alters the stability or the activity or RelA, these data implicated KDM2A as a negative regulator of NF-κB pathway through direct demethylation (Lu et al. 2009, 2010).

Similarly, Kdm2a and Kdm2b regulate the specification of body axis during *Xenopus* embryogenesis through demethylation of β-catenin. In the absence of Wnt, cytosolic β-catenin is degraded through GSK3-mediated phosphorylation. Kdm2a/b directly binds and demethylate lysine residues within the armadillo repeats of non-phosphorylated β-catenin to prime its ubiquitination and subsequent degradation (Lu et al. 2015). Mutation of those lysine residues to alanine rendered β-catenin resistant to Kdm2a/b activity and protected it from ubiquitination and subsequent degradation (Lu et al. 2015). Consistently, Kdm2a/b knockdown in *Xenopus* embryos led to increases in non-phosphorylated and methylated β-catenin, concurrent with the upregulation of β-catenin target genes (Lu et al. 2015). Notably, although this function depends on the JmjC domain, it is independent of the ZF-CXXC suggesting that Kdm2a/b binding to DNA or crosstalk with non-canonical PRC1.1 is dispensable (Lu et al. 2015).

3.5 Role of KDM2 Demethylases in Replicative Senescence, Stem Cell Biology and Somatic Cell Reprogramming

Cellular senescence in primary cells is developmentally programmed in response to telomere shortening and DNA damage accumulated over time and is a stress response that accompanies stable exit from the cell cycle (Salama et al. 2014). Oncogenic signals can also induce senescence, which protects from oncogenic transformation and plays a tumor suppressor role. In mouse embryonic fibroblasts (MEFs) and epithelial cells, passaging induces replicative senescence caused by the activation of the *Ink4α-Arf* locus which encodes two distinct proteins, $p16^{Ink4\alpha}$ and $p19^{Arf}$ that regulate the Rb and p53 pathways, respectively. $p16^{Ink4\alpha}$ inhibits cyclin-dependent kinases Cdk4 and Cdk6 that phosphorylate and inactivate Rb, whereas $p19^{Arf}$ interacts with the ubiquitin ligase MDM2 and inhibits MDM2-mediated p53 degradation. Genomic deletions or epigenetic silencing of the *Ink4α-Arf* locus frequently occur in human cancers (Salama et al. 2014).

Overexpression of KDM2 demethylases, particularly KDM2B, potently immortalized MEFs, whereas knock down of the endogenous proteins halted proliferation and induced premature senescence (Pfau et al. 2008; Tzatsos et al. 2009). In primary MEFs, downregulation of KDM2B occurs progressively through each passage, indicating it functions as a physiological barrier to replicative senescence (Pfau et al. 2008; Tzatsos et al. 2009). Immortalization driven by KDM2 demethylases was dependent both on the JmjC and ZF-CXXC domains, suggesting the need for both DNA binding and demethylation activity. On the contrary, the PHD, F-box, or LRR domains were dispensable (Pfau et al. 2008; Tzatsos et al. 2009). KDM2B directly binds and represses the expression of the *Ink4α-Arf* locus through H3K36 di-demethylation and by facilitating the recruitment of PRC2 and PRC1 to induce silencing by depositing repressive H3K27me3 and H2AK119, respectively. KDM2B overexpression in MEFs also caused a strong upregulation of EZH2, the catalytic subunit of PRC2, through repression of *let-7b*, a tumor suppressor micro-RNA that targets the 3'UTR of *EZH2* and is activated in senescence (Tzatsos et al. 2011). Forced expression of KDM2B also protected MEFs from oncogene-induced senescence, and dampened Ras-induced activation of the *Ink4α-Arf* locus, suggesting that it can cooperate with oncogenic signals to transform cells in the correct context (Pfau et al. 2008; Tzatsos et al. 2009). Unlike MEFs, forced expression of KDM2B in IMR90 human fibroblasts increased their proliferation but failed to immortalize them. This suggests that while KDM2B prevents cell cycle arrest induced by telomere shortening, it does not protect from telomere erosion per se (Pfau et al. 2008; Tzatsos et al. 2009).

Somatic cells can be reprogrammed into induced pluripotent stem cells (iPSCs) upon ectopic expression of Oct4, Klf4, Sox2, and c-Myc transcription factors (Takahashi and Yamanaka 2006). Replicative senescence has been identified as a major roadblock in the initial stages of reprogramming through activation of the *Ink4α-Arf* tumor suppressor locus (Li et al. 2009; Utikal et al. 2009). *Ink4α-Arf* or *Tp53* null cells not only exhibit increased reprogramming efficiency, but also markedly faster kinetics to iPSC conversion. In this regard, ectopic expression of Kdm2b in MEFs counteracted replicative induced senescence and increased reprogramming efficiency (Wang et al. 2011; Liang et al. 2012). Interestingly, in one report, overexpression of KDM2B along with OCT4 and vitamin C, a cofactor of the demethylation reaction, was sufficient for iPSC generation, bypassing the need for Sox2, Klf4, and c-Myc (Wang et al. 2011). Ectopic expression of the reprogramming factors also upregulated endogenous KDM2 demethylases over the course of reprogramming suggesting a physiological role in bypassing replicative senescence during reprogramming (Wang et al. 2011; Liang et al. 2012). Mutations in either the JmjC or ZF-CXXC domain of Kdm2b abrogated this effect, suggesting that H3K36me2 demethylation at target genes and binding to non-methylated CGIs are required. Interestingly, ectopic expression of Kdm2b was still able to increase reprogramming efficiency in *Ink4α-Arf* null cells indicating a role beyond antagonizing replicative senescence (Liang et al. 2012). Gene expression profiling and genome-wide ChIP-seq experiments revealed that KDM2B regulates genes during early phases of iPSC formation, including early-activated epithelial genes (Cdh1, Cldn3, −4 and −7, Epcam, Esrp1 and Ocln) and pluripotent genes (Nanog, Dppa5a and Tdgf1) (Liang et al. 2012).

Besides reprogramming Kdm2b also plays important roles in stem cells, including embryonic (ESCs) and hematopoietic (HSCs) where it is highly expressed, and levels decline upon differentiation to allow execution of lineage specification programs (He et al. 2013; Andricovich et al. 2016). *Kdm2b* is a direct target of Oct4 and Sox2 in murine ESCs, and its ablation caused genome-wide de-repression of gene programs linked to PcG-mediated silencing and primed ESCs to differentiate without compromising self-renewal per se. *Kdm2b* null ESCs formed flat and loose colonies that resemble extra-embryonic endoderm cells (He et al. 2013). Consistent with the observed morphological changes, extra-embryonic endoderm-specific genes (such as *Gata6*, *Pdgfrα*, and *Sox7*) and trophoectoderm genes (such as *Cdx2* and *Eomes*) were upregulated in the *Kdm2b* null ESCs (He et al. 2013). Surprisingly, the function of Kdm2b linked to ESC maintenance was dependent on the ZF-CXXC domain, but independent of the demethylase activity, and was accompanied by a genome-wide impairment in the targeting of Ring1B/PRC1.1 to unmethylated CGIs for repression of lineage commitment pathways (He et al. 2013; Wu et al. 2013).

3.6 KDM2 Demethylases in Normal Development and Tissue Homeostasis

Several groups have generated germline and conditional knockout mice of KDM2 demethylases, seeking to elucidate the role of those enzymes in normal embryonic development and tissue homeostasis. Consistent with a prominent role of PcG proteins in regulating developmental decisions, deletion of either KDM2A or KDM2B caused severe developmental abnormalities and embryonic lethality between E10.5 and 12.5 in mice (Fukuda et al. 2011; Boulard et al. 2015; Kawakami et al. 2015; Andricovich et al. 2016). Few reports have linked congenital abnormalities in humans stemming from loss-of-function mutations in KDM2 demethylases. In one case, a deletion mapped at chromosome 12q24.31 affecting seven genes, including *KDM2B*, has been linked to intellectual disability disorders, autistic features, and was accompanied by epilepsy and craniofacial anomalies in a limited number of patients (Labonne et al. 2016). Defective *KDM2B* has been reported as causative factor for paunch calf syndrome in *Romagnola* cattle which presents with multi-organ developmental dysplasia characterized by facial deformities, ascites, and hepatic fibrosis inherited in an autosomal monogenic recessive manner (Testoni et al. 2012). This phenotype was associated with a *KDM2B* missense mutation (c.2503G>A) leading to an amino acid exchange (p.D835N) likely affecting the integrity of ZF-CXXC domain. Considering that this domain mediates the binding of KDM2B to unmethylated CGIs, this finding strongly suggests that KDM2B mistargeting impairs developmental programs and leads to congenital abnormalities of endo- and mesodermal derived organs. No congenital diseases linked to alteration of the *KDM2A* locus have been reported so far.

Germline deletion of *Kdm2a* in mice caused embryonic lethality characterized by severe growth defects and reduced body size due to decreased cell proliferation and increased apoptosis (Kawakami et al. 2015). Some of the embryos also presented with incomplete embryonic turning and neural tube closure defects. This phenotype is consistent with the broad expression of *Kdm2a* in embryonic development, particularly in the cerebral cortex and limbs (Kawakami et al. 2015). Lack of Kdm2a resulted in downregulation of Ezh2 and PRC1-mediated H2AK119 ubiquitination, and upregulation of the cell cycle inhibitors such as $p21^{Cip1}$. Although tissue-specific knockout mice of *Kdm2a* have not yet been reported, published work has demonstrated an important role for this enzyme in regulating differentiation of mesenchymal stem cells (MSCs) through repression of epiregulin and secreted frizzled-related protein 2, an inhibitor of Wnt/β-catenin pathway, to modulate osteo-dentinogenic potential (Dong et al. 2013; Du et al. 2013; Gao et al. 2013). Thus, it is likely that some of the developmental defects seen in *Kdm2a* null embryos may result from deregulation of MSC differentiation.

Several germline and conditional knockout mice of Kdm2b lacking either the long form (LF-Kdm2b), or short form (SF-Kdm2b), or both isoforms have been reported. Kdm2b is broadly expressed during embryogenesis, with the highest expression observed in the developing brain and hemogenic endothelium within the aorta gonad mesonephros (AGM) region (Fukuda et al. 2011; Boulard et al. 2015; Andricovich et al. 2016). Selective deletion of the LF-Kdm2b led to neural tube closure defects and exencephaly in about half of the mice which died shortly after birth (Fukuda et al. 2011). Several mice also developed retinal coloboma and a curled tail with low penetrance (Fukuda et al. 2011). Deletion of LF-Kdm2b de-repressed the *Ink4α/Arf* locus and induced apoptosis affecting the number of mitotic neural progenitor cells. Interestingly, deletion of both long and short isoforms of Kdm2b either in germline (Boulard et al. 2015) or at the pre-implantation stage (Andricovich et al. 2016) led to embryonic lethality between E10.5 and 12.5 with complete penetrance, suggesting that SF-Kdm2b also contributes to embryogenesis and organismal growth although it lacks the JmjC domain. Compared to embryos lacking only the LF-Kdm2b, complete knockout embryos also presented with severe craniofacial malformations and defects in hematopoietic development (Andricovich et al. 2016). In fact, deletion of both Kdm2b isoforms specifically in hemogenic endothelium sufficed to cause embryonic lethality by disrupting definitive hematopoiesis (Andricovich et al. 2016). Similar defects were also observed in zebrafish suggesting an evolutionary conserved role of Kdm2b in regulating definitive hematopoiesis (Huang et al.

2013; Andricovich et al. 2016). On the other hand, forced expression of LF-Kdm2b in HSCs expanded the numbers of colony-forming cells with multi-lineage differentiation potential in culture, promoted lymphopoiesis in vivo, and prevented exhaustion of the long-term repopulating potential of HSCs upon serial transplantation (Konuma et al. 2011; Andricovich et al. 2016). Although the role of Kdm2b in the maintenance of HSCs is largely independent of the demethylase activity, the regulation of lymphoid commitment is (Andricovich et al. 2016). Surprisingly, deletion of only the SF-Kdm2b—in a manner that did not perturb expression of LF-Kdm2b—produced a distinct phenotype with craniofacial abnormalities, neural tube defects, and increased lethality predominately in females (Boulard et al. 2016). At the molecular level, this gender-bias was linked to a selective deregulation of genes encoded by the X chromosome, likely due to defective PcG-mediated X chromosome inactivation (Boulard et al. 2016). In that context, SF-Kdm2b was identified as an important regulator of the *Xist* non-coding RNA as well as several proteins that associate with it (Boulard et al. 2016). Overall, Kdm2b isoforms exhibit a multifaceted role in embryogenesis by regulating differentiation, cell proliferation, and survival though demethylase-dependent and independent mechanisms.

Besides development, inducible deletion of *Kdm2b* in adult mice compromised hematopoiesis, caused a precipitous drop in the numbers of long-term HSCs, and blocked lymphoid to favor myeloid commitment in a cell autonomous manner (Andricovich et al. 2016). Moreover, selective deletion of LF-Kdm2b compromised spermatogenesis, particularly in aged mice (Ozawa et al. 2016). Ex vivo culture of spermatogonia showed that testicular germ cells lacking LF-Kdm2b expressed higher levels of $p21^{Cip1}$ and $p19^{Arf}$ cyclin-dependent kinase inhibitors and cell cycle arrest at the G_0/G_1 phase. Furthermore, those mice were sensitive to chemical ablation of testicular germ cells, suggesting that Kdm2b plays important roles in long-term maintenance of spermatogenesis (Ozawa et al. 2016).

3.7 KDM2 Demethylases in Cancer

The implementation of next generation sequencing in the analysis of human cancers through the coordinated efforts of The Cancer Genome Atlas (https://cancergenome.nih.gov/) and the International Cancer Gene Consortium (http://icgc.org/) revealed that several PcG proteins carry mutations and gene copy number alterations that have been causatively linked to oncogenesis or tumor suppression in a context-dependent manner. Deregulation of PRC1 and PRC2 complexes have been implicated in establishing de novo, cancer-specific Polycomb chromatin domains to epigenetically silence cell fate and lineage commitment pathways, initially contributing to loss of cell identity facilitating transformation, and at later stages promoting de-differentiation and metastasis (Laugesen and Helin 2014).

KDM2 demethylases, particularly KDM2B, are among the PcG proteins with the most frequent alterations in human cancers, whereas both tumor-promoting and suppressing roles have been attributed. Both KDM2A and KDM2B are strongly upregulated in hematopoietic malignancies, originally cloned as putative oncogenes form MoMuLV-induced T-cell lymphomas, and in several contexts showed pro-oncogenic function by counteracting replicative and oncogene-induced senescence (Pfau et al. 2008; Tzatsos et al. 2009, 2011, 2013; Andricovich et al. 2016). Consistently, overexpression of KDM2B sufficed to immortalize and transform c-Kit^{+} hematopoietic progenitors, and it was also required for *Hox9a/Meis1*-induced myeloid transformation through direct repression of the *Ink4α-Arf-Ink4β* locus (He et al. 2011). In another experimental model, ectopic expression of KDM2B in Sca-1^{+} hematopoietic progenitors induced mixed lineage leukemias with complete penetrance in mice (Ueda et al. 2015). Knock down of KDM2B in human leukemic cell lines potently inhibited proliferation and abolished their oncogenic potential upon injection into immunodeficient mice, particularly cell lines established from B- and

T-cell acute lymphoblastic leukemias (ALL) (Andricovich et al. 2016). Surprisingly, in Kras-driven acute myeloid leukemia (AML), Kdm2b functioned as a tumor suppressor through subversion of lineage specification pathways to favor myeloid commitment, and its deletion accelerated Kras-driven AML and compromised survival in mice (Andricovich et al. 2016). Although KDM2B is neither mutated nor exhibits copy number changes in leukemias, its expression is downregulated in a subset of AML that show activation of ERK signaling (Andricovich et al. 2016). Consistently, its interacting partners, such as BCOR and components of PRC2, are frequently mutated or deleted and confer poor prognosis in the same subset of AML with active ERK signaling (Ernst et al. 2010; Grossmann et al. 2011). Besides myeloid malignancies, a tumor suppressor role has been also reported in diffuse large B-cell lymphomas which carry genomic deletions of the *KDM2B* locus and downregulate protein expression (Pasqualucci et al. 2011). ChIP-seq experiments revealed that in lymphoid malignancies, KDM2B target genes were co-bound by c-MYC and TrxG proteins, whereas in myeloid malignancies by PcG proteins, no overlap was observed between those epigenetic modules (Andricovich et al. 2016). Although counterintuitive to be associated with both PcG-repressing and c-MYC/TrxG-activating epigenetic networks, the function of KDM2B may be to orchestrate interconnected and interdependent developmental programs in a lineage-specific manner. Hence, deregulation of KDM2B may facilitate transformation of hematopoietic progenitors by blocking differentiation and expanding a pool of cells carrying stem cell-like features (Andricovich et al. 2016). Gene expression profiling in HSCs and ChIP-seq studies in human leukemia cell lines revealed a pleiotropic role for KDM2B in differentiation, quiescence, and lymphoid lineage specification—primarily through modulation of NOTCH and interferon signaling. Forced expression of Kdm2b in vivo also promoted NOTCH signaling and favored lymphoid commitment in a mechanism dependent on the demethylase activity (Andricovich et al. 2016). Clearly, further studies are needed to dissect the JmjC-dependent and independent functions of KDM2B in vivo linked to normal and malignant hematopoiesis.

KDM2A has also been implicated as both an oncogene and tumor suppressor in hematopoietic malignancies. In a *Sleeping Beauty* insertional mutagenesis screen, Kdm2a was identified as the second most frequent hit in accelerating STAT5-driven B-ALL. Insertions were mapped at the 5' end of the *Kdm2a* locus and oriented in the same direction causing its transcriptional activation and overexpression which was inversely correlated with overall survival (Heltemes-Harris et al. 2016). A likely mechanism through which Kdm2a promotes leukemogenesis is demethylation of RelA and deregulation of NFκB signaling (Lu et al. 2009, 2010). KDM2A was also shown to play a tumor suppressor role in leukemias driven by oncogenic fusions of MLL proteins (Zhu et al. 2016). Interestingly, those oncogenic fusion proteins require their wild-type MLL counterparts both for the initiation and maintenance of the ensuing leukemias (Thiel et al. 2010). At the molecular level, it was shown that KDM2A demethylates H3K36me2—an epigenetic mark written by the ASH1L methyltransferase—which serves as a docking site for LEDGF (lens epithelium-derived growth factor), a chromatin-binding protein that facilitates the recruitment of wild-type and oncogenic MLL fusion protein complexes at key target genes. Overexpression of KDM2A in *MLL–AF10* transformed hematopoietic progenitors compromised their oncogenic potential by reducing H3K36me2, displaced LEDGF and MLL protein complexes from chromatin, and reduced expression of genes involved in leukemic transformation such as *Hoxa9* (Zhu et al. 2016).

In addition to hematopoietic malignancies, KDM2 demethylases have been also implicated as oncogenes in solid tumors (Tzatsos et al. 2013; Wagner et al. 2013). KDM2B was found to be markedly overexpressed in pancreatic cancer cell lines and patient specimens, and its levels positively correlated with disease grade and stage, while the highest expression was detected in metastases. Consistently, forced expression of KDM2B in pancreatic progenitors harboring oncogenic Kras induced poorly differentiated pancreatic cancer upon orthotopic transplantation in immunodeficient mice, in a JmjC domain-dependent manner. Consistently, poorly differentiated human pancreatic cancer cell lines of the quasi-mesenchymal subtype were particularly sensitive to KDM2B knock down (Tzatsos et al. 2013). Gain- and loss-of-function experiments coupled to genome-wide gene expression and ChIP-seq studies revealed that KDM2B drives pancreatic cancer through two distinct transcriptional programs. KDM2B repressed developmental genes in the context of PcG proteins, whereas on the other hand it activated a module of metabolic genes—including mediators of protein synthesis and mitochondrial function—by cooperating with c-MYC and KDM5A, an H3K4me3 demethylase that drives drug-resistance in cancer (Tzatsos et al. 2013). The role of KDM2B in regulating metabolic pathways in pancreatic cancer was independent of the demethylase activity and remains to be further elucidated at the molecular level.

In an analogous manner, KDM2A was found to be overexpressed and amplified in a subset of patients diagnosed with non-small cell lung cancer (NSCLC), and its levels correlated with poor prognosis (Wagner et al. 2013). The demethylase activity was required for in vitro proliferation and invasion of KDM2A-overexpressing NSCLC cells, whereas knockdown of the endogenous protein abrogated tumor growth and invasion in mouse xenograft models (Wagner et al. 2013). The oncogenic functions of KDM2A were largely dependent on the repression of the expression of dual-specificity phosphatase 3 (DUSP3) via H3K36me2 demethylation. DUSP3 directly dephosphorylates ERK1/2, and thus KDM2A-mediated repression caused activation of ERK1/2 mitogenic signaling (Wagner et al. 2013). Overall, KDM2 demethylases have multifaceted roles in cancer initiation and maintenance. Considering that several oncogenic functions depend on the demethylase activity, this renders these enzymes excellent candidates for the development of small molecule inhibitors.

3.8 Targeting KDM2 Demethylases with Small Molecule Inhibitors

KDMs have emerged as interesting new targets for therapeutic intervention and a coordinated effort from academia and the pharmaceutical industry has already identified lead compounds that effectively inhibit several of these enzymes. Although the JmjC domain KDMs share highly similar catalytic domains—rendering the generation of probes that exclusively target the desired enzyme difficult—solving their three-dimensional structures along with improvements in rational drug design and computational modeling led to significant successes with the development of highly specific inhibitors against KDM6 (Kruidenier et al. 2012), KDM5 (Gale et al. 2016; Vinogradova et al. 2016), and KDM2/7 (Suzuki et al. 2013; England et al. 2014) members, among others. Thus, it is now apparent that potent inhibitors selective for small groups of KDMs is feasible, despite their significant structural homology. Notably, several of those inhibitors elicited biological responses in cultured cells and in experimental murine leukemia models, suggesting that modulation of histone methylation in vivo can trigger a therapeutic response (Kruidenier et al. 2012; Ntziachristos et al. 2014). Several of those inhibitors are expected to enter phase I/II clinical trials to assess their efficacy, tolerability, and side effects. Although, the application to non-cancer diseases currently appears more distant, potential targets may emerge from genome-wide association studies of genetic diseases in the future.

Most inhibitors of the JmjC KDMs are α-KG mimetics such as *N*-oxalylglycine (NOG). In addition, pyridine-2,4-dicarboxylate (2,4-PDCA), 8-hydroxyquinolines, hydroxamate analogues and catechol-type flavonoids have also been reported to broadly inhibit several JmjC KDMs (Rose et al. 2008; Hamada et al. 2009, 2010; King et al. 2010; Chang et al. 2011; Kristensen et al. 2012; McAllister et al. 2016). Ongoing efforts for identification of new chemical scaffolds and optimization of lead compounds are expected to increase specificity (McAllister et al. 2016). Reported compounds that inhibit KDM2A include hydroxamate analogues (compounds 9 and 13 in (Suzuki et al. 2013) with pIC_{50} 6.8 μM and 2.9 μM, respectively), and a triazolopyridine derivative (compound 35 in (England et al. 2014) with pIC_{50} 7.2 μM). Interestingly, daminozide, a chemical used to regulate plant growth, has also been shown to potently inhibit KDM2/7 subfamily with a pIC_{50} 5.8 μM for KDM2A (Rose et al. 2012). Administration of those inhibitors to cells inhibited their proliferation (Rose et al. 2012; Suzuki et al. 2013). Considering that KDM2 demethylases share almost identical domains, it is expected that those compounds also inhibit the enzymatic activity of KDM2B. Given that the activity of most, if not all, KDMs is regulated by domains other than the JmjC domain, an alternative approach to achieve specificity is to develop strategies to inhibit these domains, some of which are likely to have biological importance equal to the JmjC domain. For instance, in the case of KDM2 demethylases, the ZF-CXXC and PHD domains represent attractive candidates that could interfere with the targeting of those enzymes to chromatin.

As KDM2 demethylases have been implicated both as oncogenes and tumor suppressors (Table 3.1), in a context-dependent manner, the consequences of their inhibition need to be carefully considered in the clinical setting—particularly in hematopoietic malignancies—as the therapeutic effect may be contingent on the leukemia subtype. To this end, the currently available genetically engineered mouse models of KDM2A and KDM2B can serve as in vivo platforms for assessing the efficacy and potency of those inhibitors, alone or in combination with chemotherapies, in order to guide their application in human leukemias. In contrast, in solid tumors, such as in pancreatic cancer and NSCLC, patients will likely benefit from the inhibition of KDM2 demethylases. Although it is currently unknown what would be the impact, it is speculated that inhibition of KDM2 demethylases in vivo will reset cell identity programs and render cancer cells vulnerable to cytotoxic chemotherapies. Given that clinical oncology lacks tools to pharmacologically reprogram cancer cell identity, KDM2 demethylase inhibitors emerge as attractive candidates for modulating cell fate decisions in cancer.

Table 3.1 Context-dependent roles of KDM2 demethylases in cancer

	KDM2A	*KDM2B*	References
Hematopoietic malignancies			
ALL			
B-ALL	Oncogene		Heltemes-Harris et al. (2016)
T-ALL		Oncogene	Andricovich et al. (2016)
AML			
KRAS		Suppressor	Andricovich et al. (2016)
HOXA9A/MEIS1		Oncogene	He et al. (2011)
MLL-r	Suppressor		Zhu et al. (2016)
DLBCL		Suppressor	Pasqualucci et al. (2011)
Mixed leukemia		Oncogene	Ueda et al. (2015)
Solid tumors			
Non-Small Cell Lung Cancer	Oncogene		Wagner et al. (2013)
Pancreatic cancer		Oncogene	Tzatsos et al. (2013)

References

Andricovich J, Kai Y, Peng W, Foudi A, Tzatsos A (2016) Histone demethylase KDM2B regulates lineage commitment in normal and malignant hematopoiesis. J Clin Investig 126:905–920

Biggar KK, Li SS (2015) Non-histone protein methylation as a regulator of cellular signalling and function. Nat Rev Mol Cell Biol 16:5–17

Blackledge NP, Farcas AM, Kondo T, King HW, McGouran JF, Hanssen LL, Ito S, Cooper S, Kondo K, Koseki Y et al (2014) Variant PRC1 complex-dependent H2A ubiquitylation drives PRC2 recruitment and polycomb domain formation. Cell 157:1445–1459

Blackledge NP, Zhou JC, Tolstorukov MY, Farcas AM, Park PJ, Klose RJ (2010) CpG islands recruit a histone H3 lysine 36 demethylase. Mol Cell 38:179–190
Borgel J, Tyl M, Schiller K, Pusztai Z, Dooley CM, Deng W, Wooding C, White RJ, Warnecke T, Leonhardt H et al (2016) KDM2A integrates DNA and histone modification signals through a CXXC/PHD module and direct interaction with HP1. Nucleic Acids Res
Boulard M, Edwards JR, Bestor TH (2015) FBXL10 protects polycomb-bound genes from hypermethylation. Nat Genet 47:479–485
Boulard M, Edwards JR, Bestor TH (2016) Abnormal X chromosome inactivation and sex-specific gene dysregulation after ablation of FBXL10. Epigenetics Chromatin 9:22
Chang KH, King ON, Tumber A, Woon EC, Heightman TD, McDonough MA, Schofield CJ, Rose NR (2011) Inhibition of histone demethylases by 4-carboxy-2,2'-bipyridyl compounds. ChemMedChem 6:759–764
Cheng Z, Cheung P, Kuo AJ, Yukl ET, Wilmot CM, Gozani O, Patel DJ (2014) A molecular threading mechanism underlies jumonji lysine demethylase KDM2A regulation of methylated H3K36. Genes Dev 28:1758–1771
Clissold PM, Ponting CP (2001) JmjC: cupin metalloenzyme-like domains in jumonji, hairless and phospholipase A2beta. Trends Biochem Sci 26:7–9
Cooper S, Dienstbier M, Hassan R, Schermelleh L, Sharif J, Blackledge NP, De Marco V, Elderkin S, Koseki H, Klose R et al (2014) Targeting polycomb to pericentric heterochromatin in embryonic stem cells reveals a role for H2AK119u1 in PRC2 recruitment. Cell Rep 7:1456–1470
Cooper S, Grijzenhout A, Underwood E, Ancelin K, Zhang T, Nesterova TB, Anil-Kirmizitas B, Bassett A, Kooistra SM, Agger K et al (2016) Jarid2 binds mono-ubiquitylated H2A lysine 119 to mediate crosstalk between Polycomb complexes PRC1 and PRC2. Nat Commun 7:13661
Dong R, Yao R, Du J, Wang S, Fan Z (2013) Depletion of histone demethylase KDM2A enhanced the adipogenic and chondrogenic differentiation potentials of stem cells from apical papilla. Exp Cell Res 319:2874–2882
Du J, Ma Y, Ma P, Wang S, Fan Z (2013) Demethylation of epiregulin gene by histone demethylase FBXL11 and BCL6 corepressor inhibits osteo/dentinogenic differentiation. Stem Cells 31:126–136
England KS, Tumber A, Krojer T, Scozzafava G, Ng SS, Daniel M, Szykowska A, Che K, von Delft F, Burgess-Brown NA et al (2014) Optimisation of a triazolopyridine based histone demethylase inhibitor yields a potent and selective KDM2A (FBXL11) inhibitor. Medchemcomm 5:1879–1886
Entrevan M, Schuettengruber B, Cavalli G (2016) Regulation of genome architecture and function by polycomb proteins. Trends Cell Biol 26:511–525
Ernst T, Chase AJ, Score J, Hidalgo-Curtis CE, Bryant C, Jones AV, Waghorn K, Zoi K, Ross FM, Reiter A et al (2010) Inactivating mutations of the histone methyltransferase gene EZH2 in myeloid disorders. Nat Genet 42:722–726
Fang J, Hogan GJ, Liang G, Lieb JD, Zhang Y (2007) The Saccharomyces cerevisiae histone demethylase Jhd1 fine-tunes the distribution of H3K36me2. Mol Cell Biol 27:5055–5065
Farcas AM, Blackledge NP, Sudbery I, Long HK, McGouran JF, Rose NR, Lee S, Sims D, Cerase A, Sheahan TW et al (2012) KDM2B links the polycomb repressive complex 1 (PRC1) to recognition of CpG islands. eLife 1:e00205
Fukuda T, Tokunaga A, Sakamoto R, Yoshida N (2011) Fbxl10/Kdm2b deficiency accelerates neural progenitor cell death and leads to exencephaly. Mol Cell Neurosci 46:614–624
Gale M, Sayegh J, Cao J, Norcia M, Gareiss P, Hoyer D, Merkel JS, Yan Q (2016) Screen-identified selective inhibitor of lysine demethylase 5A blocks cancer cell growth and drug resistance. Oncotarget 7:39931–39944
Gao R, Dong R, Du J, Ma P, Wang S, Fan Z (2013) Depletion of histone demethylase KDM2A inhibited cell proliferation of stem cells from apical papilla by de-repression of p15INK4B and p27Kip1. Mol Cell Biochem 379:115–122
Gao Z, Zhang J, Bonasio R, Strino F, Sawai A, Parisi F, Kluger Y, Reinberg D (2012) PCGF homologs, CBX proteins, and RYBP define functionally distinct PRC1 family complexes. Mol Cell 45:344–356
Gearhart MD, Corcoran CM, Wamstad JA, Bardwell VJ (2006) Polycomb group and SCF ubiquitin ligases are found in a novel BCOR complex that is recruited to BCL6 targets. Mol Cell Biol 26:6880–6889
Grossmann V, Tiacci E, Holmes AB, Kohlmann A, Martelli MP, Kern W, Spanhol-Rosseto A, Klein HU, Dugas M, Schindela S et al (2011) Whole-exome sequencing identifies somatic mutations of BCOR in acute myeloid leukemia with normal karyotype. Blood 118:6153–6163
Hamada S, Kim TD, Suzuki T, Itoh Y, Tsumoto H, Nakagawa H, Janknecht R, Miyata N (2009) Synthesis and activity of N-oxalylglycine and its derivatives as jumonji C-domain-containing histone lysine demethylase inhibitors. Bioorg Med Chem Lett 19:2852–2855
Hamada S, Suzuki T, Mino K, Koseki K, Oehme F, Flamme I, Ozasa H, Itoh Y, Ogasawara D, Komaarashi H et al (2010) Design, synthesis, enzyme-inhibitory activity, and effect on human cancer cells of a novel series of jumonji domain-containing protein 2 histone demethylase inhibitors. J Med Chem 53:5629–5638
Han XR, Zha Z, Yuan HX, Feng X, Xia YK, Lei QY, Guan KL, Xiong Y (2016) KDM2B/FBXL10 targets c-Fos for ubiquitylation and degradation in response to mitogenic stimulation. Oncogene
He J, Nguyen AT, Zhang Y (2011) KDM2b/JHDM1b, an H3K36me2-specific demethylase, is required for initiation and maintenance of acute myeloid leukemia. Blood 117:3869–3880

He J, Shen L, Wan M, Taranova O, Wu H, Zhang Y (2013) Kdm2b maintains murine embryonic stem cell status by recruiting PRC1 complex to CpG islands of developmental genes. Nat Cell Biol 15:373–384

Heltemes-Harris LM, Larson JD, Starr TK, Hubbard GK, Sarver AL, Largaespada DA, Farrar MA (2016) Sleeping Beauty transposon screen identifies signaling modules that cooperate with STAT5 activation to induce B-cell acute lymphoblastic leukemia. Oncogene 35:3454–3464

Huang HT, Kathrein KL, Barton A, Gitlin Z, Huang YH, Ward TP, Hofmann O, Dibiase A, Song A, Tyekucheva S et al (2013) A network of epigenetic regulators guides developmental haematopoiesis in vivo. Nat Cell Biol 15:1516–1525

Huang J, Sengupta R, Espejo AB, Lee MG, Dorsey JA, Richter M, Opravil S, Shiekhattar R, Bedford MT, Jenuwein T et al (2007) p53 is regulated by the lysine demethylase LSD1. Nature 449:105–108

Kawakami E, Tokunaga A, Ozawa M, Sakamoto R, Yoshida N (2015) The histone demethylase Fbxl11/Kdm2a plays an essential role in embryonic development by repressing cell-cycle regulators. Mech Dev 135:31–42

King ON, Li XS, Sakurai M, Kawamura A, Rose NR, Ng SS, Quinn AM, Rai G, Mott BT, Beswick P et al (2010) Quantitative high-throughput screening identifies 8-hydroxyquinolines as cell-active histone demethylase inhibitors. PLoS ONE 5:e15535

Konuma T, Nakamura S, Miyagi S, Negishi M, Chiba T, Oguro H, Yuan J, Mochizuki-Kashio M, Ichikawa H, Miyoshi H et al (2011) Forced expression of the histone demethylase Fbxl10 maintains self-renewing hematopoietic stem cells. Exp Hematol 39(697–709):e695

Kooistra SM, Helin K (2012) Molecular mechanisms and potential functions of histone demethylases. Nat Rev Mol Cell Biol 13:297–311

Kristensen LH, Nielsen AL, Helgstrand C, Lees M, Cloos P, Kastrup JS, Helin K, Olsen L, Gajhede M (2012) Studies of H3K4me3 demethylation by KDM5B/Jarid1B/PLU1 reveals strong substrate recognition in vitro and identifies 2,4-pyridine-dicarboxylic acid as an in vitro and in cell inhibitor. FEBS J 279:1905–1914

Kruidenier L, Chung CW, Cheng Z, Liddle J, Che K, Joberty G, Bantscheff M, Bountra C, Bridges A, Diallo H et al (2012) A selective jumonji H3K27 demethylase inhibitor modulates the proinflammatory macrophage response. Nature 488:404–408

Labonne JD, Lee KH, Iwase S, Kong IK, Diamond MP, Layman LC, Kim CH, Kim HG (2016) An atypical 12q24.31 microdeletion implicates six genes including a histone demethylase KDM2B and a histone methyltransferase SETD1B in syndromic intellectual disability. Hum Genet 135:757–771

Lagarou A, Mohd-Sarip A, Moshkin YM, Chalkley GE, Bezstarosti K, Demmers JA, Verrijzer CP (2008) dKDM2 couples histone H2A ubiquitylation to histone H3 demethylation during polycomb group silencing. Genes Dev 22:2799–2810

Laugesen A, Helin K (2014) Chromatin repressive complexes in stem cells, development, and cancer. Cell Stem Cell 14:735–751

Li H, Collado M, Villasante A, Strati K, Ortega S, Canamero M, Blasco MA, Serrano M (2009) The Ink4/Arf locus is a barrier for iPS cell reprogramming. Nature 460:1136–1139

Liang G, He J, Zhang Y (2012) Kdm2b promotes induced pluripotent stem cell generation by facilitating gene activation early in reprogramming. Nat Cell Biol 14:457–466

Lu L, Gao Y, Zhang Z, Cao Q, Zhang X, Zou J, Cao Y (2015) Kdm2a/b lysine demethylases regulate canonical Wnt signaling by modulating the stability of nuclear beta-catenin. Dev Cell 33:660–674

Lu T, Jackson MW, Singhi AD, Kandel ES, Yang M, Zhang Y, Gudkov AV, Stark GR (2009) Validation-based insertional mutagenesis identifies lysine demethylase FBXL11 as a negative regulator of NFkappaB. Proc Natl Acad Sci USA 106:16339–16344

Lu T, Jackson MW, Wang B, Yang M, Chance MR, Miyagi M, Gudkov AV, Stark GR (2010) Regulation of NF-kappaB by NSD1/FBXL11-dependent reversible lysine methylation of p65. Proc Natl Acad Sci USA 107:46–51

McAllister TE, England KS, Hopkinson RJ, Brennan PE, Kawamura A, Schofield CJ (2016) Recent progress in histone demethylase inhibitors. J Med Chem 59:1308–1329

Ntziachristos P, Tsirigos A, Welstead GG, Trimarchi T, Bakogianni S, Xu L, Loizou E, Holmfeldt L, Strikoudis A, King B et al (2014) Contrasting roles of histone 3 lysine 27 demethylases in acute lymphoblastic leukaemia. Nature 514:513–517

Ozawa M, Fukuda T, Sakamoto R, Honda H, Yoshida N (2016) The histone demethylase FBXL10 regulates the proliferation of spermatogonia and ensures long-term sustainable spermatogenesis in mice. Biol Reprod 94:92

Pasqualucci L, Trifonov V, Fabbri G, Ma J, Rossi D, Chiarenza A, Wells VA, Grunn A, Messina M, Elliot O et al (2011) Analysis of the coding genome of diffuse large B-cell lymphoma. Nat Genet 43:830–837

Pfau R, Tzatsos A, Kampranis SC, Serebrennikova OB, Bear SE, Tsichlis PN (2008) Members of a family of JmjC domain-containing oncoproteins immortalize embryonic fibroblasts via a JmjC domain-dependent process. Proc Natl Acad Sci USA 105:1907–1912

Piunti A, Shilatifard A (2016) Epigenetic balance of gene expression by polycomb and COMPASS families. Science 352:aad9780

Rose NR, King HW, Blackledge NP, Fursova NA, Ember KJ, Fischer R, Kessler BM, Klose RJ (2016) RYBP stimulates PRC1 to shape chromatin-based communication between polycomb repressive complexes. eLife 5

Rose NR, Ng SS, Mecinovic J, Lienard BM, Bello SH, Sun Z, McDonough MA, Oppermann U, Schofield CJ (2008) Inhibitor scaffolds for 2-oxoglutarate-dependent histone lysine demethylases. J Med Chem 51:7053–7056

Rose NR, Woon EC, Tumber A, Walport LJ, Chowdhury R, Li XS, King ON, Lejeune C, Ng SS, Krojer T et al (2012) Plant growth regulator daminozide is a selective inhibitor of human KDM2/7 histone demethylases. J Med Chem 55:6639–6643

Salama R, Sadaie M, Hoare M, Narita M (2014) Cellular senescence and its effector programs. Genes Dev 28 99–114

Sanchez C, Sanchez I, Demmers JA, Rodriguez P, Strouboulis J, Vidal M (2007) Proteomics analysis of Ring1B/Rnf2 interactors identifies a novel complex with the Fbxl10/Jhdm1B histone demethylase and the Bcl6 interacting corepressor. Mole Cell Proteomics MCP 6:820–834

Schuettengruber B, Chourrout D, Vervoort M, Leblanc B, Cavalli G (2007) Genome regulation by polycomb and trithorax proteins. Cell 128:735–745

Shi Y, Lan F, Matson C, Mulligan P, Whetstine JR, Cole PA, Casero RA, Shi Y (2004) Histone demethylation mediated by the nuclear amine oxidase homolog LSD1. Cell 119:941–953

Simon JA, Kingston RE (2013) Occupying chromatin: polycomb mechanisms for getting to genomic targets, stopping transcriptional traffic, and staying put. Mol Cell 49:808–824

Skaar JR, Pagan JK, Pagano M (2013) Mechanisms and function of substrate recruitment by F-box proteins. Nat Rev Mol Cell Biol 14:369–381

Sorenson MR, Jha DK, Ucles SA, Flood DM, Strahl BD, Stevens SW, Kress TL (2016) Histone H3K36 methylation regulates pre-mRNA splicing in *Saccharomyces cerevisiae*. RNA Biol 13:412–426

Suzuki T, Ozasa H, Itoh Y, Zhan P, Sawada H, Mino K, Walport L, Ohkubo R, Kawamura A, Yonezawa M et al (2013) Identification of the KDM2/7 histone lysine demethylase subfamily inhibitor and its antiproliferative activity. J Med Chem 56:7222–7231

Takahashi K, Yamanaka S (2006) Induction of pluripotent stem cells from mouse embryonic and adult fibroblast cultures by defined factors. Cell 126:663–676

Testoni S, Bartolone E, Rossi M, Patrignani A, Bruggmann R, Lichtner P, Tetens J, Gentile A, Drogemuller C (2012) KDM2B is implicated in bovine lethal multi-organic developmental dysplasia. PLoS ONE 7:e45634

Thiel AT, Blessington P, Zou T, Feather D, Wu X, Yan J, Zhang H, Liu Z, Ernst P, Koretzky GA et al (2010) MLL-AF9-induced leukemogenesis requires coexpression of the wild-type Mll allele. Cancer Cell 17:148–159

Trewick SC, Minc E, Antonelli R, Urano T, Allshire RC (2007) The JmjC domain protein Epe1 prevents unregulated assembly and disassembly of heterochromatin. EMBO J 26:4670–4682

Tsukada Y, Fang J, Erdjument-Bromage H, Warren ME, Borchers CH, Tempst P, Zhang Y (2006) Histone demethylation by a family of JmjC domain-containing proteins. Nature 439:811–816

Tu S, Bulloch EM, Yang L, Ren C, Huang WC, Hsu PH, Chen CH, Liao CL, Yu HM, Lo WS et al (2007) Identification of histone demethylases in *Saccharomyces cerevisiae*. J Biol Chem 282:14262–14271

Tzatsos A, Paskaleva P, Ferrari F, Deshpande V, Stoykova S, Contino G, Wong KK, Lan F, Trojer P, Park PJ et al (2013) KDM2B promotes pancreatic cancer via Polycomb-dependent and -independent transcriptional programs. J Clin Investig 123:727–739

Tzatsos A, Paskaleva P, Lymperi S, Contino G, Stoykova S, Chen Z, Wong KK, Bardeesy N (2011) Lysine-specific demethylase 2B (KDM2B)-let-7-enhancer of zester homolog 2 (EZH2) pathway regulates cell cycle progression and senescence in primary cells. J Biol Chem 286:33061–33069

Tzatsos A, Pfau R, Kampranis SC, Tsichlis PN (2009) Ndy1/KDM2B immortalizes mouse embryonic fibroblasts by repressing the Ink4a/Arf locus. Proc Natl Acad Sci USA 106:2641–2646

Ueda T, Nagamachi A, Takubo K, Yamasaki N, Matsui H, Kanai A, Nakata Y, Ikeda K, Konuma T, Oda H et al (2015) Fbxl10 overexpression in murine hematopoietic stem cells induces leukemia involving metabolic activation and upregulation of Nsg2. Blood 125:3437–3446

Utikal J, Polo JM, Stadtfeld M, Maherali N, Kulalert W, Walsh RM, Khalil A, Rheinwald JG, Hochedlinger K (2009) Immortalization eliminates a roadblock during cellular reprogramming into iPS cells. Nature 460:1145–1148

Vinogradova M, Gehling VS, Gustafson A, Arora S, Tindell CA, Wilson C, Williamson KE, Guler GD, Gangurde P, Manieri W et al (2016) An inhibitor of KDM5 demethylases reduces survival of drug-tolerant cancer cells. Nat Chem Biol 12:531–538

Wagner KW, Alam H, Dhar SS, Giri U, Li N, Wei Y, Giri D, Cascone T, Kim JH, Ye Y et al (2013) KDM2A promotes lung tumorigenesis by epigenetically enhancing ERK1/2 signaling. J Clin Investig 123:5231–5246

Wang T, Chen K, Zeng X, Yang J, Wu Y, Shi X, Qin B, Zeng L, Esteban MA, Pan G et al (2011) The histone demethylases Jhdm1a/1b enhance somatic cell reprogramming in a vitamin-C-dependent manner. Cell Stem Cell 9:575–587

Wong SJ, Gearhart MD, Taylor AB, Nanyes DR, Ha DJ, Robinson AK, Artigas JA, Lee OJ, Demeler B, Hart PJ et al (2016) KDM2B recruitment of the polycomb group complex, PRC1.1, requires cooperation between PCGF1 and BCORL1. Structure 24:1795–1801

Wu X, Johansen JV, Helin K (2013) Fbxl10/Kdm2b recruits polycomb repressive complex 1 to CpG islands and regulates H2A ubiquitylation. Mol Cell 49:1134–1146

Wysocka J, Swigut T, Xiao H, Milne TA, Kwon SY, Landry J, Kauer M, Tackett AJ, Chait BT, Badenhorst P et al (2006) A PHD finger of NURF couples histone H3 lysine 4 trimethylation with chromatin remodelling. Nature 442:86–90

Zhu L, Li Q, Wong SH, Huang M, Klein BJ, Shen J, Ikenouye L, Onishi M, Schneidawind D, Buechele C et al (2016) ASH1L links histone H3 lysine 36 dimethylation to MLL leukemia. Cancer Discov 6:770–783

Histone Demethylase KDM3 (JMJD1) in Transcriptional Regulation and Cancer Progression

4

Lingling Fan, Khadka Sudeep and Jianfei Qi

Abstract

Methylation of histone H3 lysine 9 (H3K9) is a repressive histone mark and associated with inhibition of gene expression. KDM3 is a subfamily of the JmjC histone demethylases. It specifically removes the mono- or di-methyl marks from H3K9 and thus contributes to activation of gene expression. KDM3 subfamily includes three members: KDM3A, KDM3B and KDM3C. As KDM3A (also known as JMJD1A or JHDM2A) is the best studied, this chapter will mainly focus on the role of KDM3A-mediated gene regulation in the biology of normal and cancer cells. Knockout mouse studies have revealed that KDM3A plays a role in the physiological processes such as spermatogenesis, metabolism and sex determination. KDM3A is upregulated in several types of cancers and has been shown to promote cancer development, progression and metastasis. KDM3A can enhance the expression or activity of transcription factors through its histone demethylase activity, thereby altering the transcriptional program and promoting cancer cell proliferation and survival. We conclude that KDM3A may serve as a promising target for anti-cancer therapies.

Keywords

Histone demethylase · KDM3A · KDM3B · KDM3C · JMJD1A · JMJD1B · JMJD1C · Cancer · Epigenetics · Transcriptional regulation

4.1 Introduction

The fundamental unit of chromatin is the nucleosome, which is comprised of a segment of DNA that wraps around the octamer of core histones, which consists of two copies each of H2A, H2B, H3 and H4. The specific amino acid residues in the histone tails are subject to various types of posttranslational modifications such as phosphorylation, ubiquitination, acetylation and methylation. These modifications alter chromatin conformation and recruit additional epigenetic regulators and transcription factors, thereby regulating transcriptional gene expression in response to specific signals during various biological processes. Methylation of specific lysine residue(s) in the histone tail can activate or repress gene expression. For example,

L. Fan · K. Sudeep · J. Qi (*)
Department of Biochemistry and Molecular Biology, University of Maryland School of Medicine, 655 W Baltimore Street, Baltimore, MD, USA
e-mail: JQI@som.umaryland.edu

L. Fan · K. Sudeep · J. Qi Marlene and Stewart Greenebaum Comprehensive Cancer Center, Baltimore, MD 21201, USA

Q. Yan (ed.), *Targeting Lysine Demethylases in Cancer and Other Human Diseases*, Advances in Experimental Medicine and Biology 1433, https://doi.org/10.1007/978-3-031-38176-8_4

methylation of histone-3-lysine-4 (H3K4) is an active histone mark associated with the transcriptional gene activation, whereas methylation of histone-3-lysine-9 (H3K9) is a repressive histone mark associated with the inhibition of gene expression (Mosammaparast and Shi 2010). Methylation of H3K9 can recruit heterochromatin protein 1 (HP1) and corepressor complexes for heterochromatin formation and silencing of gene expression.

The steady state of histone methylation is determined by the balance between addition of methyl groups by histone methyl transferases (HMTs) and removal of methyl groups by histone lysine demethylases (KDMs). Based on the enzymatic mechanism, the KDMs can be categorized into two main families (Kooistra and Helin 2012). The first family includes two members, KDM1A (also known as lysine specific demethylase 1, LSD1) and KDM1B (LSD2). They are the flavin adenine dinucleotide (FAD)-dependent amine oxidases and can remove mono- and di-methyl histone marks. The second family of KDMs is characterized by presence of the Jumonji C (JmjC)-domain, which is the catalytic domain for histone demethylation. They are the Fe(II) and α-ketoglutarate (KG)-dependent dioxygenases and can remove mono-, di- and tri-methyl marks from specific histone lysines. Over 30 members of the JmjC family, histone demethylases have been identified, and they can be categorized into seven subfamilies based on the sequence or structure homologies (Labbe et al. 2013). KDM3A (also known as JMJD1A or JHDM2A) belongs to the KDM3 subfamily, which includes two other members, KDM3B (also known as JMJD1B or JHDM2B) and KDM3C (as known as JMJD1C or JHDM2C). The genes encoding KDM3A, B and C are located on human chromosomes 2p11.2, 5q31.2 and 10q21.3, respectively. The KDM3 subfamily is evolutionally conserved, with orthologs of KDM3A, B and C found among all vertebrates. The KDM3A, B and C proteins share around 50% sequence identity and have a C2HC4 zinc finger and a C-terminal JmjC domain (Fig. 4.1). They can function as coactivators for specific transcription factors, remove the repressive mono- or di-methyl marks from H3K9 (H3K9me1/2) and facilitate the binding of transcription factors to their cognate DNA sequence (Fig. 4.2) (Yamane et al. 2006; Kim et al. 2010, 2012). However, KDM3C only showed in vitro activity against H3K9me1 peptide (Chen et al. 2015). KDM3B was recently shown to also demethylate H4R3me2s and H4R3me1 (Li et al. 2018). Among the three KDM3 members, KDM3A is most extensively studied. Hereby, we will mainly review the function of KDM3A in transcriptional gene regulation, normal physiology and cancer biology.

4.2 Discovery of KDM3A as an H3K9me1/2 Demethylase

The Zhang group was the first to characterize the function of KDM3A as an H3K9me1/2 demethylase (Yamane et al. 2006). In a demethylation assay using methylated histone as substrates, they detected potential H3K9 demethylase activity in one fraction of HeLa cell nuclear extracts. This demethylase activity was dependent on cofactors Fe(II) and α-KG, a requirement of the JmjC family of demethylases. Further fractionation coupled with mass spectrometry analysis identified KDM3A as a candidate for the demethylase activity. Purified KDM3A protein possessed the histone demethylase activity but not the KDM3A mutant protein with truncation or a point mutation in its JmjC domain. In the demethylation assay using methylated lysine sites in histone H3 (K4, K9, K27, K36, K79) and H4 (K20), KDM3A only demethylated the methylated H3K9, demonstrating that KDM3A is a H3K9-specific demethylase. Lysine methylation can exist in three states as mono-, di- and tri-methylation. Using the methylated H3K9 peptides as substrates, KDM3A could demethylate both mono- and di-methyl-K9, but no the tri-methyl-K9 peptide, demonstrating that KDM3A selectively demethylates mono- and di-methylated H3K9 (H3K9me1/2) (Yamane et al. 2006).

a

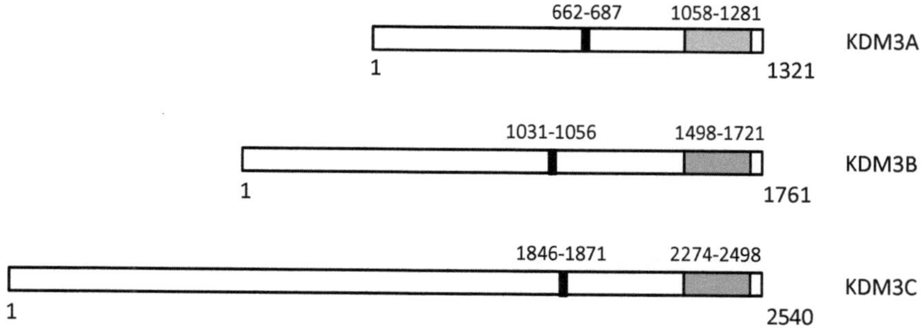

b

```
KDM3A       MPSRFDDLMANIPLPEYTRRDGKLNLASRLPNYFVRPDLGPKMYNAYGLITPEDRKYGTT
KDM3B       MPTRFEDLMENLPLPEYTKRDGRLNLASRLPSYFVRPDLGPKMYNAYGLITAEDRRVGTT
KDM3C       MPARYEDLLKSLPLPEYCNPEGKFNLASHLPGFFVRPDLGPRLCSAYGVVAAKDHDIGTT
            **:*::**: .:***** . :*::****:**.:********:: .***::: :*:  ***

KDM3A       NLHLDVSDAANVMVYVGIPKGQCEQE-EEVLKTIQDGDSDELTIKRFIEGKEKPGALWHI
KDM3B       NLHLDVSDAVNVMVYVGIPIGEGAHD-EEVLKTIDEGDADEVTKQRIHDGKEKPGALWHI
KDM3C       NLHIEVSDVVNILVYVGIAKGNGILSKAGILKKFEEEDLDDILRKRLKDSSEIPGALWHI
            ***::***..*::*****  *:   .   :**.::: * *::  :*: :..* *******

KDM3A       YAAKDTEKIREFLKKVSEEQGQENPADHDPIHDQSWYLDRSLRKRLHQEYGVQGWAIVQF
KDM3B       YAAKDAEKIRELLRKVGEEQGQENPPDHDPIHDQSWYLDQTLRKRLYEEYGVQGWAIVQF
KDM3C       YAGKDVDKIREFLQKISKEQGLEVLPEHDPIRDQSWYVNKKLRQRLLEEYGVRTCTLIQF
            **.**.:****:*:*:.:*** *   :****:*****:::.**:** :****:  :::**

KDM3A       LGDVVFIPAGAPHQVHNLYSCIKVAEDFVSPEHVKHCFWLTQEFR
KDM3B       LGDAVFIPAGAPHQVHNLYSCIKVAEDFVSPEHVKHCFRLTQEFR
KDM3C       LGDAIVLPAGALHQVQNFHSCIQVTEDFVSPEHLVESFHLTQELR
            ***.:.:**** ***:*::***:*:********: ..* ****:*
```

c

KDM3A: ^{885}LRNLL^{889}

KDM3B: ^{1293}LRDLL^{1297}

KDM3C: ^{2066}LRDLL^{2070}

Fig. 4.1 Structures of KDM3 family proteins. **a** Diagram showing human KDM3A, B and C proteins. The size of KDM3 proteins and location of C2HC4 zinc finger (black) or JmjC domain (gray) are indicated. **b** Alignment of amino acid sequences of JmjC domain from human KDM3A, B and C. **c** The LXXLL motif in the human KDM3 protein. The location of KDM3 LXXLL motif is indicated

4.3 KDM3 in the Demethylation of Non-histone Proteins

KDM3A can demethylate the substrate protein other than H3K9me1/2. For example, KDM3A can demethylate tumor suppressor p53 in breast cancer cells (Ramadoss et al. 2017). Knockdown of KDM3A in MDA-MB-231 or Hs578T cells enhanced apoptosis in response to chemotherapeutic drugs such as cisplatin or paclitaxel. Knockdown of KDM3A in these breast cancer cells increased the expression of pro-apoptotic genes such as PUMA, NOXA or BAX. Methylation of p53 at K372 was reported

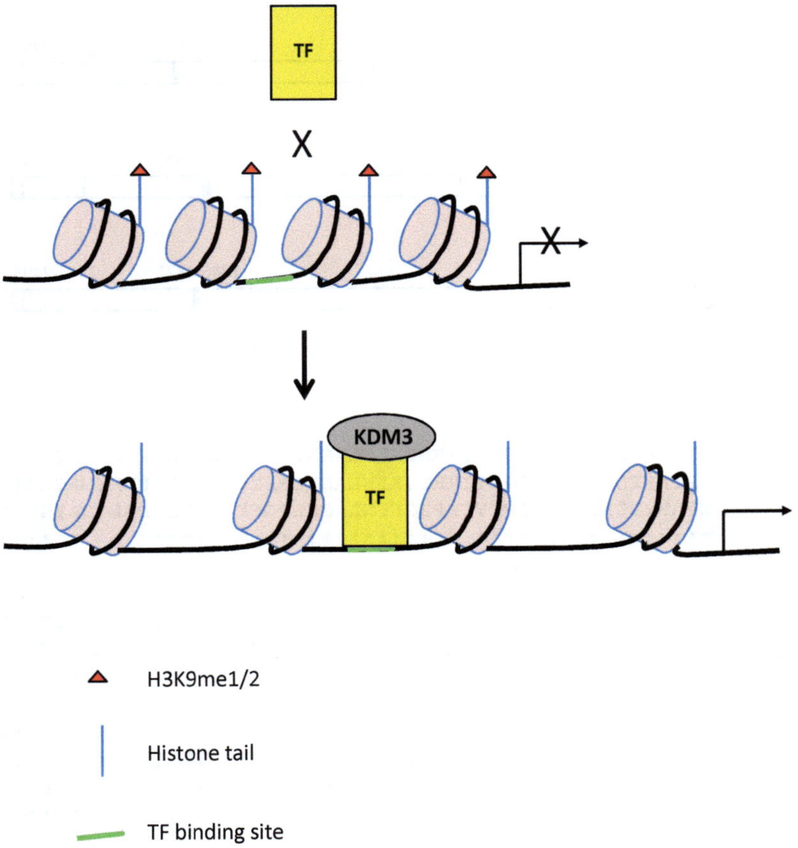

Fig. 4.2 Model of KDM3 in the regulation of gene expression. H3K9 methylation silences gene expression by compacting chromatin and blocking the access of transcription factor (TF) to its cognate DNA-binding site. KDM3A functions as coactivators of TF, removes the H3K9me1/2 marks, relaxes chromatin and allows the access of TF to its cognate DNA-binding site, leading to activation of gene expression

to enhance p53 activity (Chuikov et al. 2004). KDM3A was co-precipitated with p53 and knockdown of KDM3A increased the level of p53-K372me1 in breast cancer cells or in in vitro reaction, which suggests that KDM3A can demethylate p53 at K372. KDM3A knockdown increased the level of p53 or p53-K372me1 on PUMA and NOXA promoters. Taken together, these results suggest that knockdown of KDM3A increases p53-K372me1 levels and p53 activity for the expression of some pro-apoptotic genes.

KDM3C can also demethylate the substrate protein other than H3K9me1/2. One such example is Mediator of DNA damage checkpoint protein 1 (MDC1), which functions as a regulator of cell cycle checkpoints and recruits repair proteins to the site of DNA double-strand breaks. KDM3C was found to demethylate MDC1 at lysine 45, which, in turn, promoted MDC1-RNF8 interaction, RNF8-induced ubiquitination of MDC1, and recruitment of DNA repair protein RAP80–BRCA1 to polyubiquitinated MDC1 (Watanabe et al. 2013).

4.4 Physiological Functions of KDM3A

Five *Kdm3a*-deficient mouse lines have been established and reported thus far (Table 4.1). These mouse models offer the opportunity to evaluate the physiological role of KDM3A. The phenotypes of *Kdm3a*-deficient mice include

Table 4.1 Summary of *Kdm3a*-decificient mouse models

Knockout approach	Main phenotype	References
Deletion of the catalytic JmjC domain by an insertion in intron 10 (or intron 7 of splicing variant 2) of the *Kdm3a* gene	Spermatogenesis defect, smaller testes, fewer sperm numbers and male infertility	Okada et al. (2007)
Deletion of *Kdm3a* exons 24–27 encoding the catalytic JmjC domain using the Cre-lox system	Spermatogenesis defect, obesity and metabolism	Tateishi et al. (2009)
Deletion of *Kdm3a* exons 20–25 encoding the JmjC domain by an insertion-type vector	Obesity, metabolic syndrome, sex reversal	Inagaki et al. (2009)
Deletion of *Kdm3a* exons 17–25 encoding the JmjC domain	Spermatogenesis defect, smaller testes, fewer sperm numbers and male infertility	Liu et al. (2010)
Deletion of KDM3A full-length protein by an insertion within the *Kdm3a* intron 5–6	Spermatogenesis defect, smaller testes and male infertility	Kasioulis et al. (2014)

Five lines of *Kdm3a*-deficient mice have been established. Lists are methods used to generate the *Kdm3a*-deficient mice and main phenotypes observed

defects in spermatogenesis, fat metabolism, sex determination and stem cell activity. We will summarize the main phenotypes of *Kdm3a*-deficent mice and the possible mechanisms that underlie these mutant phenotypes.

4.4.1 Spermatogenesis

KDM3A was initially identified as a transcript that was highly expressed in the male germ cells (Hoog et al. 1991). The levels of KDM3A mRNA and protein were increased during the process of spermatogenesis in mice (Okada et al. 2007). Four out of five *Kdm3a*-deficient mouse lines (Table 4.1) showed phenotypes of spermatogenesis defect, smaller testes and male infertility (Okada et al. 2007; Tateishi et al. 2009; Liu et al. 2010; Kasioulis et al. 2014). The spermatids from the *Kdm3a*-mutant mice showed defects in the chromatin condensation (Okada et al. 2007; Kasioulis et al. 2014), an important event required for spermatogenesis. In the male germ cells, transcription factor Crem and its coactivator Act control expression of multiple genes including Tnp1, Tnp2, Prm1 and Prm2, which are required for the chromatin condensation (Nantel et al. 1996; Fimia et al. 1999). In one study, KDM3A was shown to promote the expression of Tnp1 and Prm1 by binding to and removing the H3K9 methylation marks at their promoters (Okada et al. 2007). In another study, KDM3A was shown to increase the expression of Tnp1, Tnp2, Prm1 and Prm2 by promoting Crem recruitment and Act expression (Liu et al. 2010). These studies suggest that the reduced expression of genes required for chromatin condensation may underlie the spermatogenesis defect observed in *Kdm3a*-deficient mice. Similarly, the *Kdm3c*-knockout mice showed spermatogenesis defects as well as male infertility (Kuroki et al. 2013a; Nakajima et al. 2016), which further supported the key role for the KDM3 family histone demethylases in spermatogenesis.

4.4.2 Metabolism

Two *Kdm3a*-deficient mouse lines showed phenotypes of obesity and metabolism defects (Loh et al. 2007; Tateishi et al. 2009). The *Kdm3a*-deficienct mice showed accumulation of large fat droplets in the adipose tissue, muscle and liver, as well as increased serum lipid content (Tateishi et al. 2009) and metabolic syndromes that include hypertriglyceridemia, hypercholesterolemia, hyperinsulinemia and hyperleptinemia (Loh et al. 2007). The gene expression profile studies on the wild-type and *Kdm3a*-deficient skeletal muscles (Tateishi et al. 2009) revealed downregulation of genes associated with the PPAR signaling pathway, the master regulator of adipogenesis and obesity. Reduced expression of Ppara was found in the *Kdm3a*-deficient myocytes, concomitant with an increased level of H3K9me2 at the PPAR responsive element of the Ppara gene (Tateishi et al. 2009), which indicated that KDM3A increased the expression of Ppara by H3K9 demethylation on the Ppara gene.

Ucp1 is a protein important for cold-induced heat generation in brown fat tissues. In response to β-adrenergic stimulation, KDM3A was found to increase the expression of Ucp1 in brown adipose cells by binding to and demethylating H3K9 at the enhancer of the Ucp1 gene, facilitating the recruitment of several transcription factors and coactivators (Tateishi et al. 2009). In another study, β-adrenergic stimulation was found to induce the phosphorylation of KDM3A at S265 by protein kinase A (PKA), and this promoted the interaction of KDM3A with SWI/SNF nucleosome remodeling complex and DNA-bound PPARγ. This phosphorylation is important to the KDM3A-dependent expression of β1-adrenergic receptor gene (Adrb1) and metabolic regulators including Ucp1 in brown adipose cells (Abe et al. 2015). These studies suggest that downregulation of metabolic regulators such as Ppara and Ucp1 may underlie the obesity and metabolism defect observed in the *kdm3a*-deficient mice.

4.4.3 Sex Determination

One *Kdm3a*-deficient mouse model, which was established from C57BL/6 (B6) x CBA F1 embryonic stem cells (Inagaki et al. 2009), was reported to have the male-to-female sex reversal phenotype (Kuroki et al. 2013b). Some of the *Kdm3a*-deficient XY mice were sex-reversed, either partially with one testis and one ovary or completely with two ovaries (Kuroki et al. 2013b). The *Syr* gene is located on Y chromosome and encodes a transcription factor required for male development (Koopman et al. 1991). Expression of Syr was decreased in the *Kdm3a*-deficient gonadal somatic cells, concomitant with the increased level of H3K9me2 within the *Syr* locus. Forced expression of *Sry* transgene in the *Kdm3a*-deficient mice rescued the defect of testis cord development in the XY gonads (Koopman et al. 1991). GLP/G9a methyltransferase complex was found to induce H3K9 methylation at the Sry locus and counteract the role of KDM3A in the sex determination (Kuroki et al. 2017). A heterozygous GLP mutation or a GLP/G9a inhibitor restored Sry expression and rescued the sex reversal phenotype in the *Kdm3a*-deficient mice (Kuroki et al. 2017). These studies demonstrate role of KDM3A in the expression of Syr and male development of mice.

4.4.4 Stem Cell Pluripotency

Embryonic stem cells (ESCs) are pluripotent and are able to self-renew indefinitely. KDM3A was reported to regulate the self-renewal of ESCs (Loh et al. 2007). Knockdown of KDM3A in ESCs resulted in the cell differentiation, accompanied by reduced expression of pluripotency-associated genes such as Tcl1, Tcfcp2/1 and Zfp57. ChIP-PCR analysis revealed an increased level of H3K9me2 on the Tcl1 promoter upon KDM3A knockdown. Forced restoration of Tcl1 expression in KDM3A-knockdown ES cells reversed the differentiation phenotype and maintained ES cell morphology. This study revealed that KDM3A promotes the expression of Tcl1 by H3K9 demethylation on the Tcl1 promoter and that Tcl1 is an important downstream effector of KDM3A for ESC self-renewal. Double knockout of *Kdm3a/Kdm3b* caused the elevation of

H3K9me2 marks and perturbed gene expression in ESC, resulting in rapid ESC death and embryonic lethality (Kuroki et al. 2018). This study further demonstrates a critical role for KDM3A/KDM3B-meditated H3K9 demethylation in ESC maintenance and early embryogenesis.

Somatic cells can be reprogrammed to pluripotency through fusion with ESCs, and reactivation of transcription factor Oct4 is a hallmark for effective reprograming. Ectopic overexpression of KDM3A in adult neural stem cells (NSCs) resulted in the global H3K9 demethylation and increased Oct4 reactivation upon ESC fusion, whereas overexpression of a catalytic-inactive KDM3A had no effect (Ma et al. 2008). This study revealed that KDM3A and its H3K9 demethylase activity could promote the reprogramming efficacy of NSCs upon fusion with ESCs. Somatic cells can be reprogrammed to pluripotency through the ectopic expression of Oct4, Sox2, Klf4 and c-Myc (OSKM), which results in the generation of induced pluripotent stem cells (iPSCs). The porcine iPSCs induced by OSKM and KDM3A were shown to express higher levels of pluripotency-associated genes, compared with those induced by OSKM alone (Mao et al. 2017). Thus, these studies reveal a role for KDM3A in the reprograming of somatic cells to pluripotency.

4.5 Roles of KDM3A in Gene Regulation and Cancer

KDM3A was upregulated in various types of cancers, such as neuroblastoma (Tee et al. 2014), sarcoma (Parrish et al. 2015), prostate cancer (Qi et al. 2010), breast cancer (Ramadoss et al. 2017), hepatocellular carcinoma (Yamada et al. 2012), renal cell carcinoma (Guo et al. 2011), colon cancer (Uemura et al. 2010), cervical cancer (Liu et al. 2016), gastric cancer (Yang et al. 2015) and non-small cell lung cancer (Zhan et al. 2016). KDM3A knockdown studies in various cancer cells largely point to a tumor-promoting role of KDM3A. KDM3A has been found to promote the activity and/or expression of several key transcription factors and related transcriptional programs through its demethylase activity (Fig. 4.3). Here, we will highlight

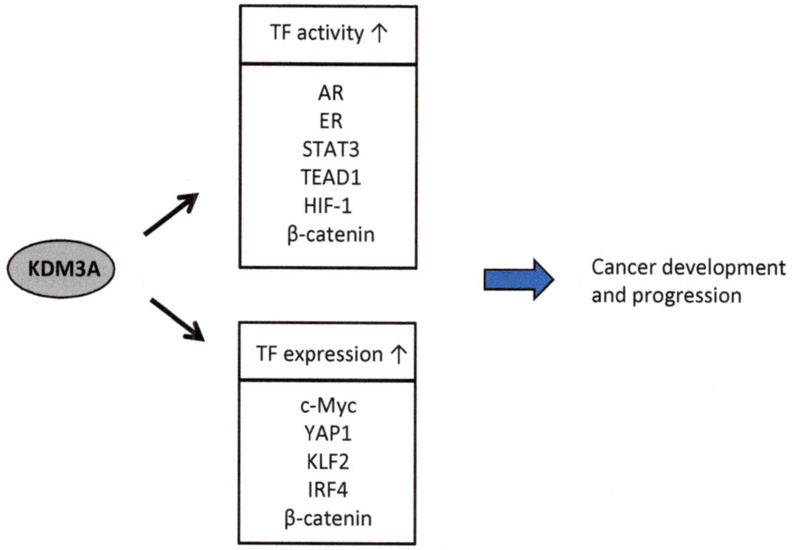

Fig. 4.3 Mechanisms of KDM3A in the transcriptional gene regulation in cancer cells. KDM3A functions as coactivators for transcription factor (TF) and/or promotes the expression of TF, resulting in the transcriptional gene alteration to drive cancer development and progression

some key transcription factors that are regulated by KDM3A and role of KDM3A-dependent gene regulation in cancer biology.

4.5.1 KDM3A is a Coactivator for the Androgen Receptor and Estrogen Receptor

The KDM3 protein contains a LXXLL sequence (Fig. 4.1c), which is a signature motif that mediates the binding of transcriptional coactivators to nuclear receptors (Heery et al. 1997). Androgen receptor (AR) belongs to the steroid nuclear receptor superfamily. It plays a key role in the progression of prostate cancer and is the primary therapeutic target for metastatic prostate cancer. Knockdown of KMD3A was found to decrease ligand-induced expression of AR target genes such as PSA, NKX3.1 and TMPRSS22 in LNCaP cells (Yamane et al. 2006). KDM3A was found to interact with AR and binds to the enhancers of PSA and NKX3.1 in a ligand-dependent manner, concomitant with a reduction of H3K9me2 levels on those enhancers. In contrast, knockdown of KDM3A reduced the recruitment of KDM3A to the enhancers of PSA and NKX3.1 and diminished the ligand-induced reduction of H3K9me2 on these enhancers (Yamane et al. 2006). Hypoxia induced the upregulation of KDM3A expression in LNCaP cells, which is associated with the elevation of PSA expression, as well as an increased recruitment of KDM3A to and H3K9 demethylation of the PSA enhancer (Lee et al. 2013). These studies showed that KDM3A promoted ligand- or hypoxia-induced expression of example AR targets in LNCaP cells through H3K9 demethylation. CWR22Rv1 cells are androgen-independent prostate cancer cells (Li et al. 2011). AR was implicated to be one of the top transcription factors regulated by KDM3A in CWR22Rv1 cells, based on the analysis of differentially expressed genes following KDM3A knockdown (Fan et al. 2016). KDM3A was shown to promote H3K9 demethylation, AR chromatin recruitment and expression of select AR target genes in CWR22Rv1 cells (Fan et al. 2016; Wilson et al. 2017). AR-V7 is a constitutively-active truncated form of AR and associated with the resistance of prostate cancer to the AR-targeted therapy (Antonarakis et al. 2014). KDM3A was found to promote the recruitment of a splicing factor HNRNPF to a cryptic exon3b and enhance the alternative splicing of AR-V7 (Fan et al. 2018). These studies revealed two mechanisms for KDM3A in the regulation of AR transcriptional activity by increasing the AR chromatin recruitment and AR-V7 generation. The future development of KDM3A inhibitors may offer an opportunity to inhibit AR activity and thus serve as a potential therapy for advanced prostate cancer.

KDM3A was also found to promote transcriptional activity of estrogen receptor (ER) in breast cancer cells (Wade et al. 2015). The profiling array analysis showed that 42% of estrogen-stimulated or repressed genes were down- or upregulated at least 1.5-fold in the KDM3A-knockdown MCF-7 breast cancer cells, which suggests that KDM3A positively regulates a significant portion of the ER transcriptional program. Re-expression of wild-type, but not the catalytically-inactive KDM3A, significantly rescued the downregulation of ER target genes such as pS2, GREB1 and CCND1 in the KDM3A-knockdown MCF-7 cells, which indicates that the demethylase activity of KDM3A is required for the expression of these ER target genes. Knockdown of KDM3A in MCF-7 cells increased the H3K9me2 and decreased the recruitment of ER to the pS2 and GREB1 genes. Knockdown of KDM3A in MCF-7 or T47D cells resulted in G1 cell cycle arrest and inhibition of cell proliferation. Hormone therapy with the estrogen receptor modulator tamoxifen is effective for the treatment of ER-positive breast cancer, but resistance to the tamoxifen invariably occurs. Knockdown of KDM3A inhibited the proliferation of MMU2 cells, which are a tamoxifen-resistant line derived from MCF-7 cells. These results suggest that targeting KDM3A may inhibit the activity of ER and thus contribute to the improved endocrine therapy for breast cancer.

Overexpression of the HER2 receptor tyrosine kinase is known to promote resistance of breast cancer to tamoxifen therapy (Clarke et al. 2015). ACK1 is a non-receptor kinase that can be activated by various receptor tyrosine kinases including HER2 (Mahajan and Mahajan 2015). One study found that heregulin-mediated ACK1 activation promoted ER activity in the presence of tamoxifen through tyrosine phosphorylation of KDM3A (Mahajan et al. 2014). HOXA1 is a potent oncogene that can transform human mammary epithelial cells upon overexpression (Zhang et al. 2003). ACK1 inhibitors blocked the heregulin-induced upregulation of HOXA expression, concomitant with the accumulation of H3K9me2 and loss of ER binding at the intron one of HOXA gene. This study suggests that ACK1 induces tyrosine phosphorylation of KDM3A to enhance ER transcriptional activity and contributes to tamoxifen resistance. Interestingly, ACK1 was also found to induce tyrosine phosphorylation of AR and promote the AR transcriptional activity under androgen deprivation conditions (Mahajan et al. 2007). It will be interesting to test whether ACK1 also induces tyrosine phosphorylation of KDM3A in prostate cancer and whether this contributes to the transcriptional activity of AR.

4.5.2 KDM3A Acts as a Coactivator for Other Transcription Factors

In addition to AR and ER, KDM3A was reported to function as coactivators for other transcription factors. JAK-STAT3 signaling is known to play an oncogenic role in various malignancies. KDM3A can contribute to the activation of JAK-STAT3 signaling, by serving as a coactivator for STAT3 to promote STAT3-mediated gene expression (Kim et al. 2018). TEAD1 is a transcription factor mediating the expression of hippo target genes in the Hippo signaling pathway. KDM3A can interact with and function as a coactivator for TEAD1 in colorectal cancer cells (Wang et al. 2019). KDM3A can also interact with and function as a coactivator for β-catenin to promote the Wnt signaling in colorectal cancer cells (Li et al. 2017; Peng et al. 2018).

4.5.3 KDM3A Regulates c-Myc Expression

c-Myc is a master regulator in cell proliferation and transformation (Dang 2012). Overexpression of c-Myc is an important factor in development of various cancers (Dang 2012). Recent studies revealed that KDM3A regulated the expression of c-Myc to drive the progression of prostate, cervical, colorectal and mammary tumors. Knockdown of KDM3A was found to reduce the level of c-Myc in prostate cancer (Fan et al. 2016). In AR-positive CWR22Rv1 or LNCaP cells, KDM3A promoted H3K9 demethylation of and recruitment of AR to the c-Myc gene enhancer.

In AR-negative PC3 and DU145 cells, KDM3A also increased the levels of c-Myc protein through its interaction with E3 ubiquitin ligase HUWE1 and inhibition of HUWE1-induced degradation of c-Myc. This stabilizing effect of KMD3A on the c-Myc protein did not require its histone demethylase activity. Of note, there are other examples for the catalytic-independent function of KDM3A. For instance, KDM3A was found to interact with and stabilize GL1 through the inhibition of its proteasomal degradation, thereby regulating the Hedgehog signaling pathway (Schneider et al. 2015).

Knockdown of KDM3A blocked the proliferation of prostate cancer cells in vitro and orthotopic tumor formation in nude mice, whereas forced re-expression of c-Myc in these cells partly reversed the growth defects caused by KDM3A knockdown (Fan et al. 2016). Thus, c-Myc is a key downstream effector of KDM3A in the growth and tumorigenesis of prostate cancer cells. Staining of KDM3A and c-Myc in a tissue microarray (TMA) of prostate cancer showed that high level of c-Myc was associated with high level of KDM3A, which implicates KDM3A in the upregulation of c-Myc in a subset of human prostate cancer (Fan et al. 2016).

Similar findings were reported in cervical and colorectal cancer cells. Knockdown of KDM3A in HeLa cells led to decreased expression of c-Myc and increased levels of H3K9me2 on the c-Myc gene promoter. In addition, knockdown of KMD3A reduced the growth, migration and invasion of Hela cells in vitro, whereas restoration of c-Myc expression in KDM3A-knockdown cells partly rescued these defects (Liu et al. 2016). Staining of cervical cancer specimens showed a positive correlation between KDM3A and c-Myc expression, whereby high levels of KDM3A and c-Myc were also strongly associated with poor patient survival (Liu et al. 2016). Similarly, KDM3A was overexpressed in colorectal cancer specimens and positively correlated with the expression of Wnt/β-catenin target genes including c-Myc (Peng et al. 2018). KDM3A was found to promote the expression of c-Myc via β-catenin in colorectal cancer cells (Peng et al. 2018).

KDM3A was found to promote the transformation of breast cells (Zhao et al. 2016). In a previously established transformation model, transduction of human primary mammary cells with Large T antigen, TERT and RAS (V12) can generate cell lines representing different stages of transformation. KDM3A was found to gradually increase during the progression of transformation, concomitant with a decrease of H3K9me2 levels. KDM3A increased the expression of cancer-related genes such as c-Myc and Pax3 through H3K9 demethylation in transformed cells. Knockdown of KDM3A, c-Myc or Pax3 reduced the proliferation of transformed cells. Thus, this study suggests that KDM3A promotes the tumorigenesis of breast cancer through the upregulation of c-Myc and Pax3 oncogene.

Together, these studies indicate that KDM3A can promote c-Myc expression and cancer progression in several types of cancers.

4.5.4 KDM3A Regulates Expression of Other Transcription Factors

KLF2 is a transcription factor of the Krüppel zinc finger family, and IRF4 is a member the interferon regulatory family of transcription factors. KDM3A was shown to promote the expression of KLF2 and IRF4 by demethylating H3K9me1/2 at the core promoter of these two genes. KDM3A-mediated expression of KLF2 and IRF4 played a key role in the survival and bone marrow homing of multiple myeloma (MM) cells (Ohguchi et al. 2016). YAP1 is a coactivator for the TEAD family of transcription factors in the Hippo signaling pathway. KDM3A promoted the expression of YAP1 via H3K9me1/2 demethylation on the YAP1 promoter and enhanced the TEAD1-mediated expression of hippo targets in colorectal cancer cells (Wang et al. 2019). KDM3A was also found to promote the expression of β -catenin by H3K9me2 demethylation of β-catenin gene promoter in colorectal cancer cells (Peng et al. 2018).

4.5.5 KDM3A in Hypoxia Response

Hypoxia is a common feature in solid tumors. HIF-1α is the master transcription factor that controls adaptive gene expression under hypoxia. The level of KDM3A is upregulated under hypoxia in various normal and cancer cells (Krieg et al. 2010; Uemura et al. 2010; Mimura et al. 2012; Osawa et al. 2013; Chakraborty et al. 2016). KDM3A has been demonstrated to be an HIF target gene (Beyer et al. 2008; Pollard et al. 2008; Wellmann et al. 2008; Krieg et al. 2010). KDM3A levels were downregulated upon knockdown of HIF-1α and upregulated upon HIF activation (Beyer et al. 2008; Pollard et al. 2008; Wellmann et al. 2008; Krieg et al. 2010). ChIP-qPCR revealed that HIF-1α could bind to the hypoxia response element (HRE) sequences located at the KDM3A promoter (Beyer et al. 2008; Pollard et al. 2008). Hypoxia or HIF-1α overexpression could increase luciferase reporter activity of a KDM3A promoter construct but not the KDM3A promoter with HRE sequence mutations (Beyer et al. 2008; Wellmann et al. 2008).

The upregulation of KDM3A by HIF contributes to the expression of a subset of hypoxia-induced genes (Krieg et al. 2010; Mimura et al. 2012; Osawa et al. 2013; Chakraborty et al. 2016). However, it remains unclear which transcription factor(s) is regulated by KDM3A under hypoxia. In one study,

KDM3A was shown to interact with HIF-1α and facilitate HIF-1α-dependent expression of GLUT3 in endothelial cells to enhance glucose uptake under hypoxia (Mimura et al. 2012). Mechanistically, KDM3A was recruited by HIF-1α to demethylate H3K9me2 at the proximal promoter and enhancers of GLUT3 gene, thereby increasing the expression of GLUT3 (Mimura et al. 2012). In another study, KDM3A was shown to mediate hypoxia/HIF-induced expression of Mmp12 to promote trophoblast cell invasion (Chakraborty et al. 2016). The regulatory sequence of Mmp12 showed KDM3A accumulation and H3K9 demethylation but did not contain the HRE motifs (Chakraborty et al. 2016). The results suggest that KDM3A may regulate a transcription factor other than HIF to promote the Mmp12 expression in trophoblast cells under hypoxia.

Targeting the VEGF/VEGFR pathways to inhibit angiogenesis serves as an anti-cancer treatment, but such cancer cells can become resistant and refractory to such antiangiogenic therapy (Ebos et al. 2009; Paez-Ribes et al. 2009). KDM3A was implicated to confer resistance of xenograft tumor cells to antiangiogenic treatment (Osawa et al. 2013). KDM3A, VEGF-A and FGF18 were upregulated in cancer cells (HeLa, HepG2, A431 and T98G) under hypoxia and nutrition deprivation condition. KDM3A mRNA expression was also upregulated in tumor tissues at the preangiogenic switch in HSML cells and B16 cells and at the refractory phase of anti-VEGF treatment. siRNA knockdown of KDM3A in HeLa and A673 cells had a minor effect on cell proliferation in vitro. In contrast, KDM3A inhibition significantly suppressed tumor growth upon injection of HeLa or A673 cells into immunodeficient mice. Expression of angiogenic factors including FGF2, HGF, and Ang2 was significantly decreased in those KDM3A-knockdown tumor tissues, which also showed reduced CD31-postive vessel formation and CD11b-positive macrophage infiltration. These results suggest that KDM3A enhances the expression of some angiogenic factors and promotes tumor angiogenesis and inflammatory cell infiltration. Importantly, KDM3A inhibition significantly enhanced the tumor-suppressive effects of the anti-VEGF antibody (bevacizumab) or antiangiogenic VEGFR inhibitor (sunitinib) in the xeonograft model. This study suggests that targeting KDM3A may enhance the efficiency of antiangiogenic therapy.

KDM3A was found to be involved in the development of neuroendocrine prostate cancer (NEPC) (Qi et al. 2010). NEPC is a rare type of prostate cancer, but its incidence is increased after treatment of prostate cancer with the new generation of AR pathway inhibitors (Li et al. 2016). Siah2 is an E3 ubiquitin ligase and plays a key role in the availability and activity of HIF-1α by ubiquitination and degradation of several HIF inhibitory proteins (Nakayama et al. 2004; Qi et al. 2013). Crossing Siah2 knockout mice with the TRAMP model reduced the formation of NEPC (Qi et al. 2010). Siah2 was found to promote the expression of a subset of HIF-1α target genes, among which are KDM3A, HES6 and SOX9. Forced expression of KDM3A, HES6 and Sox9 in Siah2-inhibited prostate tumor cells partly recued the defect of TRAMP-C cells in the formation of xenograft prostate tumors in nude mice and the defect of CWR22Rv1 cells in the expression of NE marker under hypoxia (Qi et al. 2010). Future work will be needed to determine the precise mechanisms of KDM3A in the neuroendocrine phenotype of prostate cancer.

KDM3A was upregulated in the hypoxic cells within colorectal cancer (CRC) liver metastases and was identified to be an independent prognostic factor for CRC (Uemura et al. 2010). Knockdown of KDM3A inhibited the growth of subcutaneous xenograft tumors formed by the CRC cell line HCT116 (Krieg et al. 2010; Uemura et al. 2010) and DLD1 (Uemura et al. 2010). Similarly, KDM3A was upregulated in hepatocellular carcinoma samples relative to normal liver tissues, and high expression of KDM3A in hepatocellular carcinoma was also associated with a higher rate of recurrence (Yamada et al. 2012). Hypoxia induced upregulation of KDM3A in hepatocellular carcinoma (HCC) cell line HepG2 and Hep3B, and knockdown of KDM3A in those HCC cell lines reduced their growth under hypoxia. Knockdown of KDM3A in HepG2 cells reduced the growth of xenograft tumors upon the subcutaneous injection into nude mice (Park et al. 2013).

Together, these studies reveal that KMD3A is upregulated under hypoxia and contribute to the hypoxia-associated aggressive phenotypes of various cancers.

4.5.6 KDM3A in Anoikis

Anoikis is a specialized form of apoptosis induced when epithelial cells detach from the extracellular matrix (ECM) (Buchheit et al. 2014). It plays an important role in preventing metastasis by eliminating the tumor cells that lose the proper ECM cues. In a genome-wide shRNA screen, KDM3A was identified as one of top candidates that could promote the survival of MCF10A cells, a non-tumorigenic mammary epithelial cell line, in the absence of ECM attachment (Pedanou et al. 2016). Following detachment from ECM, increased levels of KDM3A were detected in MCF10 cells but not other breast cancer cells that resist anoikis. Upregulation of KDM3A upon detachment could partly be due to the loss of integrin/FAK and EGFR/MEK signaling. KDM3A was found to promote expression of pro-apoptotic genes BNIP3 and BNIP3L by H3K9me1/2 demethylation of their promoters. Knockdown of KDM3A in non-metastatic mouse breast cancer cell lines 67NR or 4T07 promoted their lung metastasis. This study suggests that KDM3A can induce anoikis in non-transformed mammary epithelial cells or early-stage breast cancer cells to inhibit their metastatic potential.

4.6 Roles of KDM3B and KDM3C in Cancer

Acute promyelocytic leukemia (APL) can be effectively treated with differentiation therapy using all-trans-retinoic acid (ATRA), which induces terminal differentiation followed by apoptosis. KDM3B was downregulated during the differentiation of human promyelocytic leukemia cell line HL-60, and this was accompanied by the enrichment of H3K9me2 and recruitment of several corepressors to the KDM3B promoter (Kim et al. 2012). Knockdown of KDM3B in HL-60 cells enhanced differentiation, whereas overexpression of KDM3B had opposite effect. KDM3B was found to promote the expression of leukemogenic oncogene lmo2 by H3K9me1/2 demethylation of the Imo2 promoter. KDM3B and Imo2 were upregulated in blood cells from acute lymphoblastic leukemia (ALL)-type leukemia patients. This study suggests that KDM3B promotes leukemogenesis via activation of lmo2 through its H3K9 demethylase activity.

KDM3C has been shown to promote leukemogenesis as a coactivator for transcription factor RUNX1-RUNX1T1 (Chen et al. 2015) and HOXA9 (Zhu et al. 2016). RUNX1–RUNX1T1 is a transcription factor generated by the t(8;21) translocation in acute myeloid leukemia (AML), and it can increase self-renewal and inhibit the myeloid differentiation. KDM3C was found to interact with and function as a coactivator for RUNX1–RUNX1T1. KDM3C was recruited by RUNX1–RUNX1T1 to its target genes and regulated their expression by H3K9me2 demethylation. Conditional knockout of *Kdm3c* inhibited the proliferation of hematopoietic stem cells (HSCs) driven by RUNX1–RUNX1T1. Knockdown of KDM3C inhibited the proliferation of multiple AML cell lines. This study suggests that KDM3C is required for maintenance of multiple types of leukemia driven by different mutations.

KDM3C was also demonstrated to promote leukemogenesis driven by translocation of the mixed lineage leukemia (MLL) gene (Krivtsov and Armstrong 2007). The most common translocation of MLL gene in acute myeloid leukemia (AML) is t(9;11) which encodes the oncogenic MLL-AF9 fusion protein. MLL-AF9 leukemia has been shown to follow a leukemia stem cell (LSC) model in which LSCs are enriched in a subset population of leukemia cells

(Krivtsov and Armstrong 2007). Transformation by MLL-AF9 induced aberrant gene expression, which includes the canonical MLL-AF9 target genes homeobox A9 (HOXA9) and Meis homeobox 1 (MEIS1) that are important to the LSC self-renewal. The shRNA screening on the mouse LSCs identified KDM3C as one of the top MLL-AF9 target genes that are essential for MLL-AF9 leukemia (Sroczynska et al. 2014; Zhu et al. 2016). Conditional knockout of *Kdm3c* in the mouse LSCs led to a decreased self-renewal of LSC. KDM3C was found to interact with HOXA9 and may serve as a coactivator to modulate a HOXA9-dependent gene expression (Zhu et al. 2016). This study suggests that KDM3C may drive the MLL-AF9 leukemia by promoting the activity and transcriptional program of HOXA9 through its H3K9 demethylase activity.

KDM3C was found to promote the expression of YAP1 in esophageal cancer (EC) cells (Cai et al. 2017). Staining of KDM3C in 100 paired esophageal cancer tissues showed that KDM3C was highly upregulated in the cancer tissues compared to the adjacent normal tissues. Knockdown of KDM3C reduced the expression of YAP1 and inhibited the growth of two esophageal cancer cell lines, Eca109 and EC18, whereas the forced re-expression of YAP1 in the KDM3C-knockdown cells rescued the cell growth in vitro. KDM3C was shown to bind to and remove the H3K9me2 mark on the YAP1 promoter. This study indicates that KDM3C promotes the growth of esophageal cancer cells through upregulation of YAP1 expression.

4.7 Regulation of KDM3A by Posttranslational Modifications

KDM3A can be regulated by a variety of posttranslational modifications such as phosphorylation, ubiquitination and acetylation. Phosphorylation of tyrosine residues located in the JmjC domain of KDM3A can enhance its H3K9 demethylase activity. Tyrosine 1114 of KDM3A can be phosphorylated by the non-receptor tyrosine kinase ACK1, and this leads to increased H3K9 demethylation and co-activation of some ER target genes in breast cancer cells (Mahajan et al. 2014). Tyrosine 1101 of KDM3A can be phosphorylated by JAK2, and this increases the H3K9 demethylation and co-activation of STAT3 target genes in Hela cells after IL-6 treatment (Kim et al. 2018). Lysine 918 of KDM3A can be modified by ubiquitin ligase HUWE1 through a K27/K29-linked noncanonical ubiquitination, and this promotes the co-activation of c-Myc for the expression of DNA repair factors in prostate cancer cells (Fan et al. 2020). Ubiquitin ligase STUB1 can induce the canonical ubiquitination and degradation of KDM3A through the ubiquitin–proteasome pathway, and thus, the low expression of STUB1 may contribute to the upregulation of KDM3A protein in advanced prostate cancer (Xu et al. 2020). Lysine 421 of KDM3A can be acetylated by acetyltransferase p300, and this leads to recruitment of the bromodomain family member BRD4 to block KDM3A–STUB1 interaction and enhance the KMD3A protein stability (Xu et al. 2020). Importantly, inhibitors of ACK1, JAK2 or BRD4 can be used to inhibit the KDM3A activity in cancer cells (Mahajan et al. 2014; Kim et al. 2018; Xu et al. 2020). The posttranslational modifications of KMD3A may provide new targets to antagonize KDM3A activity for potential cancer therapy.

4.8 Regulation of KDM3A by MicroRNAs

MicroRNAs (miRNAs) are small non-coding RNAs that silence target gene expression through inhibition of mRNA translation or by mRNA decay. KDM3A was targeted by several tumor-suppressive miRNAs such as miR-627 (Padi et al. 2013), miR-22 (Toomey et al. 2010) and let-7c (Zhan et al. 2016). In addition, KDM3C was targeted by miR-590-3p to inhibit mitochondrial dysfunction and oxidative stress (Wang et al. 2016).

KDM3A was shown to be a target of miR-627 in colon cancer cells (Padi et al. 2013).

Overexpression of miR-627 reduced the level of KDM3A and inhibited the activity of KDM3A 3′UTR reporter construct but not the reporter construct with mutation on the potential miR-627 binding site. Calcitriol is an active form of vitamin D, which has been shown to inhibit proliferation and induce apoptosis in colon cancer cells (Deeb et al. 2007). Calcitriol treatment of colon cancer cell line HCT-116 led to upregulation of miR-627 and downregulation of KDM3A, whereas inhibition of miR-627 blocked calcitriol-induced downregulation of KDM3A. Correspondingly, calcitriol treatment inhibited the xenograft tumor formation by HCT-116 cells, and such inhibition on cell growth was blocked when miR-627 was inhibited. Moreover, knockdown of KDM3A or overexpression of miR-627 in HCT-116 cells inhibited the cell growth. This study suggests that calcitriol inhibits growth of colon cancer cells through downregulation of KDM3A via upregulation of miR-627.

KDM3A was shown to be an miR-22 target in Ewing Sarcoma cells (Parrish et al. 2015). Overexpression of miR-22 reduced the KDM3A level in the Ewing Sarcoma cell line A673, and inhibited the activity of KDM3A 3′UTR reporter construct, but not the reporter construct with mutation on the potential miR-22 binding site. Ewing Sarcoma pathogenesis is driven by oncoproteins that arise from the fusion between the EWS gene and one of Ets transcription factor genes, among which EWS/Fli1 is the most common fusion oncoprotein and underlies 80–90% of Ewing Sarcoma cases (Toomey et al. 2010). One of the miRNAs repressed by EWS/Fli1 in Ewing Sarcoma was miR-22 (McKinsey et al. 2011), which inhibited the growth of Ewing Sarcoma cell lines upon the ectopic overexpression (Parrish et al. 2015). As KDM3A is a miR-22 target, the repression of miR-22 by EWS/Fli1 may increase the level of KDM3A in Ewing Sarcoma cells. Consistently, published gene profiling data showed a positive correlation between KDM3A and EWS/Fli1 in Ewing Sarcoma. Knockdown of KDM3A in three different Ewing Sarcoma cell lines inhibited cell growth in vitro. Knockdown of KDM3A in A673 cells reduced the growth of xenograft tumors in nude mice. This study suggests that the fusion oncoprotein EWS/Fli1 promotes the growth of Ewing Sarcoma cells by upregulating KDM3A through the repression of miR-22.

A mutual regulation between KDM3A and miRNA let-7c was identified in non-small lung cancer cells (NSCLC) (Zhan et al. 2016). KDM3A was found to repress the expression of miRNA let-7c, as indicated by the increased let-7c level following KDM3A knockdown. On the other hand, KDM3A was shown to be a target of let-7c. Overexpression of let-7c in H1299 and A549 cells reduced the level of KDM3A and repressed the activity of KDM3A 3′UTR reporter construct, whereas the repression was partially alleviated after mutation of the potential let-7c-binding site in the reporter construct. Thus, this study reveals a feedback loop between KDM3A and let-7c, through which KDM3A maintains its high expression through repression of the miRNA let-7c in NSCLC.

4.9 Conclusion and Future Perspective

The KDM3 family of histone demethylases, particularly KDM3A, has been demonstrated to regulate transcription factors and transcriptional program through its H3K9me1/2 demethylase activity and thus promotes cancer development and progression. Mechanistically, KDM3A can regulate gene expression by functioning as coactivators for transcription factors and/or upregulating the expression of transcription factors (Fig. 4.3). Several issues on KDM3A-mediated gene regulation are anticipated to be resolved in future research. First is the role of KDM3 in the tumor initiation and progression. The current evidence for the tumor-promoting role of KDM3 is mainly based on the siRNA knockdown or conditional knockout in cells. Future studies to cross KDM3 knockout mice with relevant mouse transgenic tumor models are preferable and will allow better evaluation of the role of KDM3 in transcriptional gene regulation and cancer biology. The second issue is to identify the key transcriptional factor(s) and transcriptional program(s) that underlie KDM3-driven cancer progression. KDM3 may potentially regulate multiple transcription factors in cell-type, cancer-stage or context-specific manners. This issue will be better addressed with the additional studies that use the genome-wide analyzes (e.g., ChIP-seq, RNA-seq, etc.) on KDM3-inhbited cancer cell lines or models. Third, evidence suggests that KDM3A can demethylate the non-histone substrate or alter the function of its interactors independent of its catalytic activity, and further studies are needed to explore these directions. Finally, it is crucial to develop selective KDM3 inhibitors. Although selective inhibitors have been identified to target several JmjC subfamily members (Maes et al. 2015), selective inhibitors that target the KDM3 subfamily are currently unavailable. Further modifications of known JmjC KDM inhibitors or in silico screen may help identify selective KDM3 inhibitors. The structures of KDM3 have not yet been solved, and future determination of KDM3 structures is expected to facilitate the identification of selective inhibitory compounds or peptides targeting KDM3.

Acknowledgements The work was supported by NCI grant R01CA207118, R01CA244667 and DoD grant PC210437 (to J.Q.). It was also supported in part by the Maryland Department of Health's Cigarette Restitution Fund Program and the National Cancer Institute—Cancer Center Support Grant (CCSG)—P30CA134274.

References

Abe Y, Rozqie R, Matsumura Y, Kawamura T, Nakaki R, Tsurutani Y, Tanimura-Inagaki K, Shiono A, Magoori K, Nakamura K, Ogi S, Kajimura S, Kimura H, Tanaka T, Fukami K, Osborne TF, Kodama T, Aburatani H, Inagaki T, Sakai J (2015) JMJD1A is a signal-sensing scaffold that regulates acute chromatin dynamics via SWI/SNF association for thermogenesis. Nat Commun 6:7052

Antonarakis ES, Lu C, Wang H, Luber B, Nakazawa M, Roeser JC, Chen Y, Mohammad TA, Chen Y, Fedor HL, Lotan TL, Zheng Q, De Marzo AM, Isaacs JT, Isaacs WB, Nadal R, Paller CJ, Denmeade SR, Carducci MA, Eisenberger MA, Luo J (2014) AR-V7 and resistance to enzalutamide and abiraterone in prostate cancer. N Engl J Med 371:1028–1038

Beyer S, Kristensen MM, Jensen KS, Johansen JV, Staller P (2008) The histone demethylases JMJD1A and JMJD2B are transcriptional targets of hypoxia-inducible factor HIF. J Biol Chem 283:36542–36552

Buchheit CL, Weigel KJ, Schafer ZT (2014) Cancer cell survival during detachment from the ECM: multiple barriers to tumour progression. Nat Rev Cancer 14:632–641

Cai Y, Fu X, Deng Y (2017) Histone demethylase JMJD1C regulates esophageal cancer proliferation via YAP1 signaling. Am J Cancer Res 7:115–124

Chakraborty D, Cui W, Rosario GX, Scott RL, Dhakal P, Renaud SJ, Tachibana M, Rumi MA, Mason CW, Krieg AJ, Soares MJ (2016) HIF-KDM3A-MMP12 regulatory circuit ensures trophoblast plasticity and placental adaptations to hypoxia. Proc Natl Acad Sci U S A 113:E7212–E7221

Chen M, Zhu N, Liu X, Laurent B, Tang Z, Eng R, Shi Y, Armstrong SA, Roeder RG (2015) JMJD1C is required for the survival of acute myeloid leukemia by functioning as a coactivator for key transcription factors. Genes Dev 29:2123–2139

Chuikov S, Kurash JK, Wilson JR, Xiao B, Justin N, Ivanov GS, McKinney K, Tempst P, Prives C, Gamblin SJ, Barlev NA, Reinberg D (2004) Regulation of p53 activity through lysine methylation. Nature 432:353–360

Clarke R, Tyson JJ, Dixon JM (2015) Endocrine resistance in breast cancer–An overview and update. Mol Cell Endocrinol 418(Pt 3):220–234

Dang CV (2012) MYC on the path to cancer. Cell 149:22–35

Deeb KK, Trump DL, Johnson CS (2007) Vitamin D signalling pathways in cancer: potential for anticancer therapeutics. Nat Rev Cancer 7:684–700

Ebos JM, Lee CR, Cruz-Munoz W, Bjarnason GA, Christensen JG, Kerbel RS (2009) Accelerated metastasis after short-term treatment with a potent inhibitor of tumor angiogenesis. Cancer Cell 15:232–239

Fan L, Peng G, Sahgal N, Fazli L, Gleave M, Zhang Y, Hussain A, Qi J (2016) Regulation of c-Myc expression by the histone demethylase JMJD1A is essential for prostate cancer cell growth and survival. Oncogene 35:2441–2452

Fan L, Xu S, Zhang F, Cui X, Fazli L, Gleave M, Clark DJ, Yang A, Hussain A, Rassool F, Qi J (2020) Histone demethylase JMJD1A promotes expression of DNA repair factors and radio-resistance of prostate cancer cells. Cell Death Dis 11:214

Fan L, Zhang F, Xu S, Cui X, Hussain A, Fazli L, Gleave M, Dong X, Qi J (2018) Histone demethylase JMJD1A promotes alternative splicing of AR variant 7 (AR-V7) in prostate cancer cells. Proc Natl Acad Sci U S A 115:E4584–E4593

Fimia GM, De Cesare D, Sassone-Corsi P (1999) CBP-independent activation of CREM and CREB by the LIM-only protein ACT. Nature 398:165–169

Guo X, Shi M, Sun L, Wang Y, Gui Y, Cai Z, Duan X (2011) The expression of histone demethylase JMJD1A in renal cell carcinoma. Neoplasma 58:153–157

Heery DM, Kalkhoven E, Hoare S, Parker MG (1997) A signature motif in transcriptional co-activators mediates binding to nuclear receptors. Nature 387:733–736

Hoog C, Schalling M, Grunder-Brundell E, Daneholt B (1991) Analysis of a murine male germ cell-specific transcript that encodes a putative zinc finger protein. Mol Reprod Dev 30:173–181

Inagaki T, Tachibana M, Magoori K, Kudo H, Tanaka T, Okamura M, Naito M, Kodama T, Shinkai Y, Sakai J (2009) Obesity and metabolic syndrome in histone demethylase JHDM2a-deficient mice. Genes Cells 14:991–1001

Kasioulis I, Syred HM, Tate P, Finch A, Shaw J, Seawright A, Fuszard M, Botting CH, Shirran S, Adams IR, Jackson IJ, van Heyningen V, Yeyati PL (2014) Kdm3a lysine demethylase is an Hsp90 client required for cytoskeletal rearrangements during spermatogenesis. Mol Biol Cell 25:1216–1233

Kim H, Kim D, Choi SA, Kim CR, Oh SK, Pyo KE, Kim J, Lee SH, Yoon JB, Zhang Y, Baek SH (2018) KDM3A histone demethylase functions as an essential factor for activation of JAK2-STAT3 signaling pathway. Proc Natl Acad Sci U S A 115:11766–11771

Kim JY, Kim KB, Eom GH, Choe N, Kee HJ, Son HJ, Oh ST, Kim DW, Pak JH, Baek HJ, Kook H, Hahn Y, Kook H, Chakravarti D, Seo SB (2012) KDM3B is the H3K9 demethylase involved in transcriptional activation of lmo2 in leukemia. Mol Cell Biol 32:2917–2933

Kim SM, Kim JY, Choe NW, Cho IH, Kim JR, Kim DW, Seol JE, Lee SE, Kook H, Nam KI, Kook H, Bhak YY, Seo SB (2010) Regulation of mouse steroidogenesis by WHISTLE and JMJD1C through histone methylation balance. Nucleic Acids Res 38:6389–6403

Kooistra SM, Helin K (2012) Molecular mechanisms and potential functions of histone demethylases. Nat Rev Mol Cell Biol 13:297–311

Koopman P, Gubbay J, Vivian N, Goodfellow P, Lovell-Badge R (1991) Male development of chromosomally female mice transgenic for Sry. Nature 351:117–121

Krieg AJ, Rankin EB, Chan D, Razorenova O, Fernandez S, Giaccia AJ (2010) Regulation of the histone demethylase JMJD1A by hypoxia-inducible factor 1 alpha enhances hypoxic gene expression and tumor growth. Mol Cell Biol 30:344–353

Krivtsov AV, Armstrong SA (2007) MLL translocations, histone modifications and leukaemia stem-cell development. Nat Rev Cancer 7:823–833

Kuroki S, Akiyoshi M, Tokura M, Miyachi H, Nakai Y, Kimura H, Shinkai Y, Tachibana M (2013a) JMJD1C, a JmjC domain-containing protein, is required for long-term maintenance of male germ cells in mice. Biol Reprod 89:93

Kuroki S, Matoba S, Akiyoshi M, Matsumura Y, Miyachi H, Mise N, Abe K, Ogura A, Wilhelm D, Koopman P, Nozaki M, Kanai Y, Shinkai Y, Tachibana M (2013b) Epigenetic regulation of mouse sex determination by the histone demethylase Jmjd1a. Science 341:1106–1109

Kuroki S, Nakai Y, Maeda R, Okashita N, Akiyoshi M, Yamaguchi Y, Kitano S, Miyachi H, Nakato R, Ichiyanagi K, Shirahige K, Kimura H, Shinkai Y, Tachibana M (2018) Combined loss of JMJD1A and JMJD1B reveals critical roles for H3K9 demethylation in the maintenance of embryonic stem cells and early embryogenesis. Stem Cell Rep 10:1340–1354

Kuroki S, Okashita N, Baba S, Maeda R, Miyawaki S, Yano M, Yamaguchi M, Kitano S, Miyachi H, Itoh A, Yoshida M, Tachibana M (2017) Rescuing the aberrant sex development of H3K9 demethylase Jmjd1a-deficient mice by modulating H3K9 methylation balance. PLoS Genet 13:e1007034

Labbe RM, Holowatyj A, Yang ZQ (2013) Histone lysine demethylase (KDM) subfamily 4: structures, functions and therapeutic potential. Am J Transl Res 6:1–15

Lee HY, Yang EG, Park H (2013) Hypoxia enhances the expression of prostate-specific antigen by modifying the quantity and catalytic activity of Jumonji C domain-containing histone demethylases. Carcinogenesis 34:2706–2715

Li J, Yu B, Deng P, Cheng Y, Yu Y, Kevork K, Ramadoss S, Ding X, Li X, Wang CY (2017) KDM3 epigenetically controls tumorigenic potentials of human colorectal cancer stem cells through Wnt/beta-catenin signalling. Nat Commun 8:15146

Li Q, Zhang CS, Zhang Y (2016) Molecular aspects of prostate cancer with neuroendocrine differentiation. Chin J Cancer Res 28:122–129

Li S, Ali S, Duan X, Liu S, Du J, Liu C, Dai H, Zhou M, Zhou L, Yang L, Chu P, Li L, Bhatia R, Schones DE, Wu X, Xu H, Hua Y, Guo Z, Yang Y, Zheng L, Shen B (2018) JMJD1B demethylates H4R3me2s and H3K9me2 to facilitate gene expression for development of hematopoietic stem and progenitor cells. Cell Rep 23:389–403

Li Y, Alsagabi M, Fan D, Bova GS, Tewfik AH, Dehm SM (2011) Intragenic rearrangement and altered RNA splicing of the androgen receptor in a cell-based model of prostate cancer progression. Cancer Res 71:2108–2117

Liu J, Zhu M, Xia X, Huang Y, Zhang Q, Wang X (2016) Jumonji domain-containing protein 1A promotes cell growth and progression via transactivation of c-Myc expression and predicts a poor prognosis in cervical cancer. Oncotarget 7:85151–85162

Liu Z, Zhou S, Liao L, Chen X, Meistrich M, Xu J (2010) Jmjd1a demethylase-regulated histone modification is essential for cAMP-response element modulator-regulated gene expression and spermatogenesis. J Biol Chem 285:2758–2770

Loh YH, Zhang W, Chen X, George J, Ng HH (2007) Jmjd1a and Jmjd2c histone H3 Lys 9 demethylases regulate self-renewal in embryonic stem cells. Genes Dev 21:2545–2557

Ma DK, Chiang CH, Ponnusamy K, Ming GL, Song H (2008) G9a and Jhdm2a regulate embryonic stem cell fusion-induced reprogramming of adult neural stem cells. Stem Cells 26:2131–2141

Maes T, Carceller E, Salas J, Ortega A, Buesa C (2015) Advances in the development of histone lysine demethylase inhibitors. Curr Opin Pharmacol 23:52–60

Mahajan K, Lawrence HR, Lawrence NJ, Mahajan NP (2014) ACK1 tyrosine kinase interacts with histone demethylase KDM3A to regulate the mammary tumor oncogene HOXA1. J Biol Chem 289:28179–28191

Mahajan K, Mahajan NP (2015) ACK1/TNK2 tyrosine kinase: molecular signaling and evolving role in cancers. Oncogene 34:4162–4167

Mahajan NP, Liu Y, Majumder S, Warren MR, Parker CE, Mohler JL, Earp HS, Whang YE (2007) Activated Cdc42-associated kinase Ack1 promotes prostate cancer progression via androgen receptor tyrosine phosphorylation. Proc Natl Acad Sci U S A 104:8438–8443

Mao J, Zhang Q, Deng W, Wang H, Liu K, Fu H, Zhao Q, Wang X, Liu L (2017) Epigenetic modifiers facilitate induction and pluripotency of porcine iPSCs. Stem Cell Rep 8:11–20

McKinsey EL, Parrish JK, Irwin AE, Niemeyer BF, Kern HB, Birks DK, Jedlicka P (2011) A novel oncogenic mechanism in Ewing sarcoma involving IGF pathway targeting by EWS/Fli1-regulated microRNAs. Oncogene 30:4910–4920

Mimura I, Nangaku M, Kanki Y, Tsutsumi S, Inoue T, Kohro T, Yamamoto S, Fujita T, Shimamura T, Suehiro J, Taguchi A, Kobayashi M, Tanimura K, Inagaki T, Tanaka T, Hamakubo T, Sakai J, Aburatani H, Kodama T, Wada Y (2012) Dynamic change of chromatin conformation in response to hypoxia enhances the expression of GLUT3 (SLC2A3) by cooperative interaction of hypoxia-inducible factor 1 and KDM3A. Mol Cell Biol 32:3018–3032

Mosammaparast N, Shi Y (2010) Reversal of histone methylation: biochemical and molecular mechanisms of histone demethylases. Annu Rev Biochem 79:155–179

Nakajima R, Okano H, Noce T (2016) JMJD1C exhibits multiple functions in epigenetic regulation during spermatogenesis. PLoS ONE 11:e0163466

Nakayama K, Frew IJ, Hagensen M, Skals M, Habelhah H, Bhoumik A, Kadoya T, Erdjument-Bromage H, Tempst P, Frappell PB, Bowtell DD, Ronai Z (2004) Siah2 regulates stability of prolyl-hydroxylases, controls HIF1alpha abundance, and modulates physiological responses to hypoxia. Cell 117:941–952

Nantel F, Monaco L, Foulkes NS, Masquilier D, LeMeur M, Henriksen K, Dierich A, Parvinen M, Sassone-Corsi P (1996) Spermiogenesis deficiency and germ-cell apoptosis in CREM-mutant mice. Nature 380:159–162

Ohguchi H, Hideshima T, Bhasin MK, Gorgun GT, Santo L, Cea M, Samur MK, Mimura N, Suzuki R, Tai YT, Carrasco RD, Raje N, Richardson PG, Munshi NC, Harigae H, Sanda T, Sakai J, Anderson KC (2016) The KDM3A-KLF2-IRF4 axis maintains myeloma cell survival. Nat Commun 7:10258

Okada Y, Scott G, Ray MK, Mishina Y, Zhang Y (2007) Histone demethylase JHDM2A is critical for Tnp1 and Prm1 transcription and spermatogenesis. Nature 450:119–123

Osawa T, Tsuchida R, Muramatsu M, Shimamura T, Wang F, Suehiro J, Kanki Y, Wada Y, Yuasa Y, Aburatani H, Miyano S, Minami T, Kodama T, Shibuya M (2013) Inhibition of histone demethylase JMJD1A improves anti-angiogenic therapy and reduces tumor-associated macrophages. Cancer Res 73:3019–3028

Padi SK, Zhang Q, Rustum YM, Morrison C, Guo B (2013) MicroRNA-627 mediates the epigenetic mechanisms of vitamin D to suppress proliferation of human colorectal cancer cells and growth of xenograft tumors in mice. Gastroenterology 145:437–446

Paez-Ribes M, Allen E, Hudock J, Takeda T, Okuyama H, Vinals F, Inoue M, Bergers G, Hanahan D, Casanovas O (2009) Antiangiogenic therapy elicits malignant progression of tumors to increased local invasion and distant metastasis. Cancer Cell 15:220–231

Park SJ, Kim JG, Son TG, Yi JM, Kim ND, Yang K, Heo K (2013) The histone demethylase JMJD1A regulates adrenomedullin-mediated cell proliferation in hepatocellular carcinoma under hypoxia. Biochem Biophys Res Commun 434:722–727

Parrish JK, Sechler M, Winn RA, Jedlicka P (2015) The histone demethylase KDM3A is a microRNA-22-regulated tumor promoter in Ewing Sarcoma. Oncogene 34:257–262

Pedanou VE, Gobeil S, Tabaries S, Simone TM, Zhu LJ, Siegel PM, Green MR (2016) The histone H3K9 demethylase KDM3A promotes anoikis by transcriptionally activating pro-apoptotic genes BNIP3 and BNIP3L. Elife 5

Peng K, Su G, Ji J, Yang X, Miao M, Mo P, Li M, Xu J, Li W, Yu C (2018) Histone demethylase JMJD1A promotes colorectal cancer growth and metastasis by enhancing Wnt/beta-catenin signaling. J Biol Chem 293:10606–10619

Pollard PJ, Loenarz C, Mole DR, McDonough MA, Gleadle JM, Schofield CJ, Ratcliffe PJ (2008) Regulation of Jumonji-domain-containing histone demethylases by hypoxia-inducible factor (HIF)-1alpha. Biochem J 416:387–394

Qi J, Kim H, Scortegagna M, Ronai ZA (2013) Regulators and effectors of Siah ubiquitin ligases. Cell Biochem Biophys 67:15–24

Qi J, Nakayama K, Cardiff RD, Borowsky AD, Kaul K, Williams R, Krajewski S, Mercola D, Carpenter PM, Bowtell D, Ronai ZA (2010) Siah2-dependent concerted activity of HIF and FoxA2 regulates formation of neuroendocrine phenotype and neuroendocrine prostate tumors. Cancer Cell 18:23–38

Ramadoss S, Guo G, Wang CY (2017) Lysine demethylase KDM3A regulates breast cancer cell invasion and apoptosis by targeting histone and the non-histone protein p53. Oncogene 36:47–59

Schneider P, Bayo-Fina JM, Singh R, Kumar Dhanyamraju P, Holz P, Baier A, Fendrich V, Ramaswamy A, Baumeister S, Martinez ED, Lauth M (2015) Identification of a novel actin-dependent signal transducing module allows for the targeted degradation of GLI1. Nat Commun 6:8023

Sroczynska P, Cruickshank VA, Bukowski JP, Miyagi S, Bagger FO, Walfridsson J, Schuster MB, Porse B, Helin K (2014) shRNA screening identifies JMJD1C as being required for leukemia maintenance. Blood 123:1870–1882

Tateishi K, Okada Y, Kallin EM, Zhang Y (2009) Role of Jhdm2a in regulating metabolic gene expression and obesity resistance. Nature 458:757–761

Tee AE, Ling D, Nelson C, Atmadibrata B, Dinger ME, Xu N, Mizukami T, Liu PY, Liu B, Cheung B, Pasquier E, Haber M, Norris MD, Suzuki T, Marshall GM, Liu T (2014) The histone demethylase JMJD1A induces cell migration and invasion by up-regulating the expression of the long noncoding RNA MALAT1. Oncotarget 5:1793–1804

Toomey EC, Schiffman JD, Lessnick SL (2010) Recent advances in the molecular pathogenesis of Ewing's sarcoma. Oncogene 29:4504–4516

Uemura M, Yamamoto H, Takemasa I, Mimori K, Hemmi H, Mizushima T, Ikeda M, Sekimoto M, Matsuura N, Doki Y, Mori M (2010) Jumonji domain containing 1A is a novel prognostic marker for colorectal cancer: in vivo identification from hypoxic tumor cells. Clin Cancer Res 16:4636–4646

Wade MA, Jones D, Wilson L, Stockley J, Coffey K, Robson CN, Gaughan L (2015) The histone demethylase enzyme KDM3A is a key estrogen receptor regulator in breast cancer. Nucleic Acids Res 43:196–207

Wang HY, Long QY, Tang SB, Xiao Q, Gao C, Zhao QY, Li QL, Ye M, Zhang L, Li LY, Wu M (2019) Histone demethylase KDM3A is required for enhancer activation of hippo target genes in colorectal cancer. Nucleic Acids Res

Wang J, Le T, Wei R, Jiao Y (2016) Knockdown of JMJD1C, a target gene of hsa-miR-590-3p, inhibits mitochondrial dysfunction and oxidative stress in MPP+-treated MES23.5 and SH-SY5Y cells. Cell Mol Biol (Noisy-le-grand) 62:39–45

Watanabe S, Watanabe K, Akimov V, Bartkova J, Blagoev B, Lukas J, Bartek J (2013) JMJD1C demethylates MDC1 to regulate the RNF8 and BRCA1-mediated chromatin response to DNA breaks. Nat Struct Mol Biol 20:1425–1433

Wellmann S, Bettkober M, Zelmer A, Seeger K, Faigle M, Eltzschig HK, Buhrer C (2008) Hypoxia upregulates the histone demethylase JMJD1A via HIF-1. Biochem Biophys Res Commun 372:892–897

Wilson S, Fan L, Sahgal N, Qi J, Filipp FV (2017) The histone demethylase KDM3A regulates the transcriptional program of the androgen receptor in prostate cancer cells. Oncotarget 8:30328–30343

Xu S, Fan L, Jeon HY, Zhang F, Cui X, Mickle MB, Peng G, Hussain A, Fazli L, Gleave ME, Dong X, Qi J (2020) p300-mediated acetylation of histone demethylase JMJD1A prevents its degradation by ubiquitin ligase STUB1 and enhances its activity in prostate cancer. Cancer Res 80:3074–3087

Yamada D, Kobayashi S, Yamamoto H, Tomimaru Y, Noda T, Uemura M, Wada H, Marubashi S, Eguchi H, Tanemura M, Doki Y, Mori M, Nagano H (2012) Role of the hypoxia-related gene, JMJD1A, in hepatocellular carcinoma: clinical impact on recurrence after hepatic resection. Ann Surg Oncol 19(Suppl 3):S355-364

Yamane K, Toumazou C, Tsukada Y, Erdjument-Bromage H, Tempst P, Wong J, Zhang Y (2006) JHDM2A, a JmjC-containing H3K9 demethylase, facilitates transcription activation by androgen receptor. Cell 125:483–495

Yang H, Liu Z, Yuan C, Zhao Y, Wang L, Hu J, Xie D, Wang L, Chen D (2015) Elevated JMJD1A is a novel predictor for prognosis and a potential therapeutic target for gastric cancer. Int J Clin Exp Pathol 8:11092–11099

Zhan M, Wen F, Liu L, Chen Z, Wei H, Zhou H (2016) JMJD1A promotes tumorigenesis and forms a feedback loop with EZH2/let-7c in NSCLC cells. Tumour Biol 37:11237–11247

Zhang X, Zhu T, Chen Y, Mertani HC, Lee KO, Lobie PE (2003) Human growth hormone-regulated HOXA1 is a human mammary epithelial oncogene. J Biol Chem 278:7580–7590

Zhao QY, Lei PJ, Zhang X, Zheng JY, Wang HY, Zhao J, Li YM, Ye M, Li L, Wei G, Wu M (2016) Global histone modification profiling reveals the epigenomic dynamics during malignant transformation in a four-stage breast cancer model. Clin Epigenet 8:34

Zhu N, Chen M, Eng R, DeJong J, Sinha AU, Rahnamay NF, Koche R, Al-Shahrour F, Minehart JC, Chen CW, Deshpande AJ, Xu H, Chu SH, Ebert BL, Roeder RG, Armstrong SA (2016) MLL-AF9- and HOXA9-mediated acute myeloid leukemia stem cell self-renewal requires JMJD1C. J Clin Invest 126:997–1011

KDM4 Demethylases: Structure, Function, and Inhibitors

5

Yuanyuan Jiang, Lanxin Liu and Zeng-Quan Yang

Abstract

KDM4 histone demethylases mainly catalyze the removal of methyl marks from H3K9 and H3K36 to epigenetically regulate chromatin structure and gene expression. KDM4 expression is strictly regulated to ensure proper function in a myriad of biological processes, including transcription, cellular proliferation and differentiation, DNA damage repair, immune response, and stem cell self-renewal. Aberrant expression of KDM4 demethylase has been documented in many types of blood and solid tumors, and thus, KDM4s represent promising therapeutic targets. In this chapter, we summarize the current knowledge of the structures and regulatory mechanisms of KDM4 proteins and our understanding of their alterations in human pathological processes with a focus on development and cancer. We also review the reported KDM4 inhibitors and discuss their potential as therapeutic agents.

Keywords

KDM4 · Histone demethylase · Cancer · Inhibitors

5.1 Introduction

Histone lysine methylation, governed by the opposing activities of histone methyltransferases and demethylases, serves as the principal chromatin-regulatory mechanism that influences fundamental nuclear processes and has a central role in various cellular processes, including transcription, proliferation, cell fate, DNA damage repair, immune response, and stem cell self-renewal. These methylation marks, which localize not only to the flexible histone tails, but also to a lesser extent to core histone residues, alter DNA compaction and recruit transcription factors and transcriptional machinery. The KDM4 proteins mainly catalyze demethylation on tri- and di-methylated histone H3 lysine 9 (H3K9me3/me2), histone marks associated with gene repression and found in the heterochromatin. In addition, KDM4A-C catalyzes the demethylation of H3K36me3/me2, H3K27me3/me2, and possibly non-histone proteins, albeit at a lower rate. The accumulated evidence demonstrates a link between improper histone methylation and dysregulation of cellular processes underlying several human diseases. For instance,

Y. Jiang · L. Liu · Z.-Q. Yang (✉)
Department of Oncology, Karmanos Cancer Institute, Wayne State University, 4100 John R Street, HWCRC 815, Detroit, MI 48201, USA
e-mail: yangz@karmanos.org

Q. Yan (ed.), *Targeting Lysine Demethylases in Cancer and Other Human Diseases*, Advances in Experimental Medicine and Biology 1433, https://doi.org/10.1007/978-3-031-38176-8_5

members of the KDM4 demethylases are commonly overexpressed in human cancers, where they were implicated in disrupting normal cellular proliferative balance (Berry and Janknecht 2013; Labbe et al. 2014; Wu et al. 2022; Lee et al. 2020). Furthermore, the KDM4 demethylases are considered interesting targets for the development of anti-cancer therapies. Notably, a potent small-molecule inhibitor of KDM4, called TACH101, has recently entered clinical trial in 2022 for advanced and/or metastatic cancers. Here, we summarize the current knowledge on the KDM4 demethylases and their involvement in human pathological processes, focusing on development and cancer. We also review the recently reported KDM4 inhibitors and discuss their potential and applications as therapeutic agents.

5.2 Structural Domain and Biochemistry of KDM4 Demethylases

The histone lysine demethylases are a diverse group of proteins which can be broadly grouped into two functional enzymatic families (Klose and Zhang 2007; Murn and Shi 2017; Agger et al. 2008). The first family of histone lysine demethylases includes the lysine-specific demethylase 1 (LSD1, also known as KDM1A) and LSD2 (KDM1B), which are flavin adenine dinucleotide (FAD)-dependent amine oxidases that remove mono- and dimethyl histone lysine marks (Shi et al. 2004; Metzger et al. 2005). The second family consists of the Jumonji C (JmjC)-domain-containing proteins, which use an oxygenase mechanism to remove histone mono-, di-, and tri-methyllysine residues (Labbe et al. 2014; Agger et al. 2008; Klose et al. 2006a). The KDM4 family is the largest subfamily of JmjC-domain-containing histone demethylases, and in the human genome, there are five functional KDM4 genes (KDM4A-E). KDM4A, KDM4B, and KDM4C localize to human chromosomes 1p34.1, 19p13.3, and 9p24.1, respectively, while KDM4D localizes to human chromosome 11q21 and forms a cluster with two additional intronless KDM4 genes, KDM4E, and KDM4F (Labbe et al. 2014; Katoh and Katoh 2007; Yang et al. 2000; Whetstine et al. 2006). It was previously believed that KDM4E and F were pseudogenes; however, studies have shown that KDM4E is expressed in normal human tissues and may have a functional role (Whetstine et al. 2006; Hillringhaus et al. 2011; Fritzsche et al. 2013; Liu et al. 2018; Jack et al. 2013). In this chapter, we will focus on the KDM4A-D members, because of the relatively low expression of KDM4E in normal human tissues and tumor samples (Uhlen et al. 2015, 2017).

The KDM4A, KDM4B, and KDM4C proteins, which share more than 50% sequence identity, contain multiple functional domains, including N-terminal JmjN and JmjC domains, as well as C-terminal plant homeodomains (PHD) and Tudor domains (Whetstine et al. 2006). KDM4D and KDM4E are shorter proteins lacking the C-terminal region (Fig. 5.1). The JmjC domain is the catalytic core for lysine demethylation and requires cofactors α-ketoglutarate (α-KG) and iron Fe(II) (Klose et al. 2006a; Whetstine et al. 2006; Couture et al. 2007; Ng et al. 2007). Although the JmjC domain is highly conserved across the KDM4 family, biochemical and structural studies have shown that substrates of the KDM4s are different (Lee et al. 2020; Hillringhaus et al. 2011; Pilka et al. 2015; Williams et al. 2014). Phylogenetic analysis of the N-terminal JmjN and JmjC domains of KDM4A-D reveals that KDM4A and KDM4C have greater similarity to each other than to either KDM4B or KDM4D (Whetstine et al. 2006). KDM4A, KDM4B, and KDM4C catalyze the demethylation of di- and tri-methylated H3K9 and H3K36, whereas KDM4D demethylates H3K9me3/me2/me1 and KDM4E demethylates H3K9me3 and H3K56me3 (Whetstine et al. 2006; Cloos et al. 2006; Klose et al. 2006b; Chen et al. 2006). Crystal structures of KDM4A bound to different methylated forms of H3K9 and H3K36 peptides reveal that, when bound to KDM4A, H3K9me3 lysine side chain

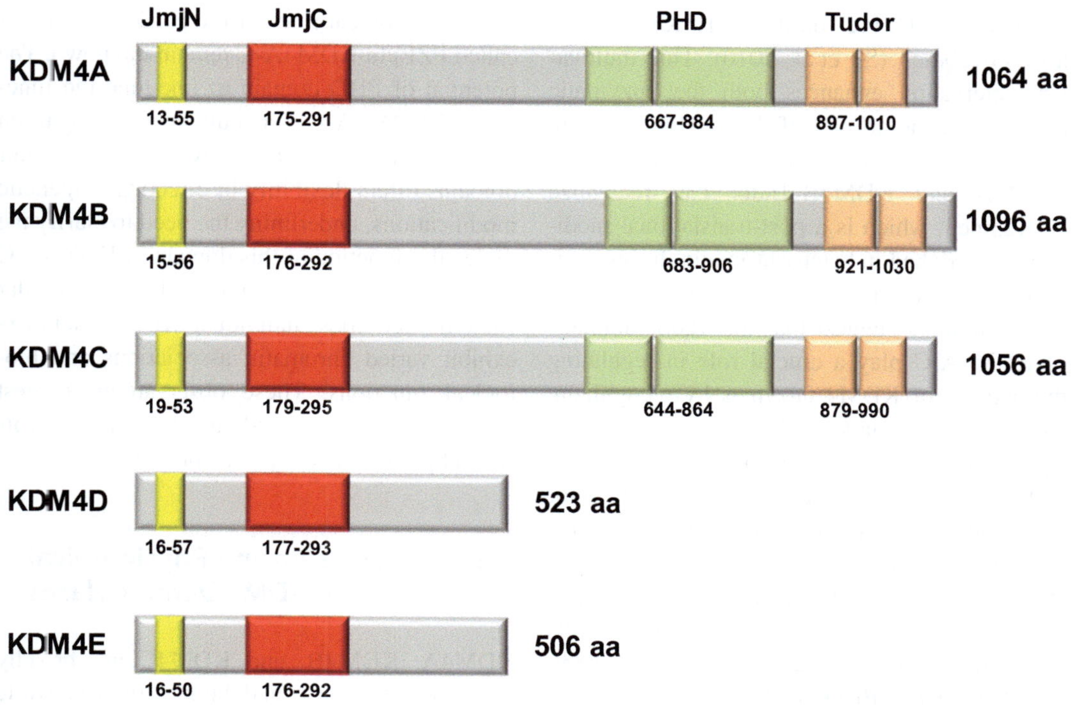

Fig. 5.1 Schematic representation of KDM4A-E protein domains. The protein size and amino acid locations of JmjN, JmjC, two PHD, and two Tudor domains for each KDM4 demethylase are indicated

adopts a "W"-shaped conformation, whereas H3K36me3 forms a "U"-shaped conformation (Ng et al. 2007). The JmjN domain interacts extensively with JmjC and provides structural integrity and stability. Additionally, there is evidence that KDM4A and KDM4C, but not KDM4B, dimerize via their JmjN domain, and this dimerization is a pre-requisite for their H3K9me3 demethylase activity (Levin et al. 2018). Genome-wide occupancy studies also reveal that KDM4A and KDM4C both localize to H3K4me3-positive promoter, while KDM4B likely localizes to enhanced regions (Das et al. 2014; Pedersen et al. 2014, 2016; Singh et al. 2022). Furthermore, loss of one KDM4 family member is not sufficient to distort total histone methylation, indicating that each KDM4 member might regulate a specific set of genes in a specific cell type or condition (Das et al. 2014; Pedersen et al. 2016).

The C-terminal PHD and Tudor domains of KDM4A-C play a critical role in histone recognition and binding (Gayatri and Bedford 2014; Park et al. 2022). KDM4A-C proteins contain two Tudor domains that form an interdigitated double Tudor structure (Huang et al. 2006; Su et al. 2016). Extensive structural and biochemical studies have revealed that the Tudor domains of KDM4A recognize and bind two different histone marks, H3K4me3/me2 and H4K20me3/me2, using distinct binding mechanisms. The KDM4A-Tudor domains contain three aromatic residues, F932, W967, and Y973, which form an open cage to accommodate H3K4me3 binding. Conversely, the binding of KDM4A to H4K20me3 involves the Tudor domains adopting opposite relative orientations, utilizing the same three aromatic residues to interact with distinct surfaces (Lee et al. 2008). KDM4A-Tudor's recognition of methylated H3K4 may play a role in recruiting KDM4A to chromatin, where H3K9me3 markers can be removed and gene promoters activated (Pedersen et al. 2014). The Tudor domain of KDM4C binds to H3K4me3, but not H3K20me3 (Su et al. 2016). This multivalent interaction enhances both the enzymatic activity and the affinity of the catalytic domain for H3K9me3 (Pack et al. 2016). Furthermore, KDM4A and KDM4B-Tudor can recognize H3K23me3, which is a post-translational modification enriched in heterochromatin during meiosis in primary spermatocytes (Su et al. 2016). These findings suggest that the Tudor domains of KDM4A-C play a crucial role in regulating the activity of KDM4 enzymes by recognizing specific histone marks and enhancing their ability to demethylate target residues.

PHD domain is an epigenetic effector or reader domain that can recognize various histone markers, such as unmodified H3, H3K4me3, H3K9me3, H3K36me3, and H3K14ac, on one or more histone tails (Musselman and Kutateladze 2011, 2009; Yu et al. 2017; Black and Kutateladze 2023; Sanchez and Zhou 2011). Interestingly, PHD domain, in combination with different histone reader domains, such as bromodomains, chromodomains, and Tudor domains, recognizes distinct histone markers and mediates the recruitment of a particular complex to a specific genomic site (Musselman and Kutateladze 2011; Yu et al. 2017; Black and Kutateladze 2023). Notably, phylogenetic analysis of KDM4A-C with AF10/17, BRPF, and JADE proteins indicated that two PHD fingers linked by a single zinc finger form an integrated module, called PZP (PHD-Zn-knuckle-PHD) module (Black and Kutateladze 2023; Chen et al. 2015; Klein et al. 2016, 2020, 2021; Zheng et al. 2021). Structural studies of PZPs derived from AF10, BRPF1, and PHF14 have shown that these domains possess a very similar saddle-like globular fold, and all PZPs have been shown to bind to unmodified histone H3 tail, but not identically (Black and Kutateladze 2023; Chen et al. 2015; Klein et al. 2016, 2020, 2021; Zheng et al. 2021). Additionally, PZP of AF10 engages the nucleosome through multivalent interactions with the entire H3 tail as well as DNA (Klein et al. 2021). However, the biochemical and physiological roles of the PHD domains (or called PZP) in KDM4A-C remain unknown. The potential of PHD domain to fine-tune the function of KDM4A-C via multivalent recognition and combinatorial readout with other effector domains offers flexibility in directing epigenetic modifications, underlining the need to clarify the molecular function of this domain in KDM4A-C demethylases. Furthermore, despite similar catalytic activities, individual KDM4 members exhibit varied chromatin associations and biological functions. These observations suggest that an uncharacterized mechanism controls KDM4 protein functions on chromatin.

5.3 Expression and Physiological Roles of KDM4 Demethylases

KDM4A, KDM4B, and KDM4C are broadly expressed in mouse and human tissues, while KDM4D is predominantly expressed in the testis (Labbe et al. 2014; Yang et al. 2000; Zhang et al. 2011; Iwamori et al. 2011). Analysis of next-generation sequencing profiles for normal tissues using the Human Protein Atlas (HPA) database confirms this (Uhlen et al. 2017, 2015) (Fig. 5.2). In addition, KDM4E expression level is dramatically lower [< 1 "Transcript Per Million" (TPM)] in all tissues. However, KDM4E appears to express in a specific stage of embryos and regulate embryonic genome activation (EGA)-coupled molecular events (Liu et al. 2018; Hendrickson et al. 2017). Based on the structural domains and expression patterns of KDM4, it seems clear that the KDM4 members have both distinct and overlapping functions, particularly in tissue-specific differentiation, DNA repair, and hormone-mediated gene expression.

KDM4 members likely play important roles in maintaining the open chromatin state required in embryonic stem cells (ESCs) to ensure efficient proliferation and readiness for differentiation (Das et al. 2014; Pedersen et al. 2014; Tomaz et al. 2017). At an epigenetic level, this euchromatic state relies on the absence of H3K9

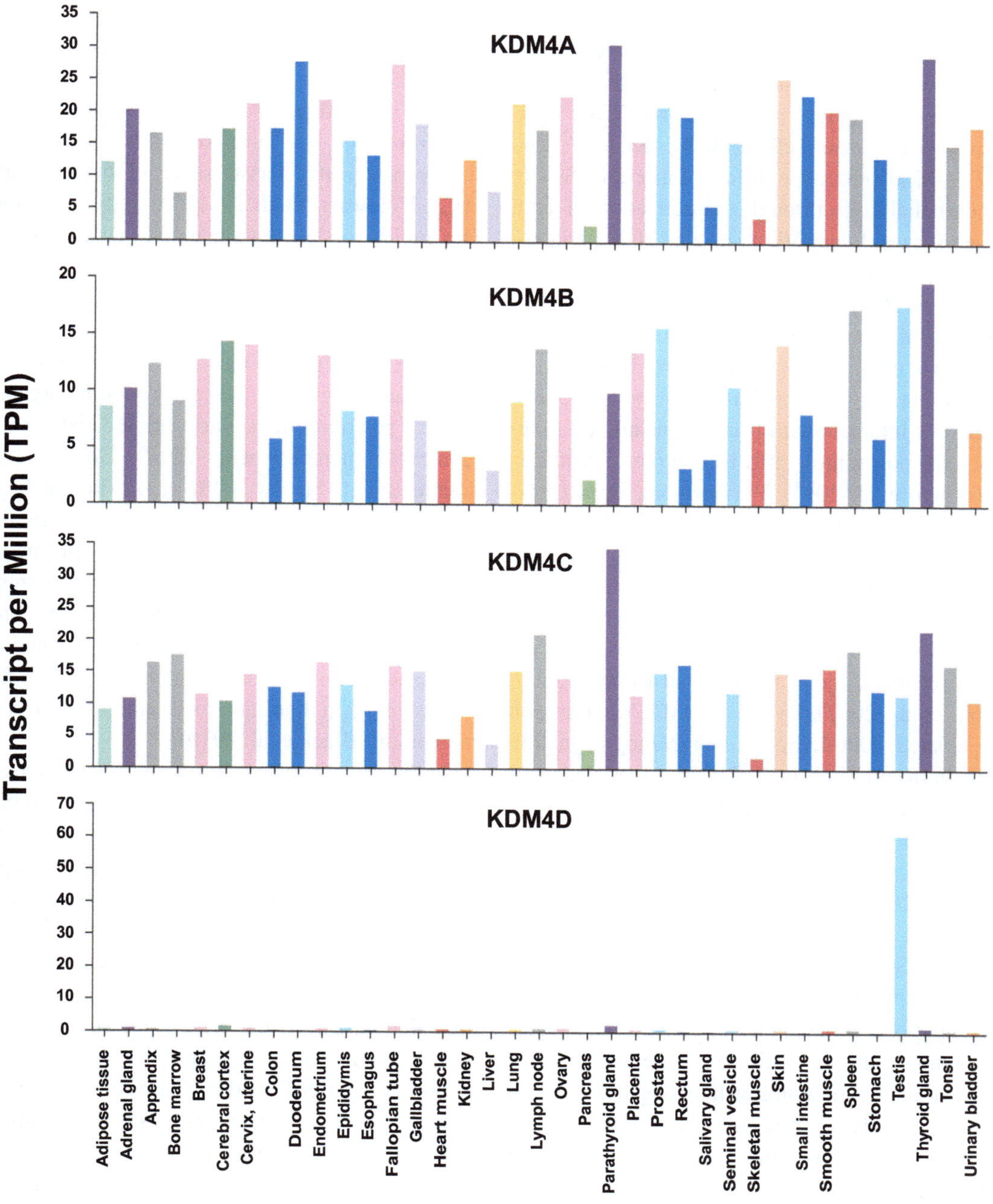

Fig. 5.2 Expression levels for KDM4A-D in 37 normal human tissues using the Human Protein Atlas (HPA). Transcript abundance is indicated as mean transcripts per million (TPM), corresponding to mean values of the different individual samples from each tissue. Color-coding is based on tissue groups, each consisting of tissues with functional features in common

methylation, which is ensured by KDM4 demethylase activity (Das et al. 2014). In mouse development, *Kdm4a*, *b*, and *c* are expressed early in the fertilized egg and in undifferentiated ESCs (Katoh and Katoh 2007; Wang et al. 2010). Knockout of *Kdm4a*, *b*, and *c* individually or combinatorially in mouse ESC demonstrated that while individual KDM4 family members are dispensable for ESC maintenance and embryogenesis, combined deficiency for specifically Kdm4a and Kdm4c leads to early embryonic lethality and impaired ESC self-renewal (Pedersen et al. 2016). KDM4A and KDM4C also regulate differentiation of ESCs to endothelial cells through the activation of fetal liver kinase 1 and VE (vascular endothelial)—cadherin promoters, respectively (Wu et al. 2015). KDM4A directly regulates canonical replicative histone gene networks during cell cycle (Rechem et al. 2020). Furthermore, KDM4A has a non-chromatin-related role in the cytoplasm where it interacts with translation initiation factors on polysomes, affecting protein synthesis (Rechem et al. 2015). Furthermore, overexpression of KDM4A and KDM4B improves somatic cell reprogramming into pluripotency (Chung et al. 2015; Wei et al. 2017).

Evidence also supports the participation of KDM4C in the Oct-4/Sox2/Nanog expression feedback loop (Wagner and Cooney 2009; Loh et al. 2007). When KDM4C expression is ablated, Oct-4, Sox2, and Nanog signaling is eliminated (Loh et al. 2007). In this context, H3K9me3 demethylation by KDM4C directs the expression of pluripotency factors with critical implications in cellular reprogramming (Wang et al. 2010; Loh et al. 2007). In another study, Tomaz et al. revealed that Kdm4c is required in mouse ESCs to initiate appropriate gene expression programs upon somatic multi-lineage differentiation (Tomaz et al. 2017). In the absence of Kdm4c, differentiation is stalled at an early post-implantation epiblast-like stage. Dissection of the underlying molecular basis revealed that Kdm4c is re-distributed to lineage-specific enhancers during ESC priming for differentiation (Tomaz et al. 2017). KDM4A and KDM4C demethylases also regulate the activation of B cells (Hung et al. 2018). Together, the interactions between KDM4 proteins with several other molecular regulators likely play important roles in directing stem cell functions during organismal development.

To investigate the role of KDM4, knockout and/or transgenic models have been established in several model organisms, including *Drosophila melanogaster*, *Caenorhabditis elegans*, and mice. Double homozygous mutants of both *Drosophila* KDM4 orthologs, dKDM4A and 4B, are not viable and die in the second instar larval stage (Tsurumi et al. 2013; Holowatyj et al. 2015). A study using the *Drosophila* models demonstrated that dKDM4A (the closest mammalian homolog of which is KDM4D despite its name, since both lack the PHD and Tudor domains found in human KDM4A) is highly enriched in heterochromatin and regulates heterochromatin organization, position-effect variegation, and DNA repair (Colmenares et al. 2017). Specifically, double-strand breaks (DSBs) in heterochromatin, but not in euchromatin, require specific DSB-induced dKDM4A-dependent chromatin changes to promote timely DSB repair progression (Janssen et al. 2019). Depletion of the single *C. elegans* KDM4, which similarly contains PHD and Tudor domains as human KDM4A-C, results in germ line apoptosis and slows DNA replication (Black et al. 2010).

In mice, several studies have revealed that individual *Kdm4* knockout mice are viable and have not resulted in gross abnormalities (Eppig et al. 2012). However, double homozygous mutants of *Kdm4a* and *Kdm4c* cause early embryonic lethality (Pedersen et al. 2016). Studies in mice using conditional heart-specific *Kdm4a* knockout as well as transgenic mice have demonstrated that KDM4A promotes cardiac hypertrophy in response to hypertrophic stimuli (Zhang et al. 2011; Skarnes et al. 2011). Another study with *Kdm4a* knockout mice revealed that KDM4A as a maternal factor plays a key role in embryo survival and is vital for female fertility (Sankar et al. 2017). This is due to a role for KDM4A in uterine function, where its loss causes reduced expression of key genes involved in ion transport, nutrient supply, and cytokine signaling, which impact embryo survival (Sankar et al. 2017). Conditional ablation of *Kdm4a* in skeletal muscle caused impairment of embryonic and postnatal muscle formation (Zhu et al. 2021). KDM4A also plays a crucial role in preserving the maternal epigenome integrity required for proper zygotic genome activation and transfer of developmental control to the embryo (Sankar et al. 2020). Conditional knockout of *Kdm4b* in mammary epithelial cells exhibits delayed mammary gland development with reduced branching (Kawazu et al. 2011). Neuron-specific *Kdm4b* knockout mice displayed neurodevelopmental disorders including spinal malformations and hippocampal impairment (Fujiwara et al. 2016). More recently, Duncan et al. found that heterozygous variants in *KDM4B* lead to global developmental delay and neuroanatomical defects by identification of a cohort of nine individuals with mono-allelic de novo or inherited variants in *KDM4B* as well as analysis of brain anatomy and behavior through an in vivo heterozygous mouse model (Duncan et al. 2020). Another study revealed that *Kdm4b* knockout mice exhibit age- and diet-induced obesity (Cheng et al. 2018). Mechanically, KDM4B directly and epigenetically controls metabolic genes in adipose tissues; thus, the loss of KDM4B impairs energy expenditure, adaptive thermogenesis, and adipose tissue lipolysis, subsequently resulting in metabolic dysfunction and obesity (Cheng et al. 2018).

Kdm4c hypomorphic mutant mice exhibit abnormal behaviors including hyperactivity, persistence, and many types of learning and memory deficits and abnormal synaptic functions such as prolonged long-term potentiation; some of these phenotypes resemble the phenotypic characteristics of neurodevelopmental disorders such as autism spectrum disorder (Sudo et al. 2016). Interestingly, SNPs in KDM4C genes are associated with autism and alcohol withdrawal symptoms (Kantojarvi et al. 2010; Wang et al. 2012; Kato et al. 2020). A study with *Kdm4c* knockout zebrafish and mice models revealed that KDM4C might play a critical role in maintaining cell survival in acute kidney injury (Pan et al. 2022). Though absent or less expressed in other tissues, KDM4D is highly expressed in spermatocytes and spermatids (Iwamori et al. 2011). Mutant *Kdm4d* male mice have globally higher levels of H3K9me3 than control mice (Iwamori et al. 2011). However, adult *Kdm4d* mutant mice are as fertile as control mice, possibly through *Kdm4b* compensation. In summary, each of these KDM4 proteins is likely to perform distinct as well as overlapping functions in different contexts or physiological processes.

5.4 Regulatory Mechanisms of KDM4 Expression and Activation

Cells have developed various mechanisms for regulating KDM4 demethylase localization, expression, and activity. Despite having high sequence homology, KDM4A-C exhibit distinct subcellular distributions in cells. KDM4A is expressed at similar levels in both the nucleus and cytoplasm, KDM4B is mainly expressed in the nucleus, and KDM4C is closely associated with chromatin (Lee et al. 2020). Expression of KDM4 demethylase is regulated by several transcription factors, particularly hormonal receptors and hypoxia-inducible factor 1 (HIF1), in physiological and/or pathological conditions. Previous studies indicated that KDM4B is a bona fide target of estrogen receptor α (ERα). The first intron of KDM4B contains an ERα binding site (Yang et al. 2010). Additionally, KDM4B is highly expressed in ER-positive primary breast cancers and breast cancer cell lines whose expression can be driven by estradiol treatment in ER-positive breast cancer cell lines (Kawazu et al. 2011; Yang et al. 2010; Ye et al. 2015). Furthermore, four KDM4 members (A–D) have been identified or proposed as estrogen receptor (ER) coactivators that form an ER-KDM4 complex, by which the overexpression of KDM4 demethylases increases estrogen-dependent transcription (Kawazu et al. 2011; Yang et al. 2010). KDM4B also influences androgen receptor (AR) transcriptional activity not only via demethylation but also by modulation of AR ubiquitination (Coffey et al. 2013). KDM4B is furthermore a direct transcriptional target of p53 (Castellini et al. 2017). Additionally, the cytokine TGF-β dramatically induced the expression of KDM4B in human mesenchymal stem cells (MSCs) and indicates the critical role of KDM4B in the epigenetic regulation of TGF-β-mediated chondrogenic differentiation of MSCs (Lee et al. 2016). HIF1, a master regulator of cellular and systemic homeostatic responses to hypoxia can induce the expression of KDM4B and KDM4C in both normoxic and hypoxic conditions (Tausendschon et al. 2011). Furthermore, KDM4C selectively interacts with HIF1α, which mediates its recruitment to the HIF1α target gene response elements in breast cancer (Luo et al. 2012).

Several studies have shed light on the regulation of KDM4 family members by post-translational modifications and protein–protein interactions. For example, KDM4A is regulated by S-phase kinase-associated protein 1 (SKP1)–Cullin1 (CUL1)–F-box protein (SCF) ubiquitin ligase complexes, which control its turnover and ubiquitination during cell cycle progression (Tan et al. 2011; Rechem et al. 2011). Similarly, FBXO22 (F-box only protein 22)-mediated KDM4B degradation plays a crucial role in determining selective estrogen receptor modulator activity in breast cancer (Johmura et al. 2018). In response to DNA damage, KDM4A and KDM4B, but not C or D, are regulated by E3 ubiquitin-protein ligase RNF8 and RNF168 complexes (Mallette et al. 2012). These ubiquitin ligases catalyze the K48-linked ubiquitination of KDM4A and KDM4B, which stimulates their proteasomal degradation, thus allowing the recruitment of 53BP1 to H4K20me2 and the formation of 53BP1 foci (Mallette et al. 2012). Additionally, a molecular chaperon Hsp90 interacts with and stabilizes KDM4B protein, but not KDM4C (Ipenberg et al. 2013). Furthermore, KDM4A is SUMOylated on lysine 471 by KSHV K-bZIP, a viral SUMO-2/3-specific E3 ligase, in a SUMO-interacting motif (SIM)-dependent manner (Yang et al. 2017a). Yang et al. demonstrated that SUMOylation modulates the chromatin binding and histone demethylase activity of KDM4A (Yang et al. 2017a). Together, these studies highlight the importance of the ubiquitination and SUMOylation pathways in regulating the abundance and activity of KDM4 demethylases in various biological processes, including cell cycle progression, DNA damage response, and viral infection.

5.5 Alterations and Roles of the KDM4 Demethylases in Cancer Development

In cancer, dysregulation of histone demethylases can result in the activation of oncogenes, repression of tumor suppressors, disruption of DNA mismatch repair, alterations in chromosomal stability, and interaction with key hormonal receptors that control cellular proliferation or influence the tumor immunogenicity (Labbe et al. 2014; Lee et al. 2020; Young et al. 2013; Black et al. 2013; Young and Hendzel 2013; Pfister and Ashworth 2017; Sterling et al. 2020). Mounting studies have demonstrated that *KDM4* genes are amplified and overexpressed in various tumor types, including lung, breast, esophageal, prostate cancers, and lymphoma (Yang et al. 2000; Coffey et al. 2013; Italiano et al. 2006; Liu et al. 2009; Vinatzer et al. 2008). To determine the spectrum of genetic alterations in KDM4 genes in human cancers, we queried copy number alterations (CNAs) and mutations of four KDM4 (A-D) genes compiled from more than 10,000 tumor samples spanning 32 tissue types in TCGA via cBioPortal (September 2017) (Gao et al. 2013; Cerami et al. 2012). An overview of this data reveals that KDM4A-D is genetically altered across many tumor types (Fig. 5.3). Despite the similarities between enzymes of the KDM4 subfamily, their roles in carcinogenesis appear distinct, as only some family members are found to be misregulated in each cancer type (Zack et al. 2013).

5.5.1 KDM4A

Based on the TCGA datasets, *KDM4A* amplification is highly prevalent in ovarian serous cystadenocarcinoma (8.8% of 579 cases), uterine carcinosarcoma (5.4% of 56 cases), bladder urothelial carcinoma (3.9% of 408 cases), and

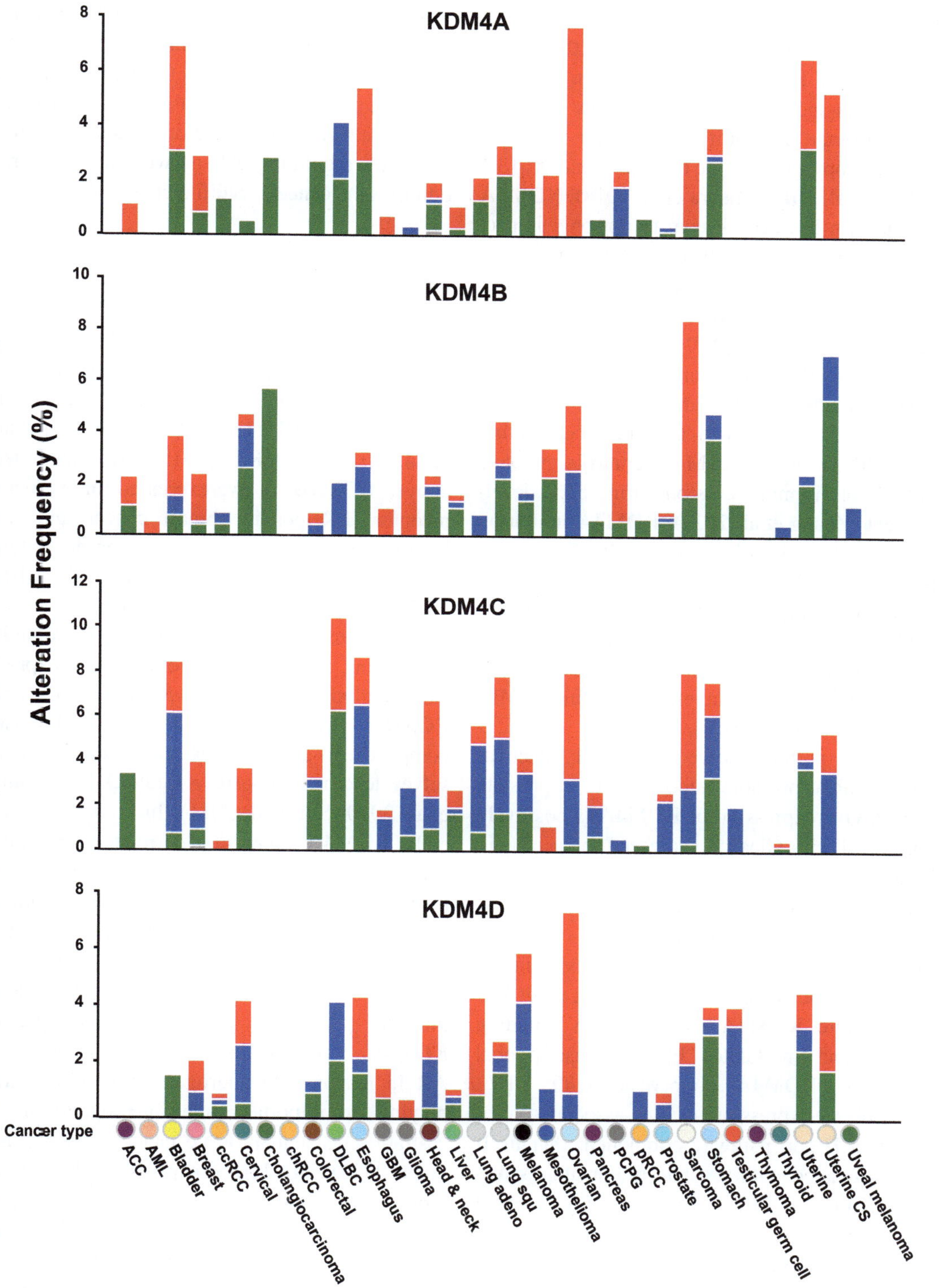

Fig. 5.3 Alteration frequencies of KDM4A-D genes identified in more than 10,000 tumor samples spanning 32 tissue types in TCGA via the cBioPortal. Alteration frequencies are displayed for each of four categories, including: genetic amplifications (red), deletions (blue), mutations (green), or multiple alterations (gray)

uterine corpus endometrial carcinoma (3.0% of 539 cases) (Fig. 5.3) (Black et al. 2013; Ding et al. 2013). KDM4A overexpression in ovarian tumors specifically triggers highly localized chromosomal instability, consisting of site-specific copy gains at 1q12, 1q21, and Xq13.1 (Black et al. 2013; Mishra et al. 2018). KDM4A knockdown has been shown to not only impact cell growth but also metastasis of squamous cell carcinoma (SCC) in vitro and in mouse models (Ding et al. 2013). KDM4A interacts with the activating protein 1 (AP1) transcription factor and induces the expression of AP1 downstream genes including *JUN* and *FOSL1*, which promote tumor cell growth and metastasis (Ding et al. 2013). Also, KDM4A controls invasive growth and immune evasion during SCC development (Zhang et al. 2021). KDM4A inhibition not only significantly repressed SCC invasive growth but also epigenetically activated anti-tumor immunity (Zhang et al. 2021). Another study found that selective loss of KDM4A is sufficient to induce apoptosis in a broad spectrum of human acute myeloid leukemia (AML) cells (Massett et al. 2021).

KDM4 proteins serve as critical coactivators of AR to promote tumor growth in prostate cancer. Overexpression of KDM4A is positively correlated with Gleason score and metastasis in human prostate tumors (Kim et al. 2016). Kim et al. demonstrated that KDM4A overexpression induces prostatic neoplasia in a transgenic mouse model, establishing KDM4A as an initiator of prostate tumorigenesis (Kim et al. 2016). Furthermore, KDM4A is a novel ETV1-binding protein and modulates ETV1 transcriptional responses. KDM4A cooperated with ETV1 to increase expression of yes-associated protein 1, a Hippo pathway component that itself was associated with prostate tumor aggressiveness (Kim et al. 2016). Another study revealed a functional role of KDM4A in prostate tumor metabolism (Wang et al. 2016). Wang et al. revealed that KDM4A functions as an E2F1 coactivator, and the KDM4A-E2F complex regulates metabolism by upregulating pyruvate dehydrogenase kinases (PDKs) PDK1 and PDK3, thereby promoting the switch of oxidative phosphorylation to glycolytic metabolism, offering proliferative and survival advantages to prostate cancer cells (Wang et al. 2016). KDM4A also links ribosomal RNA transcription to nutrients and growth factors availability, subsequently regulating cell growth and proliferation in some cancers (Salifou et al. 2016).

5.5.2 KDM4B

Among KDM4 demethylases, KDM4B is highly expressed in hormone-related cancers such as breast, prostate, and ovarian cancers (Yang et al. 2010; Ye et al. 2015; Duan et al. 2019; Chu et al. 2014; Wilson and Krieg 2019). As mentioned above, KDM4B is overexpressed in estrogen receptor (ER)-positive breast cancer and can be induced by ER in an estrogen-dependent manner (Kawazu et al. 2011; Yang et al. 2010). KDM4B binds to ER to demethylate repressive H3K9me3 marks and recruit chromatin remodeling complexes to promote gene expression, including oncogenic MYB, MYC, and CCND1 (Kawazu et al. 2011). KDM4B-ER complex also activates ER and KDM4B themselves, leading to a positive feedback loop (Yang et al. 2010; Shi et al. 2011). In prostate cancer cells, KDM4B expression correlates with cancer severity and cooperates with the androgen receptor (AR) to promote the AR transcriptional response (Coffey et al. 2013). KDM4B also stabilizes AR by inhibiting its degradation and regulates gene transcription in an AR-independent manner (Coffey et al. 2013). Additionally, KDM4B regulates the alternative splicing of AR in response to androgen deprivation, thus playing an important role in progression of castration-resistant prostate cancer (Duan et al. 2019, 2023). KDM4B also plays a role in promoting metastatic genes and pathways required for peritoneal seeding in epithelial ovarian cancer (Wilson et al. 2017). Together, the interaction between KDM4B and nuclear hormone receptors in hormone-related cancers consists of major drivers that can dictate the aggressiveness of diseases.

KDM4B also contributes to tumor growth and metastasis in other cancers. In colorectal cancer, KDM4B overexpression induces the expression of the plasma membrane signaling protein, PRL-3, which triggers lymph node metastasis (Liu et al. 2013). In renal cancer cells, KDM4B promotes a pro-survival gene expression response by accumulating HIF1α under hypoxic conditions (Beyer et al. 2008). Additionally, in neuroblastoma, KDM4B interacts with N-Myc to promote brain tumor progression by maintaining low levels of the repressive transcription mark, H3K9me3/me2 (Yang et al. 2015, 2017b). Recently, Singh et al. revealed that KDM4B interacts with a pathognomonic Paired Box 3-Forkhead Box O1 (PAX3-FOXO1) fusion protein, which governs a core regulatory circuitry transcription factor network in alveolar rhabdomyosarcoma (Singh et al. 2022). Genetic and pharmacologic inhibition of KDM4B substantially delayed rhabdomyosarcoma growth in vitro and in vivo (Singh et al. 2022). Thus, KDM4B is a therapeutic vulnerability for PAX3-FOXO1-positive rhabdomyosarcoma patients (Singh et al. 2022).

5.5.3 KDM4C

KDM4C, also referred to as Gene Amplified in Squamous Cell Carcinoma (GASC1), was originally identified and cloned from esophageal squamous cell carcinoma (Yang et al. 2000). Accumulated evidence demonstrated that KDM4C is amplified and/or overexpressed in numerous cancers including breast and prostate cancers, medulloblastoma, metastatic lung sarcomatoid carcinoma, primary mediastinal B-cell lymphoma and Hodgkin's lymphoma, and acute myeloid leukemia (Yang et al. 2000; Cloos et al. 2006; Italiano et al. 2006; Liu et al. 2009; Ehrbrecht et al. 2006; Helias et al. 2008; Northcott et al. 2009; Sun et al. 2013; Shao et al. 2021). In TCGA datasets, *KDM4C* amplification is highly prevalent in sarcoma (5.2% of 248 cases), ovarian serous cystadenocarcinoma (4.8% of 311 cases), head and neck squamous cell carcinoma (4.4% of 504 cases), and lymphoid neoplasm diffuse large B-cell lymphoma (DLBC) (4.2% of 48 cases) (Fig. 5.3). Notably, we found that DLBCs contain KDM4C amplification, but showed KDM4A, B, and D deletions (Fig. 5.3). In breast cancer, 2.5% of 963 cases have KDM4C amplification. Breast cancer is a heterogeneous disease that has five molecular subtypes: estrogen receptor-positive Luminal A and B, epidermal growth factor receptor 2-enriched (HER2+), basal-like (commonly known as triple-negative), and normal-like breast cancers (Carey et al. 2006; The Cancer Genome Atlas Network 2012). Basal-like breast cancer usually occurs in young women and presents aggressively with recurrence, an early pattern of metastasis, and poor prognosis (Carey et al. 2006; Bertucci et al. 2012; Burstein et al. 2015). We found that KDM4C is highly amplified in approximately 10% of basal-like breast cancers (Ye et al. 2015). In a high-resolution SNP analysis of 212 medulloblastoma genomes, KDM4C was among several histone-modifying enzymes aberrantly expressed, specifically enriched, in a significant 15% of genomes (Northcott et al. 2009). Accordingly, high levels of chromosome 9 gains observed correspond to hypomethylation of H3K9 residues in medulloblastoma tumors, supporting the substantial role played by the methylome in aberrant gene transcription (Ehrbrecht et al. 2006; Northcott et al. 2009). A novel germline variant (H217R) of KDM4C, which is predicated to be a gain-of-function mutation, was recently found to segregate with seven affected individuals in a striking early-onset multi-cancer family (Katainen et al. 2022). Furthermore, *Kdm4c*-heterozygous (*Kdm4c*±) mice displayed a significantly lower incidence and multiplicity of both benign and malignant tumors induced by carcinogenesis than wild-type mice (Ozaki et al. 2015). Multiple studies strongly indicate that KDM4C serves to regulate processes fundamental to tumorigenesis.

In vitro and in vivo studies demonstrated that KDM4C promotes tumorigenesis, via various molecular pathways (Cloos et al. 2006; Ye et al. 2015; Luo et al. 2012; Liu et al. 2009; Shao et al. 2021; Ozaki et al. 2015; Cheung et al. 2016; Rui et al. 2010; Ishimura et al. 2009; Zhao et al. 2016; Agger et al. 2016; Yu et al. 2018; Lee et al. 2021). Early studies revealed that KDM4C activates expression of oncogenes such as MDM2, a regulator of p53, and binds to the AR to stimulate androgen-dependent gene expression and tumor cell proliferation (Ishimura et al. 2009; Wissmann et al. 2007). In breast cancer, KDM4C amplification and overexpression are prevalent in aggressive basal subtypes (Liu et al. 2009). Several studies indicated that KDM4C is a transforming breast oncogene: stable KDM4C overexpression in non-tumorigenic cells induces transformed phenotypes, whereas KDM4C knockdown inhibits tumor proliferation and metastasis (Luo et al. 2012; Liu et al. 2009; Wu et al. 2012; Bhan et al. 2021). HIF1 activates transcription of genes encoding proteins that play key roles in breast cancer biology. Luo et al. demonstrated that KDM4C functions as a coactivator for HIF1 and stimulates transcription of HIF1 target genes including SLC2A1, LDHA, and PDK1 by decreasing H3K9me3 levels of these target genes (Luo et al. 2012). KDM4C overexpression also confers stem cell-like characteristics, such as the ability to form mammospheres in culture, and induces expression of NOTCH1, a pro-survival factor in breast cancer stem cells (Liu et al. 2009; Farnie and Clarke 2007). Additionally, KDM4C transcriptionally activates amino acid biosynthesis and transport, leading to a significant increase in intracellular amino acid levels (Zhao et al. 2016). This ability of KDM4C requires ATF4, a transcriptional master regulator of amino acid metabolism and stress responses. KDM4C activates ATF4 transcription and interacts with ATF4 to target serine pathway genes for transcriptional activation and cell proliferation (Zhao et al. 2016). In acute myeloid leukemia (AML), KDM4C is required for maintenance of transcriptional programs by MLL fusions, and pharmacological inhibition of KDM4C suppresses leukemia development in both syngeneic mouse model and human AML xenograft model (Cheung et al. 2016). Using *Kdm4a*, *Kdm4b*, and *Kdm4c* conditional triple-knockout mice, Agger et al. show that KDM4 activities are required for MLL-AF9-translocated AML in vivo and in vitro (Agger et al. 2016). Another study revealed that KDM4C is a major driver of melanomagenesis by enabling melanocytes to overcome senescence (Yu et al. 2018). Notably, KDM4C is a specific dependency and therapeutic target in JAK2-mutated cancer cells that is essential for oncogenic signaling and prevents induction of senescence (Ernst et al. 2022; Staehle et al. 2023). Overall, KDM4C can act to promote tumorigenesis through several mechanisms.

5.5.4 KDM4D

In contrast to other KDM4 members, KDM4D and KDM4E are structurally divergent proteins, lacking both C-terminal PHD and Tudor domains (Fig. 5.1). In addition, KDM4D and KDM4E expressions are very low or below detection in most normal tissues, with the notable exception of KDM4D expression in testis (Fig. 5.2). Our unpublished data also revealed that KDM4D and KDM4E expressions at mRNA levels were lower or below detection in the majority of cancer cell lines. However, the oncogenic role of KDM4D in several cancer types, including prostate, colorectal, and liver cancers, has recently been recognized (Chen et al. 2022a, 2022b; Deng et al. 2021; Li et al. 2020; Peng et al. 2019, 2020). KDM4D can interact with nuclear receptors such as the AR, suggesting that it may function to regulate gene expression in prostate cancer (Shin and Janknecht 2007). Immunohistochemistry assays revealed that strong KDM4D expression associates with radioresistance and aggressive phenotype in classical Hodgkin's lymphoma (Bur et al. 2016). KDM4D is significantly upregulated in gastrointestinal stromal tumors (GIST) compared with matched normal tissues and promotes GIST progression through HIF1β/VEGFA signaling (Hu et al. 2018). KDM4D serves as a coactivator of β-catenin, HIF1α, SP-1, STAT3, and IRF1 to promote the progression of colorectal cancer and immune escape (Chen et al. 2022b; Peng et al. 2019, 2020). By enhancing EpCAM and Sox9 expression, KDM4D promotes the self-renewal of liver cancer stem-like cells (Deng et al. 2021). Additionally, KDM4D can bind to p53 to block its transcriptional activity, thereby reducing the expression of p21 and PUMA tumor suppressors in liver cancer (Li et al. 2020). KDM4D also has a role in DNA damage response, furthering the links between the cancer-relevant networks of epigenetic regulation and genome stability (Khoury-Haddad et al. 2014).

Based on TCGA datasets, mutations of KDM4A-D also exist in multiple tumor types (Fig. 5.3). In approximately 10,000 sequenced TCGA tumor samples, KDM4A has 86 mutations, including 70 missense, 1 in-frame deletion, 13 truncating, and 2 other mutations. KDM4B has 87 mutations, including 77 missense, 2 in-frame deletion, 7 truncating, and 1 other mutation. KDM4C has 93 mutations, including 77 missense, 14 truncating, and 2 other mutations. KDM4D has 42 missense, 1 in-frame deletion, and 14 truncating. The most frequent KDM4A-D mutations in human cancers are missense mutations, and these mutations are distributed throughout the entire coding region for each of the KDM4 genes. However, the functional significance of these mutations in cancer development and progression has not yet been investigated.

5.6 Targeting KDM4 Demethylases with Small-Molecule Inhibitors

Considering the widespread upregulation of KDM4s across human cancers, KDM4 demethylases represent good targets for drug development. Over the years, a number of KDM4 inhibitors have been developed. These inhibitors can be categorized into three major groups: α-KG cofactor mimics and disruptors, metal cofactor mimics, and histone substrate analogs (Fig. 5.4) (Labbe et al. 2014; Wu et al. 2022; Lee et al. 2020; Jambhekar et al. 2017; Das et al. 2023; Baby et al. 2021). Here, we will focus on inhibitors reported in the academic literature to have shown activity in cellular or animal model studies of cancer, as these compounds show the most potential for development into therapeutics.

5.6.1 Cofactor Mimics and Disruptors

All JmjC-domain-containing demethylases, including KDM4 subfamily, require α-KG and Fe(II) as cofactors in the demethylation reaction (Labbe et al. 2014; Wu et al. 2022; Lee et al. 2020; Jambhekar et al. 2017; Das et al. 2023). A range of small-molecule inhibitors of KDM4 demethylases has been reported, the majority of which are α-KG-competitive and coordinate to Fe(II) in the catalytic site. In 2008, Rose et al. reported their research on identifying N-oxalylglycine (NOG), an α-KG analog, as one of the inhibitors of JmjC KDMs (Rose et al. 2008). Hamada et al. designed and synthesized a set of NOG derivatives and subsequently presented hydroxamate analogs such as NCDM-32, which has a 500-fold better KDM4C inhibitory activity compared to NOG (Fig. 5.4) (Hamada et al. 2009, 2010). NCDM-32 suppressed growth of breast and prostate cancer in vitro (Ye et al. 2015; Suzuki and Miyata 2011).

Another KDM4 subfamily cofactor disruptor identified by Rose et al. is 2,4-pyridinedicarboxylic acid (PDCA), which is a nonspecific α-KG oxygenase inhibitor (Fig. 5.4) (Wu et al. 2022; Rose et al. 2008). The binding mode of PDCA is similar to α-KG, in which the pyridine nitrogen and carbonyl oxygen chelate the Fe(II) ion in a bidentate manner (Rose et al. 2008). On the basis of PDCA scaffold, Westaway et al. at the GlaxoSmithKline reported two series of cell penetrant inhibitors of KDM4 and KDM5 families: one is 3-amino-4-pyridine carboxylate derivatives (e.g., Compound 34, Fig. 5.4) and another is pyrido[3,4-d]pyrimidin-4(3H)-one derivatives (e.g., Compound 41, Fig. 5.4) (Westaway et al. 2016a, b). Compound 34 possesses interesting activity in a target specific, cellular mechanistic assay against overexpressed

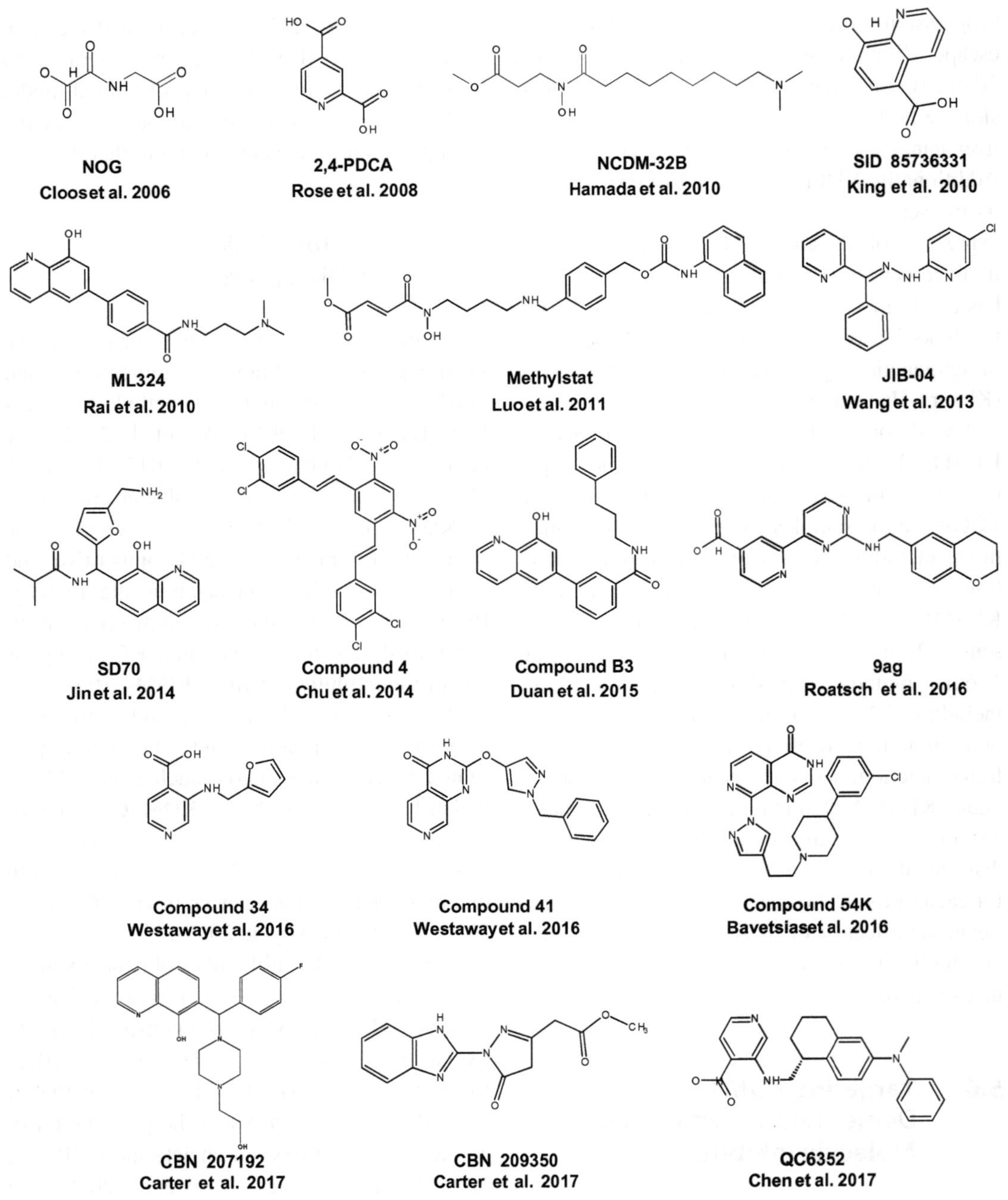

Fig. 5.4 Chemical structure for representative KDM4 inhibitors. References describing their development or use are provided

KDM4C with IC50 values of < 10 μM in cell assays (Westaway et al. 2016b). In addition, Bavetsias et al. performed a high throughput screening (HTS) of a 150k compound collection using human recombinant KDM4B (amino acid residues 1–500 with an N-terminal GST tag) and discovered 8-substituted pyrido[3,4-d]pyrimidin-4(3H)-one derivatives (e.g., Compound

54K, Fig. 5.4) as KDM4 and KDM5 inhibitors (Bavetsias et al. 2016). However, compound 54K demonstrated equipotent activity versus the KDM4 and KDM5 subfamily demethylases and inhibition of H3K9me3 and H3K4me3 demethylation in a cell-based assay (Bavetsias et al 2016). In a subsequent study, a derivative of 54K was found to have improved affinity for KDM4A through engagement of residues E169 and V313 (Bihan et al. 2019). Very recently, starting with 2,4-PDCA, Chen et al. discovered a series of potent KDM4 inhibitors that are both cell permeable and anti-proliferative in cancer models (Chen et al. 2017). One potent KDM4 inhibitor QC6352 has excellent physical properties and drug-like characteristics (Chen et al. 2017). Importantly, QC6352 blocked breast cancer stem-like cell proliferation, sphere formation, and xenograft tumor formation (Chen et al. 2017; Metzger et al. 2017). QC6352 also abrogated expression of EGFR which drives the growth of therapy-resistant triple-negative breast cancer cells (Metzger et al. 2017). Recent in vitro and in vivo studies also revealed QC6352 has anti-cancer activity in squamous cell carcinoma and rhabdomyosarcoma (Singh et al. 2022; Zhang et al. 2021). More significantly, TACH101 (formerly QC8222), a selective and potent inhibitor of KDM4, has recently entered clinical trial in 2022 for advanced and/or metastatic cancers (NCT05076552).

In addition to these inhibitors, compounds structurally unrelated to α-KG were also found to bind and inhibit the KDM4 catalytic site. In many screens, 8-hydroxyquinoline derivatives emerged as lead compounds (Warshakoon et al. 2006; King et al. 2010). Among 236,000 compounds assayed in a high throughput screen by King et al. were 8-hydroxyquinoline derivatives such as SID_85736331 (King et al. 2010). Roatsch et al. identified 20 potential KDM4 inhibitors by screening the ZINC drug-like database and docking to known crystal structures (Roatsch et al. 2016). Further optimization efforts resulted in the development of submicromolar potent KDM4 cosubstrate competitors, with 9ag being one of them (Fig. 5.4). Within this class of inhibitors, Liang et al. showed that the related compound, ML324, effectively inhibited intermediate early viral gene replication mediated by KDM4A in herpes virus-infected cells (King et al. 2010; Liang et al. 2013; Rai et al. 2010). ML324 was also used to demonstrate inhibition of KDM4A activity as a strategy to suppress interleukin-6 production and attenuate colitis induction (Ishiguro et al. 2017). Based on a virtual structure-guided screening method, Chu et al. identified a KDM4 inhibitor, Compound 4 (Fig. 5.4), that selectively blocks in vitro demethylation activity (H3K9me3 and H3K36me3) by KDM4A/KDM4B (Chu et al. 2014). Compound 4 significantly inhibits histone demethylase activity on H3K9me3 and induces apoptosis in cultured prostate cancer cells (Chu et al. 2014). Duan et al. identified three KDM4 inhibitors (B3, A1, and I9) derived from 8-hydroxyquinoline. Among them, compound B3 (Fig. 5.4) is the most potent; it is highly selective for androgen-independent prostate cancer PC3 cells (Duan et al. 2015).

To identify KDM4C demethylase inhibitors, several targeted and large-scale screens, including virtual screens, have been conducted. Leurs et al. screened a heterocyclic ring system library against the histone demethylase KDM4C and identified a 4-hydroxypyrazole scaffold (Leurs et al. 2012). A novel Chem–seq (chemical affinity capture and massively parallel DNA sequencing) approach identified SD70 as a potential inhibitor of KDM4C (Jin et al. 2014). Notably, SD70 also contains an 8-hydroxyquinoline moiety (King et al. 2010) (Fig. 5.4). SD70 could inhibit the prostate cancer cell transcriptional program as well as cell growth in vitro and in vivo, at least in part by inhibition of KDM4C demethylase function (Jin et al. 2014). SD70 also suppresses transcription and transformation ability of MLL fusions and MOZ-TIF2 in AML (Cheung et al. 2016). Recently, Le et al. reported that SD49-7, a derivative of SD70, impairs the progression of leukemia stem cells (LSCs) in vitro and suppresses leukemia development in the mouse model and patient-derived xenograft model of leukemia (Li et al. 2022).

Additionally, the catalytic activity of KDM4 protein can be inhibited by disrupting its iron cofactor, and this can be achieved using non-iron metals and organic molecules (Sekirnik et al. 2009; Giri et al. 2013; Ruger et al. 2015; Malecki et al. 2019). Nickel is one such metal that can disable the catalytic activity of KDM4A and KDM4C by occupying the iron binding pocket, providing an alternative inhibitory mechanism that may selectively target KDM4 demethylases (Giri et al. 2013). Particularly, a Cys3-His Zn(II) binding site is exclusive to KDM4s among other α-KG dioxygenases (Ng et al. 2007). This site is located near the catalytic binding pocket of KDM4A and plays a crucial role in its stability. Zn-ejectors such as disulfiram analogs can destabilize and inhibit KDM4A protein (Sekirnik et al. 2009; Kim et al. 2019). To identify novel KDM4 inhibitors, Carter et al. screened the ChemBioNet small-molecule library and identified several compounds with IC50 values in the low micromolar range. Two hits, CBN 207192 and CBN 209350, were validated as active by an orthogonal enzyme-linked immunosorbent assay (Carter et al. 2017). Interestingly, X-ray crystallography and kinetics-based analysis of a set of derivatives of CBN 209350 revealed that the mechanism of inhibition is complex, in part by active-site metal removal and possibly via binding to a distal binding pocket (Carter et al. 2021). Additionally, a compound with tenfold increased potency relative to CBN 209350 inhibiting intracellular KDM4 activity coincides with the down-regulation of genes expressed during prostate cancer progression (Carter et al. 2021). Thus, these metal cofactor disruptors could be an alternative avenue for future research on inhibiting KDM4 demethylases.

5.6.2 Histone Substrate Competitive Inhibitors

Substrate mimics have been developed as inhibitors of KDM4, including truncated or modified histone peptides (Nielsen et al. 2016; Passioura et al. 2018; Kawamura et al. 2017). For example, Kawamura et al. developed a potent macrocyclic peptide inhibitor, CP2, with high selectivity for KDM4A-C over other KDMs (Kawamura et al. 2017). The crystal structure of KDM4A complexed with CP2 revealed that it occupies the histone-binding groove of KDM4A (Kawamura et al. 2017). To identify KDM4C inhibitors, three series of peptides were synthesized by modifying the lysine residue at H3K9 (Nielsen et al. 2016). One of the 14 peptides demonstrated inhibitory activity at KDM4C (Nielsen et al. 2016). While peptide inhibitors have shown selectivity and potency toward KDM4s over other KDMs, their poor cell permeability and instability present significant challenges in achieving desired cellular activity (Wu et al. 2022).

Based on crystal structures and the enzymatic mechanism of KDMs, Luo et al. designed and synthesized a potential KDM inhibitor, which contains a methyllysine (substrate) mimic linked to an α-KG (cofactor) mimic (Luo et al. 2011). In vitro assays have demonstrated that while this molecule and its prodrug, Methylstat, potently inhibit KDM4A, C, and E, its inhibition of non-target oxygenases is much weaker (Luo et al. 2011). However, Methylstat induces hypermethylation of lysine residues including H3K4, H3K9, H3K27, and H3K36 at almost all methylation states investigated in a concentration-dependent manner in KDM4C-amplified KYSE150 esophageal cancer cell line, indicating Methylstat as the pan-KDM inhibitor (Luo et al. 2011).

Another pan-KDM inhibitor, JIB-04, was identified in an unbiased cellular screen (Wang et al. 2013; Cascella et al. 2017; Bayo et al. 2018). In biochemical assays, JIB-04 potently inhibited the catalytic activity of KDM4 member proteins including KDM4A, B, C, and E (Wang et al. 2013; Cascella et al. 2017). JIB-04 has an unprecedented capacity to specifically inhibit KDM4 protein function in cancer cells, as well as in tumors in vivo (Wang et al. 2013). Structural analysis indicates that JIB-04 disrupts the binding of O_2 and histone substrates in the KDM4A active site (Cascella et al. 2017). JIB-04 has been tested in various cancer models and shows antitumor growth in vitro and in vivo (Bayo et al.

2018; Romani et al. 2019; Kim et al. 2018). A recent study revealed that JIB-04, through inhibiting KDM4A and KDM4C activity, suppresses HER2+ breast leptomeningeal carcinomatosis growth in vitro and in patient-derived xenograft mouse models (Bhan et al. 2021).

Finally, targeting the non-catalytic (PHD and Tudor) domains of KDM4A-C proteins with inhibitors may offer more selective potential, although these studies are still in the early stages (Park et al. 2022; Ortiz et al. 2023). Tudor domains present in the C-terminal half of the KDM4A-C bind to different tri-methylated lysine residues on histone H3 (H3K4me3, H3K23me3) and histone H4 (H4K20me3), thus playing important roles in regulating their chromatin localizations and substrate specificities (Pedersen et al. 2014; Su et al. 2016). More recently, Upadhyay et al. used a two-dimensional nuclear magnetic resonance spectroscopy (2D-NMR)-based fragment screening approach to identify a novel fragment (1a), which binds to the KDM4A-Tudor domain and shows modest competition with H3K4me3 binding in biochemical as well as in vitro cell-based assays (Upadhyay et al. 2018). However, no inhibitors targeting the PHD domains of KDM4A-C proteins have been reported, likely due to a lack of detailed understanding of their structure and biochemical functions.

5.7 Conclusions

KDM4 demethylases play crucial roles in various cellular processes during ESC maintenance, embryogenesis, organismal development, and homeostasis. While their H3K9 and H3K36 demethylase activities are known to regulate gene expression and chromatin architecture, much remains to be learned about their recruitment to genomic loci and downstream gene regulation in different cell types. Furthermore, KDM4 alterations are implicated in human diseases, particularly cancer, but the molecular mechanisms underlying their oncogenicity and cancer progression require further investigation. Therefore, gaining a deep understanding of the biology and mechanisms of KDM4 demethylases is crucial for future research.

Accumulating evidence suggests that KDM4 inhibitors can successfully decrease the growth of various types of cancer cells in vitro and in vivo. However, one caveat remains that most KDM4 inhibitor scaffolds are borrowed from studies of structurally or mechanistically related enzymes (other demethylases as well as enzymes using the same catalytic strategy) and are often possibly active against related non-target proteins. Encouragingly, the KDM4 inhibitor TACH101 has entered clinical trials (NCT05076552) for advanced/metastatic cancer patients, and we await the results. Notably, numerous academic and pharmaceutical labs are continuing research to identify potent, cell-permeable, and selective KDM4 inhibitors to study their role in cancer biology and their potential as anti-cancer agents.

Acknowledgements This work was partially supported by grants from the NIH/NCI R21CA175244-01A1 and the Office of Research on Women's Health (OWRH) of NIH and the Department of Defense (DoD) Prostate Cancer Program PC130259 and Breast Cancer Program BC201476 to Dr. Zeng-Quan Yang (Note: partial sections and results of this chapter have been submitted to DOD as progress reports). We thank Shomita Rode for critical reading of the manuscript.

References

Agger K, Christensen J, Cloos PA, Helin K (2008) The emerging functions of histone demethylases. Curr Opin Genet Dev 18(2):159–168

Agger K, Miyagi S, Pedersen MT, Kooistra SM, Johansen JV, Helin K (2016) Jmjd2/Kdm4 demethylases are required for expression of Il3ra and survival of acute myeloid leukemia cells. Genes Dev 30(11):1278–1288

Baby S, Gurukkala Valapil D, Shankaraiah N (2021) Unravelling KDM4 histone demethylase inhibitors for cancer therapy. Drug Discov Today 26(8):1841–1856

Bavetsias V, Lanigan RM, Ruda GF, Atrash B, McLaughlin MG, Tumber A, Mok NY, Le Bihan YV, Dempster S, Boxall KJ et al (2016) 8-Substituted pyrido[3,4-d]pyrimidin-4(3H)-one derivatives as potent, cell permeable, KDM4 (JMJD2) and KDM5 (JARID1) histone lysine demethylase inhibitors. J Med Chem 59(4):1388–1409

Bayo J, Tran TA, Wang L, Pena-Llopis S, Das AK, Martinez ED (2018) Jumonji inhibitors overcome radioresistance in cancer through changes in H3K4 methylation at double-strand breaks. Cell Rep 25(4):1040–1050 e1045

Berry WL, Janknecht R (2013) KDM4/JMJD2 histone demethylases: epigenetic regulators in cancer cells. Can Res 73(10):2936–2942

Bertucci F, Finetti P, Birnbaum D (2012) Basal breast cancer: a complex and deadly molecular subtype. Curr Mol Med 12(1):96–110

Beyer S, Kristensen MM, Jensen KS, Johansen JV, Staller P (2008) The histone demethylases JMJD1A and JMJD2B are transcriptional targets of hypoxia-inducible factor HIF. J Biol Chem 283(52):36542–36552

Bhan A, Ansari KI, Chen MY, Jandial R (2021) Inhibition of Jumonji histone demethylases selectively suppresses HER2(+) breast leptomeningeal carcinomatosis growth via inhibition of GMCSF expression. Can Res 81(12):3200–3214

Black JC, Allen A, Van Rechem C, Forbes E, Longworth M, Tschop K, Rinehart C, Quiton J, Walsh R, Smallwood A et al (2010) Conserved antagonism between JMJD2A/KDM4A and HP1gamma during cell cycle progression. Mol Cell 40(5):736–748

Black JC, Manning AL, Van Rechem C, Kim J, Ladd B, Cho J, Pineda CM, Murphy N, Daniels DL, Montagna C et al (2013) KDM4A lysine demethylase induces site-specific copy gain and rereplication of regions amplified in tumors. Cell 154(3):541–555

Black JC, Kutateladze TG (2023) Atypical histone targets of PHD fingers. J Biol Chem 299(4):104601

Bur H, Haapasaari KM, Turpeenniemi-Hujanen T, Kuittinen O, Auvinen P, Marin K, Soini Y, Karihtala P (2016) Strong KDM4B and KDM4D expression associates with radioresistance and aggressive phenotype in classical Hodgkin lymphoma. Anticancer Res 36(9):4677–4683

Burstein MD, Tsimelzon A, Poage GM, Covington KR, Contreras A, Fuqua SA, Savage MI, Osborne CK, Hilsenbeck SG, Chang JC et al (2015) Comprehensive genomic analysis identifies novel subtypes and targets of triple-negative breast cancer. Clin Cancer Res 21(7):1688–1698

Carey LA, Perou CM, Livasy CA, Dressler LG, Cowan D, Conway K, Karaca G, Troester MA, Tse CK, Edmiston S et al (2006) Race, breast cancer subtypes, and survival in the Carolina Breast Cancer Study. JAMA 295(21):2492–2502

Carter DM, Specker E, Przygodda J, Neuenschwander M, von Kries JP, Heinemann U, Nazare M, Gohlke U (2017) Identification of a novel benzimidazole pyrazolone scaffold that inhibits KDM4 lysine demethylases and reduces proliferation of prostate cancer cells. Slas Discov 22(7):801–812

Carter DM, Specker E, Malecki PH, Przygodda J, Dudaniec K, Weiss MS, Heinemann U, Nazare M, Gohlke U (2021) Enhanced properties of a benzimidazole benzylpyrazole lysine demethylase inhibitor: mechanism-of-action, binding site analysis, and activity in cellular models of prostate cancer. J Med Chem 64(19):14266–14282

Cascella B, Lee SG, Singh S, Jez JM, Mirica LM (2017) The small molecule JIB-04 disrupts O(2) binding in the Fe-dependent histone demethylase KDM4A/JMJD2A. Chem Commun (Camb) 53(13):2174–2177

Castellini L, Moon EJ, Razorenova OV, Krieg AJ, von Eyben R, Giaccia AJ (2017) KDM4B/JMJD2B is a p53 target gene that modulates the amplitude of p53 response after DNA damage. Nucleic Acids Res 45(7):3674–3692

Cerami E, Gao J, Dogrusoz U, Gross BE, Sumer SO, Aksoy BA, Jacobsen A, Byrne CJ, Heuer ML, Larsson E et al (2012) The cBio cancer genomics portal: an open platform for exploring multidimensional cancer genomics data. Cancer Discov 2(5):401–404

Chen Z, Zang J, Whetstine J, Hong X, Davrazou F, Kutateladze TG, Simpson M, Mao Q, Pan CH, Dai S et al (2006) Structural insights into histone demethylation by JMJD2 family members. Cell 125(4):691–702

Chen S, Yang Z, Wilkinson AW, Deshpande AJ, Sidoli S, Krajewski K, Strahl BD, Garcia BA, Armstrong SA, Patel DJ et al (2015) The PZP domain of AF10 senses unmodified H3K27 to regulate DOT1L-mediated methylation of H3K79. Mol Cell 60(2):319–327

Chen YK, Bonaldi T, Cuomo A, Del Rosario JR, Hosfield DJ, Kanouni T, Kao SC, Lai C, Lobo NA, Matuszkiewicz J et al (2017) Design of KDM4 inhibitors with antiproliferative effects in cancer models. ACS Med Chem Lett 8(8):869–874

Chen Q, Zhuang S, Hong Y, Yang L, Guo P, Mo P, Peng K, Li W, Xiao N, Yu C (2022b) Demethylase JMJD2D induces PD-L1 expression to promote colorectal cancer immune escape by enhancing IFNGR1-STAT3-IRF1 signaling. Oncogene 41(10):1421–1433

Chen Q, Peng K, Mo P, Yu C (2022a) Histone demethylase JMJD2D: a novel player in colorectal and hepatocellular cancers. Cancers (Basel) 14(12)

Cheng Y, Yuan Q, Vergnes L, Rong X, Youn JY, Li J, Yu Y, Liu W, Cai H, Lin JD et al (2018) KDM4B protects against obesity and metabolic dysfunction. Proc Natl Acad Sci U S A 115(24):E5566–E5575

Cheung N, Fung TK, Zeisig BB, Holmes K, Rane JK, Mowen KA, Finn MG, Lenhard B, Chan LC, So CW (2016) Targeting aberrant epigenetic networks mediated by PRMT1 and KDM4C in acute myeloid leukemia. Cancer Cell 29(1):32–48

Chu CH, Wang LY, Hsu KC, Chen CC, Cheng HH, Wang SM, Wu CM, Chen TJ, Li LT, Liu R et al (2014) KDM4B as a target for prostate cancer: structural analysis and selective inhibition by a novel inhibitor. J Med Chem 57(14):5975–5985

Chung YG, Matoba S, Liu Y, Eum JH, Lu F, Jiang W, Lee JE, Sepilian V, Cha KY, Lee DR et al (2015) Histone demethylase expression enhances human somatic cell nuclear transfer efficiency and promotes derivation of pluripotent stem cells. Cell Stem Cell 17(6):758–766

Cloos PA, Christensen J, Agger K, Maiolica A, Rappsilber J, Antal T, Hansen KH, Helin K (2006) The putative oncogene GASC1 demethylates tri- and dimethylated lysine 9 on histone H3. Nature 442(7100):307–311

Coffey K, Rogerson L, Ryan-Munden C, Alkharaif D, Stockley J, Heer R, Sahadevan K, O'Neill D, Jones D, Darby S et al (2013) The lysine demethylase, KDM4B, is a key molecule in androgen receptor signalling and turnover. Nucleic Acids Res 41(8):4433–4446

Colmenares SU, Swenson JM, Langley SA, Kennedy C, Costes SV, Karpen GH (2017) Drosophila histone demethylase KDM4A has enzymatic and non-enzymatic roles in controlling heterochromatin integrity. Dev Cell 42(2):156–169 e155

Couture JF, Collazo E, Ortiz-Tello PA, Brunzelle JS, Trievel RC (2007) Specificity and mechanism of JMJD2A, a trimethyllysine-specific histone demethylase. Nat Struct Mol Biol 14(8):689–695

Das PP, Shao Z, Beyaz S, Apostolou E, Pinello L, De Los AA, O'Brien K, Atsma JM, Fujiwara Y, Nguyen M et al (2014) Distinct and combinatorial functions of Jmjd2b/Kdm4b and Jmjd2c/Kdm4c in mouse embryonic stem cell identity. Mol Cell 53(1):32–48

Das ND, Niwa H, Umehara T (2023) Chemical inhibitors targeting the histone lysine demethylase families with potential for drug discovery. Epigenomes 7(1):7

Deng Y, Li M, Zhuo M, Guo P, Chen Q, Mo P, Li W, Yu C (2021) Histone demethylase JMJD2D promotes the self-renewal of liver cancer stem-like cells by enhancing EpCAM and Sox9 expression. J Biol Chem 296:100121

Ding X, Pan H, Li J, Zhong Q, Chen X, Dry SM, Wang CY (2013) Epigenetic activation of AP1 promotes squamous cell carcinoma metastasis. Sci Signal 6(273):ra28 21-13, S20-15

Duan L, Rai G, Roggero C, Zhang QJ, Wei Q, Ma SH, Zhou Y, Santoyo J, Martinez ED, Xiao G et al (2015) KDM4/JMJD2 histone demethylase inhibitors block prostate tumor growth by suppressing the expression of AR and BMYB-regulated genes. Chem Biol 22(9):1185–1196

Duan L, Chen Z, Lu J, Liang Y, Wang M, Roggero CM, Zhang QJ, Gao J, Fang Y, Cao J et al (2019) Histone lysine demethylase KDM4B regulates the alternative splicing of the androgen receptor in response to androgen deprivation. Nucleic Acids Res 47(22):11623–11636

Duan L, Chen YA, Liang Y, Chen Z, Lu J, Fang Y, Cao J, Lu J, Zhao H, Pong RC et al (2023) Therapeutic targeting of histone lysine demethylase KDM4B blocks the growth of castration-resistant prostate cancer. Biomed Pharmacother 158:114077

Duncan AR, Vitobello A, Collins SC, Vancollie VE, Lelliott CJ, Rodan L, Shi J, Seman AR, Agolini E, Novelli A et al (2020) Heterozygous variants in KDM4B lead to global developmental delay and neuroanatomical defects. Am J Hum Genet 107(6):1170–1177

Ehrbrecht A, Muller U, Wolter M, Hoischen A, Koch A, Radlwimmer B, Actor B, Mincheva A, Pietsch T, Lichter P et al (2006) Comprehensive genomic analysis of desmoplastic medulloblastomas: identification of novel amplified genes and separate evaluation of the different histological components. J Pathol 208(4):554–563

Eppig JT, Blake JA, Bult CJ, Kadin JA, Richardson JE, Mouse Genome Database G (2012) The Mouse Genome Database (MGD): comprehensive resource for genetics and genomics of the laboratory mouse. Nucleic Acids Res 40(Database issue):D881–D886

Ernst P, Schnoder TM, Huber N, Perner F, Jayavelu AK, Eifert T, Hsu CJ, Tubio-Santamaria N, Crodel CC, Ungelenk M et al (2022) Histone demethylase KDM4C is a functional dependency in JAK2-mutated neoplasms. Leukemia 36(7):1843–1849

Farnie G, Clarke RB (2007) Mammary stem cells and breast cancer–role of Notch signalling. Stem Cell Reviews 3(2):169–175

Fritzsche R, Karra D, Bennett KL, Ang FY, Heraud-Farlow JE, Tolino M, Doyle M, Bauer KE, Thomas S, Planyavsky M et al (2013) Interactome of two diverse RNA granules links mRNA localization to translational repression in neurons. Cell Rep 5(6):1749–1762

Fujiwara K, Fujita Y, Kasai A, Onaka Y, Hashimoto H, Okada H, Yamashita T (2016) Deletion of JMJD2B in neurons leads to defective spine maturation, hyperactive behavior and memory deficits in mouse. Transl Psychiatry 6(3):e766

Gao J, Aksoy BA, Dogrusoz U, Dresdner G, Gross B, Sumer SO, Sun Y, Jacobsen A, Sinha R, Larsson E et al (2013) Integrative analysis of complex cancer genomics and clinical profiles using the cBioPortal. Sci Signal 6(269):pl1

Gayatri S, Bedford MT (2014) Readers of histone methylarginine marks. Biochim Biophys Acta 1839(8):702–710

Giri NC, Passantino L, Sun H, Zoroddu MA, Costa M, Maroney MJ (2013) Structural investigations of the nickel-induced inhibition of truncated constructs of the JMJD2 family of histone demethylases using X-ray absorption spectroscopy. Biochemistry 52(24):4168–4183

Hamada S, Kim TD, Suzuki T, Itoh Y, Tsumoto H, Nakagawa H, Janknecht R, Miyata N (2009) Synthesis and activity of N-oxalylglycine and its derivatives as Jumonji C-domain-containing histone lysine demethylase inhibitors. Bioorg Med Chem Lett 19(10):2852–2855

Hamada S, Suzuki T, Mino K, Koseki K, Oehme F, Flamme I, Ozasa H, Itoh Y, Ogasawara D, Komaarashi H et al (2010) Design, synthesis, enzyme-inhibitory activity, and effect on human cancer cells of a novel series of jumonji

domain-containing protein 2 histone demethylase inhibitors. J Med Chem 53(15):5629–5638
Helias C, Struski S, Gervais C, Leymarie V, Mauvieux L, Herbrecht R, Lessard M (2008) Polycythemia vera transforming to acute myeloid leukemia and complex abnormalities including 9p homogeneously staining region with amplification of MLLT3, JMJD2C, JAK2, and SMARCA2. Cancer Genet Cytogenet 180(1):51–55
Hendrickson PG, Dorais JA, Grow EJ, Whiddon JL, Lim JW, Wike CL, Weaver BD, Pflueger C, Emery BR, Wilcox AL et al (2017) Conserved roles of mouse DUX and human DUX4 in activating cleavage-stage genes and MERVL/HERVL retrotransposons. Nat Genet 49(6):925–934
Hillringhaus L, Yue WW, Rose NR, Ng SS, Gileadi C, Loenarz C, Bello SH, Bray JE, Schofield CJ, Oppermann U (2011) Structural and evolutionary basis for the dual substrate selectivity of human KDM4 histone demethylase family. J Biol Chem 286(48):41616–41625
Holowatyj A, Yang ZQ, Pile LA (2015) Histone lysine demethylases in Drosophila melanogaster. Fly (austin) 9(1):36–44
Hu F, Li H, Liu L, Xu F, Lai S, Luo X, Hu J, Yang X (2018) Histone demethylase KDM4D promotes gastrointestinal stromal tumor progression through HIF1beta/VEGFA signalling. Mol Cancer 17(1):107
Huang Y, Fang J, Bedford MT, Zhang Y, Xu RM (2006) Recognition of histone H3 lysine-4 methylation by the double tudor domain of JMJD2A. Science 312(5774):748–751
Hung KH, Woo YH, Lin IY, Liu CH, Wang LC, Chen HY, Chiang BL, Lin KI (2018) The KDM4A/KDM4C/NF-kappaB and WDR5 epigenetic cascade regulates the activation of B cells. Nucleic Acids Res 46(11):5547–5560
Ipenberg I, Guttmann-Raviv N, Khoury HP, Kupershmit I, Ayoub N (2013) Heat shock protein 90 (Hsp90) selectively regulates the stability of KDM4B/JMJD2B histone demethylase. J Biol Chem 288(21):14681–14687
Ishiguro K, Watanabe O, Nakamura M, Yamamura T, Matsushita M, Goto H, Hirooka Y (2017) Inhibition of KDM4A activity as a strategy to suppress interleukin-6 production and attenuate colitis induction. Clin Immunol 180:120–127
Ishimura A, Terashima M, Kimura H, Akagi K, Suzuki Y, Sugano S, Suzuki T (2009) Jmjd2c histone demethylase enhances the expression of Mdm2 oncogene. Biochem Biophys Res Commun 389(2):366–371
Italiano A, Attias R, Aurias A, Perot G, Burel-Vandenbos F, Otto J, Venissac N, Pedeutour F (2006) Molecular cytogenetic characterization of a metastatic lung sarcomatoid carcinoma: 9p23 neocentromere and 9p23-p24 amplification including JAK2 and JMJD2C. Cancer Genet Cytogenet 167(2):122–130
Iwamori N, Zhao M, Meistrich ML, Matzuk MM (2011) The testis-enriched histone demethylase, KDM4D, regulates methylation of histone H3 lysine 9 during spermatogenesis in the mouse but is dispensable for fertility. Biol Reprod 84(6):1225–1234
Jack AP, Bussemer S, Hahn M, Punzeler S, Snyder M, Wells M, Csankovszki G, Solovei I, Schotta G, Hake SB (2013) H3K56me3 is a novel, conserved heterochromatic mark that largely but not completely overlaps with H3K9me3 in both regulation and localization. PLoS ONE 8(2):e51765
Jambhekar A, Anastas JN, Shi Y (2017) Histone lysine demethylase inhibitors. Cold Spring Harb Perspect Med 7(1):a026484
Janssen A, Colmenares SU, Lee T, Karpen GH (2019) Timely double-strand break repair and pathway choice in pericentromeric heterochromatin depend on the histone demethylase dKDM4A. Genes Dev 33(1–2):103–115
Jin C, Yang L, Xie M, Lin C, Merkurjev D, Yang JC, Tanasa B, Oh S, Zhang J, Ohgi KA et al (2014) Chem-seq permits identification of genomic targets of drugs against androgen receptor regulation selected by functional phenotypic screens. Proc Natl Acad Sci U S A 111(25):9235–9240
Johmura Y, Maeda I, Suzuki N, Wu W, Goda A, Morita M, Yamaguchi K, Yamamoto M, Nagasawa S, Kojima Y et al (2018) Fbxo22-mediated KDM4B degradation determines selective estrogen receptor modulator activity in breast cancer. J Clin Investig 128(12):5603–5619
Kantojarvi K, Onkamo P, Vanhala R, Alen R, Hedman M, Sajantila A, Nieminen-von Wendt T, Jarvela I (2010) Analysis of 9p24 and 11p12-13 regions in autism spectrum disorders: rs1340513 in the JMJD2C gene is associated with ASDs in Finnish sample. Psychiatr Genet 20(3):102–108
Katainen R, Donner I, Raisanen M, Berta D, Kuosmanen A, Kaasinen E, Hietala M, Aaltonen LA (2022) Novel germline variant in the histone demethylase and transcription regulator KDM4C induces a multicancer phenotype. J Med Genet 59(7):644–651
Kato H, Kushima I, Mori D, Yoshimi A, Aleksic B, Nawa Y, Toyama M, Furuta S, Yu Y, Ishizuka K et al (2020) Rare genetic variants in the gene encoding histone lysine demethylase 4C (KDM4C) and their contributions to susceptibility to schizophrenia and autism spectrum disorder. Transl Psychiatry 10(1):421
Katoh Y, Katoh M (2007) Comparative integromics on JMJD2A, JMJD2B and JMJD2C: preferential expression of JMJD2C in undifferentiated ES cells. Int J Mol Med 20(2):269–273
Kawamura A, Munzel M, Kojima T, Yapp C, Bhushan B, Goto Y, Tumber A, Katoh T, King ON, Passioura T et al (2017) Highly selective inhibition of histone demethylases by de novo macrocyclic peptides. Nat Commun 8:14773
Kawazu M, Saso K, Tong KI, McQuire T, Goto K, Son DO, Wakeham A, Miyagishi M, Mak TW, Okada H (2011) Histone demethylase JMJD2B functions as a co-factor of estrogen receptor in breast cancer proliferation and mammary gland development. PLoS ONE 6(3):e17830

Khoury-Haddad H, Guttmann-Raviv N, Ipenberg I, Huggins D, Jeyasekharan AD, Ayoub N (2014) PARP1-dependent recruitment of KDM4D histone demethylase to DNA damage sites promotes double-strand break repair. Proc Natl Acad Sci U S A 111(7):E728-737

Kim TD, Jin F, Shin S, Oh S, Lightfoot SA, Grande JP, Johnson AJ, van Deursen JM, Wren JD, Janknecht R (2016) Histone demethylase JMJD2A drives prostate tumorigenesis through transcription factor ETV1. J Clin Investig 126(2):706–720

Kim MS, Cho HI, Yoon HJ, Ahn YH, Park EJ, Jin YH, Jang YK (2018) JIB-04, a small molecule histone demethylase inhibitor, selectively targets colorectal cancer stem cells by inhibiting the Wnt/beta-catenin signaling pathway. Sci Rep 8(1):6611

Kim YJ, Lee DH, Choi YS, Jeong JH, Kwon SH (2019) Benzo[b]tellurophenes as a potential histone H3 lysine 9 demethylase (KDM4) inhibitor. Int J Mol Sci 20(23):5908

King ON, Li XS, Sakurai M, Kawamura A, Rose NR, Ng SS, Quinn AM, Rai G, Mott BT, Beswick P et al (2010) Quantitative high-throughput screening identifies 8-hydroxyquinolines as cell-active histone demethylase inhibitors. PLoS ONE 5(11):e15535

Klein BJ, Muthurajan UM, Lalonde ME, Gibson MD, Andrews FH, Hepler M, Machida S, Yan K, Kurumizaka H, Poirier MG et al (2016) Bivalent interaction of the PZP domain of BRPF1 with the nucleosome impacts chromatin dynamics and acetylation. Nucleic Acids Res 44(1):472–484

Klein BJ, Deshpande A, Cox KL, Xuan F, Zandian M, Barbosa K, Khanal S, Tong Q, Zhang Y, Zhang P et al (2021) The role of the PZP domain of AF10 in acute leukemia driven by AF10 translocations. Nat Commun 12(1):4130

Klein BJ, Cox KL, Jang SM, Cote J, Poirier MG, Kutateladze TG (2020) Molecular basis for the PZP domain of BRPF1 association with chromatin. Structure 28(1):105–110 e103

Klose RJ, Zhang Y (2007) Regulation of histone methylation by demethylimination and demethylation. Nat Rev Mol Cell Biol 8(4):307–318

Klose RJ, Kallin EM, Zhang Y (2006a) JmjC-domain-containing proteins and histone demethylation. Nat Rev Genet 7(9):715–727

Klose RJ, Yamane K, Bae Y, Zhang D, Erdjument-Bromage H, Tempst P, Wong J, Zhang Y (2006b) The transcriptional repressor JHDM3A demethylates trimethyl histone H3 lysine 9 and lysine 36. Nature 442(7100):312–316

Labbe RM, Holowatyj A, Yang ZQ (2014) Histone lysine demethylase (KDM) subfamily 4: structures, functions and therapeutic potential. Am J Transl Res 6(1):1–15

Le Bihan YV, Lanigan RM, Atrash B, McLaughlin MG, Velupillai S, Malcolm AG, England KS, Ruda GF, Mok NY, Tumber A et al (2019) C8-substituted pyrido[3,4-d]pyrimidin-4(3H)-ones: Studies towards the identification of potent, cell penetrant Jumonji C domain containing histone lysine demethylase 4 subfamily (KDM4) inhibitors, compound profiling in cell-based target engagement assays. Eur J Med Chem 177:316–337

Lee J, Thompson JR, Botuyan MV, Mer G (2008) Distinct binding modes specify the recognition of methylated histones H3K4 and H4K20 by JMJD2A-tudor. Nat Struct Mol Biol 15(1):109–111

Lee HL, Yu B, Deng P, Wang CY, Hong C (2016) Transforming growth factor-beta-induced KDM4B promotes chondrogenic differentiation of human mesenchymal stem cells. Stem Cells 34(3):711–719

Lee DH, Kim GW, Jeon YH, Yoo J, Lee SW, Kwon SH (2020) Advances in histone demethylase KDM4 as cancer therapeutic targets. FASEB J 34(3):3461–3484

Lee DH, Kim GW, Yoo J, Lee SW, Jeon YH, Kim SY, Kang HG, Kim DH, Chun KH, Choi J et al (2021) Histone demethylase KDM4C controls tumorigenesis of glioblastoma by epigenetically regulating p53 and c-Myc. Cell Death Dis 12(1):89

Leurs U, Clausen RP, Kristensen JL, Lohse B (2012) Inhibitor scaffold for the histone lysine demethylase KDM4C (JMJD2C). Bioorg Med Chem Lett 22(18):5811–5813

Levin M, Stark M, Assaraf YG (2018) The JmjN domain as a dimerization interface and a targeted inhibitor of KDM4 demethylase activity. Oncotarget 9(24):16861–16882

Li M, Deng Y, Zhuo M, Zhou H, Kong X, Xia X, Su Z, Chen Q, Guo P, Mo P et al (2020) Demethylase-independent function of JMJD2D as a novel antagonist of p53 to promote liver cancer initiation and progression. Theranostics 10(19):8863–8879

Li Y, Wang C, Gao H, Gu J, Zhang Y, Zhang Y, Xie M, Cheng X, Yang M, Zhang W et al (2022) KDM4 inhibitor SD49-7 attenuates leukemia stem cell via KDM4A/MDM2/p21(CIP1) axis. Theranostics 12(11):4922–4934

Liang Y, Vogel JL, Arbuckle JH, Rai G, Jadhav A, Simeonov A, Maloney DJ, Kristie TM (2013) Targeting the JMJD2 histone demethylases to epigenetically control herpesvirus infection and reactivation from latency. Sci Transl Med 5(167):167ra165

Liu G, Bollig-Fischer A, Kreike B, van de Vijver MJ, Abrams J, Ethier SP, Yang ZQ (2009) Genomic amplification and oncogenic properties of the GASC1 histone demethylase gene in breast cancer. Oncogene 28(50):4491–4500

Liu Y, Zheng P, Liu Y, Ji T, Liu X, Yao S, Cheng X, Li Y, Chen L, Xiao Z et al (2013) An epigenetic role for PRL-3 as a regulator of H3K9 methylation in colorectal cancer. Gut 62(4):571–581

Liu X, Wang Y, Gao Y, Su J, Zhang J, Xing X, Zhou C, Yao K, An Q, Zhang Y (2018) H3K9 demethylase KDM4E is an epigenetic regulator for bovine embryonic development and a defective factor for nuclear reprogramming. Development 145(4)

Loh YH, Zhang W, Chen X, George J, Ng HH (2007) Jmjd1a and Jmjd2c histone H3 Lys 9 demethylases regulate self-renewal in embryonic stem cells. Genes Dev 21(20):2545–2557

Luo X, Liu Y, Kubicek S, Myllyharju J, Tumber A, Ng S, Che KH, Podoll J, Heightman TD, Oppermann U et al (2011) A selective inhibitor and probe of the cellular functions of Jumonji C domain-containing histone demethylases. J Am Chem Soc 133(24):9451–9456

Luo W, Chang R, Zhong J, Pandey A, Semenza GL (2012) Histone demethylase JMJD2C is a coactivator for hypoxia-inducible factor 1 that is required for breast cancer progression. Proc Natl Acad Sci U S A 109(49):E3367-3376

Malecki PH, Ruger N, Roatsch M, Krylova O, Link A, Jung M, Heinemann U, Weiss MS (2019) Structure-based screening of tetrazolylhydrazide Inhibitors versus KDM4 histone demethylases. ChemMedChem 14(21):1828–1839

Mallette FA, Mattiroli F, Cui G, Young LC, Hendzel MJ, Mer G, Sixma TK, Richard S (2012) RNF8- and RNF168-dependent degradation of KDM4A/JMJD2A triggers 53BP1 recruitment to DNA damage sites. Embo J 31(8):1865–1878

Massett ME, Monaghan L, Patterson S, Mannion N, Bunschoten RP, Hoose A, Marmiroli S, Liskamp RMJ, Jorgensen HG, Vetrie D et al (2021) A KDM4A-PAF1-mediated epigenomic network is essential for acute myeloid leukemia cell self-renewal and survival. Cell Death Dis 12(6):573

Metzger E, Wissmann M, Yin N, Muller JM, Schneider R, Peters AH, Gunther T, Buettner R, Schule R (2005) LSD1 demethylates repressive histone marks to promote androgen-receptor-dependent transcription. Nature 437(7057):436–439

Metzger E, Stepputtis SS, Strietz J, Preca BT, Urban S, Willmann D, Allen A, Zenk F, Iovino N, Bronsert P et al (2017) KDM4 inhibition targets breast cancer stem-like cells. Can Res 77(21):5900–5912

Mishra S, Van Rechem C, Pal S, Clarke TL, Chakraborty D, Mahan SD, Black JC, Murphy SE, Lawrence MS, Daniels DL et al (2018) Cross-talk between lysine-modifying enzymes controls site-specific DNA amplifications. Cell 174(4):803–817 e816

Murn J, Shi Y (2017) The winding path of protein methylation research: milestones and new frontiers. Nat Rev Mol Cell Biol 18(8):517–527

Musselman CA, Kutateladze TG (2009) PHD fingers: epigenetic effectors and potential drug targets. Mol Interv 9(6):314–323

Musselman CA, Kutateladze TG (2011) Handpicking epigenetic marks with PHD fingers. Nucleic Acids Res 39(21):9061–9071

Ng SS, Kavanagh KL, McDonough MA, Butler D, Pilka ES, Lienard BM, Bray JE, Savitsky P, Gileadi O, von Delft F et al (2007) Crystal structures of histone demethylase JMJD2A reveal basis for substrate specificity. Nature 448(7149):87–91

Nielsen SD, Leurs U, Bergner M, Barris SA, Devkota K, Meyer K, Iaria D, McCaughan J, Lohse B, Kristensen JL et al (2016) Synthesis and characterisation of substrate-based peptides as inhibitors of histone demethylase KDM4C. Protein Pept Lett 23(9):772–776

Northcott PA, Nakahara Y, Wu X, Feuk L, Ellison DW, Croul S, Mack S, Kongkham PN, Peacock J, Dubuc A et al (2009) Multiple recurrent genetic events converge on control of histone lysine methylation in medulloblastoma. Nat Genet 41(4):465–472

Ortiz G, Kutateladze TG, Fujimori DG (2023) Chemical tools targeting readers of lysine methylation. Curr Opin Chem Biol 74:102286

Ozaki Y, Fujiwara K, Ikeda M, Ozaki T, Terui T, Soma M, Inazawa J, Nagase H (2015) The oncogenic role of GASC1 in chemically induced mouse skin cancer. Mamm Genome 26(11–12):591–597

Pack LR, Yamamoto KR, Fujimori DG (2016) Opposing chromatin signals direct and regulate the activity of lysine demethylase 4C (KDM4C). J Biol Chem 291(12):6060–6070

Pan HC, Chen YH, Fang WC, Wu VC, Sun CY (2022) Essential roles of the histone demethylase KDM4C in renal development and acute kidney injury. Int J Mol Sci 23(16)

Park IG, Jeon M, Kim H, Lee JM (2022) Coordinated methyl readers: Functional communications in cancer. Semin Cancer Biol 83:88–99

Passioura T, Bhushan B, Tumber A, Kawamura A, Suga H (2018) Structure-activity studies of a macrocyclic peptide inhibitor of histone lysine demethylase 4A. Bioorg Med Chem 26(6):1225–1231

Pedersen MT, Agger K, Laugesen A, Johansen JV, Cloos PA, Christensen J, Helin K (2014) The demethylase JMJD2C localizes to H3K4me3-positive transcription start sites and is dispensable for embryonic development. Mol Cell Biol 34(6):1031–1045

Pedersen MT, Kooistra SM, Radzisheuskaya A, Laugesen A, Johansen JV, Hayward DG, Nilsson J, Agger K, Helin K (2016) Continual removal of H3K9 promoter methylation by Jmjd2 demethylases is vital for ESC self-renewal and early development. Embo J 35(14):1550–1564

Peng K, Kou L, Yu L, Bai C, Li M, Mo P, Li W, Yu C (2019) Histone Demethylase JMJD2D interacts with beta-catenin to induce transcription and activate colorectal cancer cell proliferation and tumor growth in mice. Gastroenterology 156(4):1112–1126

Peng K, Zhuo M, Li M, Chen Q, Mo P, Yu C (2020) Histone demethylase JMJD2D activates HIF1 signaling pathway via multiple mechanisms to promote colorectal cancer glycolysis and progression. Oncogene 39(47):7076–7091

Pfister SX, Ashworth A (2017) Marked for death: targeting epigenetic changes in cancer. Nat Rev Drug Discov 16(4):241–263

Pilka ES, James T, Lisztwan JH (2015) Structural definitions of Jumonji family demethylase selectivity. Drug Discov Today 20(6):743–749

Rai G, Kawamura A, Tumber A, Liang Y, Vogel JL, Arbuckle JH, Rose NR, Dexheimer TS, Foley TL,

King ON et al (2010) Discovery of ML324, a JMJD2 demethylase inhibitor with demonstrated antiviral activity. In: Probe reports from the NIH Molecular Libraries Program. Bethesda, MD

Roatsch M, Robaa D, Pippel M, Nettleship JE, Reddivari Y, Bird LE, Hoffmann I, Franz H, Owens RJ, Schule R et al (2016) Substituted 2-(2-aminopyrimidin-4-yl)pyridine-4-carboxylates as potent inhibitors of JumonjiC domain-containing histone demethylases. Future Med Chem 8(13):1553–1571

Romani M, Daga A, Forlani A, Pistillo MP, Banelli B (2019) Targeting of histone demethylases KDM5A and KDM6B inhibits the proliferation of temozolomide-resistant glioblastoma cells. Cancers (Basel) 11(6)

Rose NR, Ng SS, Mecinovic J, Lienard BM, Bello SH, Sun Z, McDonough MA, Oppermann U, Schofield CJ (2008) Inhibitor scaffolds for 2-oxoglutarate-dependent histone lysine demethylases. J Med Chem 51(22):7053–7056

Ruger N, Roatsch M, Emmrich T, Franz H, Schule R, Jung M, Link A (2015) Tetrazolylhydrazides as selective fragment-like inhibitors of the JumonjiC-domain-containing histone demethylase KDM4A. ChemMedChem 10(11):1875–1883

Rui L, Emre NC, Kruhlak MJ, Chung HJ, Steidl C, Slack G, Wright GW, Lenz G, Ngo VN, Shaffer AL et al (2010) Cooperative epigenetic modulation by cancer amplicon genes. Cancer Cell 18(6):590–605

Salifou K, Ray S, Verrier L, Aguirrebengoa M, Trouche D, Panov KI, Vandromme M (2016) The histone demethylase JMJD2A/KDM4A links ribosomal RNA transcription to nutrients and growth factors availability. Nat Commun 7:10174

Sanchez R, Zhou MM (2011) The PHD finger: a versatile epigenome reader. Trends Biochem Sci 36(7):364–372

Sankar A, Kooistra SM, Gonzalez JM, Ohlsson C, Poutanen M, Helin K (2017) Maternal expression of the histone demethylase Kdm4a is crucial for pre-implantation development. Development 144(18):3264–3277

Sankar A, Lerdrup M, Manaf A, Johansen JV, Gonzalez JM, Borup R, Blanshard R, Klungland A, Hansen K, Andersen CY et al (2020) KDM4A regulates the maternal-to-zygotic transition by protecting broad H3K4me3 domains from H3K9me3 invasion in oocytes. Nat Cell Biol 22(4):380–388

Sekirnik R, Rose NR, Thalhammer A, Seden PT, Mecinovic J, Schofield CJ (2009) Inhibition of the histone lysine demethylase JMJD2A by ejection of structural Zn(II). Chem Commun (Camb) 42:6376–6378

Shao N, Cheng J, Huang H, Gong X, Lu Y, Idris M, Peng X, Ong BX, Zhang Q, Xu F et al (2021) GASC1 promotes hepatocellular carcinoma progression by inhibiting the degradation of ROCK2. Cell Death Dis 12(3):253

Shi Y, Lan F, Matson C, Mulligan P, Whetstine JR, Cole PA, Casero RA, Shi Y (2004) Histone demethylation mediated by the nuclear amine oxidase homolog LSD1. Cell 119(7):941–953

Shi L, Sun L, Li Q, Liang J, Yu W, Yi X, Yang X, Li Y, Han X, Zhang Y et al (2011) Histone demethylase JMJD2B coordinates H3K4/H3K9 methylation and promotes hormonally responsive breast carcinogenesis. Proc Natl Acad Sci U S A 108(18):7541–7546

Shin S, Janknecht R (2007) Activation of androgen receptor by histone demethylases JMJD2A and JMJD2D. Biochem Biophys Res Commun 359(3):742–746

Singh S, Abu-Zaid A, Jin H, Fang J, Wu Q, Wang T, Feng H, Quarni W, Shao Y, Maxham L et al (2022) Targeting KDM4 for treating PAX3-FOXO1-driven alveolar rhabdomyosarcoma. Sci Transl Med 14(653):eabq2096

Skarnes WC, Rosen B, West AP, Koutsourakis M, Bushell W, Iyer V, Mujica AO, Thomas M, Harrow J, Cox T et al (2011) A conditional knockout resource for the genome-wide study of mouse gene function. Nature 474(7351):337–342

Staehle AM, Peeken JC, Vladimirov G, Hoeness ME, Bojtine Kovacs S, Karantzelis N, Gruender A, Koellerer C, Jutzi JS, Pahl HL et al (2023) The histone demethylase JMJD2C constitutes a novel NFE2 target gene that is required for the survival of JAK2(V617F) mutated cells. Leukemia 37(4):919–923

Sterling J, Menezes SV, Abbassi RH, Munoz L (2020) Histone lysine demethylases and their functions in cancer. Int J Cancer 148:2375–2388

Su Z, Wang F, Lee JH, Stephens KE, Papazyan R, Voronina E, Krautkramer KA, Raman A, Thorpe JJ, Boersma MD et al (2016) Reader domain specificity and lysine demethylase-4 family function. Nat Commun 7:13387

Sudo G, Kagawa T, Kokubu Y, Inazawa J, Taga T (2016) Increase in GFAP-positive astrocytes in histone demethylase GASC1/KDM4C/JMJD2C hypomorphic mutant mice. Genes Cells 21(3):218–225

Sun LL, Holowatyj A, Xu XE, Wu JY, Wu ZY, Shen JH, Wang SH, Li EM, Yang ZQ, Xu LY (2013) Histone demethylase GASC1, a potential prognostic and predictive marker in esophageal squamous cell carcinoma. Am J Cancer Res 3(5):509–517

Suzuki T, Miyata N (2011) Lysine demethylases inhibitors. J Med Chem 54(24):8236–8250

Tan MK, Lim HJ, Harper JW (2011) SCF(FBXO22) regulates histone H3 lysine 9 and 36 methylation levels by targeting histone demethylase KDM4A for ubiquitin-mediated proteasomal degradation. Mol Cell Biol 31(18):3687–3699

Tausendschon M, Dehne N, Brune B (2011) Hypoxia causes epigenetic gene regulation in macrophages by attenuating Jumonji histone demethylase activity. Cytokine 53(2):256–262

The Cancer Genome Atlas Network (2012) Comprehensive molecular portraits of human breast tumours. Nature 490(7418):61–70
Tomaz RA, Harman JL, Karimlou D, Weavers L, Fritsch L, Bou-Kheir T, Bell E, Del Valle TI, Niakan KK, Fisher C et al (2017) Jmjd2c facilitates the assembly of essential enhancer-protein complexes at the onset of embryonic stem cell differentiation. Development 144(4):567–579
Tsurumi A, Dutta P, Shang R, Yan SJ, Li WX (2013) Drosophila Kdm4 demethylases in histone H3 lysine 9 demethylation and ecdysteroid signaling. Sci Rep 3:2894
Uhlen M, Fagerberg L, Hallstrom BM, Lindskog C, Oksvold P, Mardinoglu A, Sivertsson A, Kampf C, Sjostedt E, Asplund A et al (2015) Proteomics. Tissue-based map of the human proteome. Science 347(6220):1260419
Uhlen M, Zhang C, Lee S, Sjostedt E, Fagerberg L, Bidkhori G, Benfeitas R, Arif M, Liu Z, Edfors F et al: A pathology atlas of the human cancer transcriptome. Science 2017, 357(6352).
Upadhyay AK, Judge RA, Li L, Pithawalla R, Simanis J, Bodelle PM, Marin VL, Henry RF, Petros AM, Sun C (2018) Targeting lysine specific demethylase 4A (KDM4A) tandem TUDOR domain—a fragment based approach. Bioorg Med Chem Lett 28(10):1708–1713
Van Rechem C, Black JC, Abbas T, Allen A, Rinehart CA, Yuan GC, Dutta A, Whetstine JR (2011) The SKP1-Cul1-F-box and leucine-rich repeat protein 4 (SCF-FbxL4) ubiquitin ligase regulates lysine demethylase 4A (KDM4A)/Jumonji domain-containing 2A (JMJD2A) protein. J Biol Chem 286(35):30462–30470
Van Rechem C, Black JC, Boukhali M, Aryee MJ, Graslund S, Haas W, Benes CH, Whetstine JR (2015) Lysine demethylase KDM4A associates with translation machinery and regulates protein synthesis. Cancer Discov 5(3):255–263
Van Rechem C, Ji F, Mishra S, Chakraborty D, Murphy SE, Dillingham ME, Sadreyev RI, Whetstine JR (2020) The lysine demethylase KDM4A controls the cell-cycle expression of replicative canonical histone genes. Biochim Biophys Acta Gene Regul Mech 1863(10):194624
Vinatzer U, Gollinger M, Mullauer L, Raderer M, Chott A, Streubel B (2008) Mucosa-associated lymphoid tissue lymphoma: novel translocations including rearrangements of ODZ2, JMJD2C, and CNN3. Clin Cancer Res 14(20):6426–6431
Wagner RT, Cooney AJ (2009) OCT4: less is more. Cell Res 19(5):527–528
Wang J, Zhang M, Zhang Y, Kou Z, Han Z, Chen DY, Sun QY, Gao S (2010) The histone demethylase JMJD2C is stage-specifically expressed in preimplantation mouse embryos and is required for embryonic development. Biol Reprod 82(1):105–111
Wang L, Chang J, Varghese D, Dellinger M, Kumar S, Best AM, Ruiz J, Bruick R, Pena-Llopis S, Xu J et al (2013) A small molecule modulates Jumonji histone demethylase activity and selectively inhibits cancer growth. Nat Commun 4:2035
Wang LY, Hung CL, Chen YR, Yang JC, Wang J, Campbell M, Izumiya Y, Chen HW, Wang WC, Ann DK et al (2016) KDM4A coactivates E2F1 to regulate the PDK-dependent metabolic switch between mitochondrial oxidation and glycolysis. Cell Rep 16(11):3016–3027
Wang KS, Liu X, Zhang Q, Wu LY, Zeng M (2012) Genome-wide association study identifies 5q21 and 9p24.1 (KDM4C) loci associated with alcohol withdrawal symptoms. J Neural Transm (Vienna) 119(4):425–433
Warshakoon NC, Wu S, Boyer A, Kawamoto R, Sheville J, Renock S, Xu K, Pokross M, Zhou S, Winter C et al (2006) Structure-based design, synthesis, and SAR evaluation of a new series of 8-hydroxyquinolines as HIF-1alpha prolyl hydroxylase inhibitors. Bioorg Med Chem Lett 16(21):5517–5522
Wei J, Antony J, Meng F, MacLean P, Rhind R, Laible G, Oback B (2017) KDM4B-mediated reduction of H3K9me3 and H3K36me3 levels improves somatic cell reprogramming into pluripotency. Sci Rep 7(1):7514
Westaway SM, Preston AG, Barker MD, Brown F, Brown JA, Campbell M, Chung CW, Drewes G, Eagle R, Garton N et al (2016a) Cell penetrant inhibitors of the KDM4 and KDM5 families of histone lysine demethylases. 2. Pyrido[3,4-d]pyrimidin-4(3H)-one derivatives. J Med Chem 59(4):1370–1387
Westaway SM, Preston AG, Barker MD, Brown F, Brown JA, Campbell M, Chung CW, Diallo H, Douault C, Drewes G et al (2016b) Cell penetrant inhibitors of the KDM4 and KDM5 families of histone lysine demethylases. 1.3-Amino-4-pyridine carboxylate derivatives. J Med Chem 59(4):1357–1369
Whetstine JR, Nottke A, Lan F, Huarte M, Smolikov S, Chen Z, Spooner E, Li E, Zhang G, Colaiacovo M et al (2006) Reversal of histone lysine trimethylation by the JMJD2 family of histone demethylases. Cell 125(3):467–481
Williams ST, Walport LJ, Hopkinson RJ, Madden SK, Chowdhury R, Schofield CJ, Kawamura A (2014) Studies on the catalytic domains of multiple JmjC oxygenases using peptide substrates. Epigenetics 9(12):1596–1603
Wilson C, Qiu L, Hong Y, Karnik T, Tadros G, Mau B, Ma T, Mu Y, New J, Louie RJ et al (2017) The histone demethylase KDM4B regulates peritoneal seeding of ovarian cancer. Oncogene 36(18):2565–2576
Wilson C, Krieg AJ (2019) KDM4B: a nail for every hammer? Genes (Basel) 10(2):134
Wissmann M, Yin N, Muller JM, Greschik H, Fodor BD, Jenuwein T, Vogler C, Schneider R, Gunther T, Buettner R et al (2007) Cooperative demethylation by JMJD2C and LSD1 promotes androgen receptor-dependent gene expression. Nat Cell Biol 9(3):347–353

Wu J, Liu S, Liu G, Dombkowski A, Abrams J, Martin-Trevino R, Wicha MS, Ethier SP, Yang ZQ (2012) Identification and functional analysis of 9p24 amplified genes in human breast cancer. Oncogene 31(3):333–341

Wu L, Wary KK, Revskoy S, Gao X, Tsang K, Komarova YA, Rehman J, Malik AB (2015) Histone demethylases KDM4A and KDM4C regulate differentiation of embryonic stem cells to endothelial cells. Stem Cell Rep 5(1):10–21

Wu Q, Young B, Wang Y, Davidoff AM, Rankovic Z, Yang J (2022) Recent advances with KDM4 inhibitors and potential applications. J Med Chem 65(14):9564–9579

Yang ZQ, Imoto I, Fukuda Y, Pimkhaokham A, Shimada Y, Imamura M, Sugano S, Nakamura Y, Inazawa J (2000) Identification of a novel gene, GASC1, within an amplicon at 9p23-24 frequently detected in esophageal cancer cell lines. Can Res 60(17):4735–4739

Yang J, Jubb AM, Pike L, Buffa FM, Turley H, Baban D, Leek R, Gatter KC, Ragoussis J, Harris AL (2010) The histone demethylase JMJD2B is regulated by estrogen receptor alpha and hypoxia, and is a key mediator of estrogen induced growth. Can Res 70(16):6456–6466

Yang WS, Campbell M, Chang PC (2017a) SUMO modification of a heterochromatin histone demethylase JMJD2A enables viral gene transactivation and viral replication. Plos Pathog 13(2):e1006216

Yang J, Milasta S, Hu D, AlTahan AM, Interiano RB, Zhou J, Davidson J, Low J, Lin W, Bao J et al (2017b) Targeting histone demethylases in MYC-driven neuroblastomas with ciclopirox. Can Res 77(17):4626–4638

Yang J, AlTahan AM, Hu D, Wang Y, Cheng PH, Morton CL, Qu C, Nathwani AC, Shohet JM, Fotsis T et al (2015) The role of histone demethylase KDM4B in Myc signaling in neuroblastoma. JNCI J Natl Cancer I 107(6):djv080

Ye Q, Holowatyj A, Wu J, Liu H, Zhang L, Suzuki T, Yang ZQ (2015) Genetic alterations of KDM4 subfamily and therapeutic effect of novel demethylase inhibitor in breast cancer. Am J Cancer Res 5(4):1519–1530

Young LC, Hendzel MJ (2013) The oncogenic potential of Jumonji D2 (JMJD2/KDM4) histone demethylase overexpression. Biochem Cell Biol 91(6):369–377

Young LC, McDonald DW, Hendzel MJ (2013) Kdm4b histone demethylase is a DNA damage response protein and confers a survival advantage following gamma-irradiation. J Biol Chem 288(29):21376–21388

Yu H, Jiang Y, Liu L, Shan W, Chu X, Yang Z, Yang ZQ (2017) Integrative genomic and transcriptomic analysis for pinpointing recurrent alterations of plant homeodomain genes and their clinical significance in breast cancer. Oncotarget 8(8):13099–13115

Yu Y, Schleich K, Yue B, Ji S, Lohneis P, Kemper K, Silvis MR, Qutob N, van Rooijen E, Werner-Klein M et al (2018) Targeting the senescence-overriding cooperative activity of structurally unrelated H3K9 demethylases in melanoma. Cancer Cell 33(2):322–336 e328

Zack TI, Schumacher SE, Carter SL, Cherniack AD, Saksena G, Tabak B, Lawrence MS, Zhsng CZ, Wala J, Mermel CH et al (2013) Pan-cancer patterns of somatic copy number alteration. Nat Genet 45(10):1134–1140

Zhang QJ, Chen HZ, Wang L, Liu DP, Hill JA, Liu ZP (2011) The histone trimethyllysine demethylase JMJD2A promotes cardiac hypertrophy in response to hypertrophic stimuli in mice. J Clin Investig 121(6):2447–2456

Zhang W, Liu W, Jia L, Chen D, Chang I, Lake M, Bentolila LA, Wang CY (2021) Targeting KDM4A epigenetically activates tumor-cell-intrinsic immunity by inducing DNA replication stress. Mol Cell 81(10):2148–2165 e2149

Zhao E, Ding J, Xia Y, Liu M, Ye B, Choi JH, Yan C, Dong Z, Huang S, Zha Y et al (2016) KDM4C and ATF4 cooperate in transcriptional control of amino acid metabolism. Cell Rep 14(3):506–519

Zheng S, Bi Y, Chen H, Gong B, Jia S, Li H (2021) Molecular basis for bipartite recognition of histone H3 by the PZP domain of PHF14. Nucleic Acids Res 49(15):8961–8973

Zhu Q, Liang F, Cai S, Luo X, Duo T, Liang Z, He Z, Chen Y, Mo D (2021) KDM4A regulates myogenesis by demethylating H3K9me3 of myogenic regulatory factors. Cell Death Dis 12(6):514

KDM5 Lysine Demethylases in Pathogenesis, from Basic Science Discovery to the Clinic

6

Shang-Min Zhang, Jian Cao and Qin Yan

Abstract

The histone lysine demethylase 5 (KDM5) family proteins are Fe^{2+} and α-ketoglutarate-dependent dioxygenases, with jumonji C (JmjC) domain as their catalytic core and several plant homeodomains (PHDs) to bind different histone methylation marks. These enzymes are capable of demethylating tri-, di- and mono-methylated lysine 4 in histone H3 (H3K4me3/2/1), the key epigenetic marks for active chromatin. Thus, this H3K4 demethylase family plays critical roles in cell fate determination during development as well as malignant transformation. KDM5 demethylases have both oncogenic and tumor suppressive functions in a cancer type-dependent manner. In solid tumors, KDM5A/B are generally oncogenic, whereas KDM5C/D have tumor suppressive roles. Their involvement in de-differentiation, cancer metastasis, drug resistance, and tumor immunoevasion indicated that KDM5 family proteins are promising drug targets for cancer therapy. Significant efforts from both academia and industry have led to the development of potent and selective KDM5 inhibitors for preclinical experiments and phase I clinical trials. However, a better understanding of the roles of KDM5 demethylases in different physiological and pathological conditions is critical for further developing KDM5 modulators for clinical applications.

Keywords

KDM5 · Jumonji · Histone demethylase · Cancer · Stem cell · Drug resistance · Antitumor immunity

6.1 Introduction

Emerging evidence has shown that epigenetic alterations contribute to disease initiation and progression. As epigenetic changes are reversible, epigenetic regulators are attractive drug

S.-M. Zhang (✉)
School of Life Science and Technology, ShanghaiTech University, Shanghai 201210, China
e-mail: zhangshm@shanghaitech.edu.cn

J. Cao (✉)
Rutgers Cancer Institute of New Jersey, New Brunswick, NJ 08901, USA
e-mail: jian.cao@rutgers.edu

J. Cao
Department of Medicine, Robert Wood Johnson Medical School, Rutgers, The State University of New Jersey, New Brunswick, NJ 08901, USA

Q. Yan (✉)
Department of Pathology, Yale Cancer Center, Yale Stem Cell Center, Yale Center for Immuno-Oncology, Yale Center for Research on Aging, Yale School of Medicine, P.O. Box 208023, New Haven, CT 06520-8023, USA
e-mail: qin.yan@yale.edu

Q. Yan (ed.), *Targeting Lysine Demethylases in Cancer and Other Human Diseases*, Advances in Experimental Medicine and Biology 1433, https://doi.org/10.1007/978-3-031-38176-8_6

targets. One major class of epigenetic modifications are covalent posttranslational modifications of the histone tails, including histone acetylation, phosphorylation, and methylation (Blair and Yan 2012). These modifications can change the charges of histone tails, promote chromatin structure changes, or modulate the binding affinity of chromatin regulatory proteins (Berger 2007; Campos and Reinberg 2009). Therefore, different histone marks are linked to various biological processes including transcription, RNA processing, and DNA repair, e.g., trimethylation of histone H3 lysine 4 (H3K4me3), in general, is enriched at transcription start sites (TSSs) and correlated with active transcription (Santos-Rosa et al. 2002; Ruthenburg et al. 2007). H3K4me3 creates a binding site for epigenetic readers with PHD finger, chromodomain, or Tudor domain, which can mediate the downstream epigenetic signaling to modulate transcription (Berger 2007; Ruthenburg et al. 2007; Campos and Reinberg 2009).

Histone methylation was initially considered irreversible until the first-in-class histone demethylase, KDM1A (LSD1), was identified by Yang Shi's group in 2004 (Shi et al. 2004). Following this discovery, Robin Allshire's group predicted that Jumonji C (JmjC) domain can catalyze the removal of methyl groups from histones through a hydroxylation mechanism (Trewick et al. 2005), which allows for the demethylation of trimethylated histones that LSD1 cannot catalyze. Meanwhile, Yi Zhang's group independently purified several histone demethylases using an unbiased biochemical method around the same time and found them to be JmjC domain-containing proteins (Tsukada et al. 2006). These breakthroughs completely opened up the demethylase field. Most of the JmjC domain-containing proteins, now named from KDM2 to KDM9 (Nowak et al. 2016), were later shown as lysine demethylases with diverse substrate specificities.

In 2007, the KDM5 enzymes were discovered to be lysine demethylases specific for H3K4me3/2/1 in several organisms by multiple groups including ours (Christensen et al. 2007; Iwase et al. 2007; Klose et al. 2007; Lee et al. 2007; Liang et al. 2007; Seward et al. 2007; Tahiliani et al. 2007; Xiang et al. 2007). The only KDM5 protein in *Saccharomyces cerevisiae*, *Caenorhabditis elegans*, and *Drosophila melanogaster* is called JmjC domain-containing histone demethylase 2 (Jhd2) (Tu et al. 2007), retinoblastoma-related protein 2 (Rbr-2) (Christensen et al. 2007), and little imaginal disks (Lid) (Seward et al. 2007; Lloret-Llinares et al. 2008), respectively (Fig. 6.1). In mammals, there are four KDM5 members, also called Jumonji AT-Rich interactive domain (JARID1) proteins, and named KDM5A/JARID1A, KDM5B/JARID1B, KDM5C/JARID1C, and KDM5D/JARID1D, respectively (reviewed in Blair et al. (2011)) (Fig. 6.1).

KDM5A was first identified as retinoblastoma binding protein 2 (RBP2), through a cDNA expression library screen for partners of pRB (retinoblastoma) in 1991 (Defeo-Jones et al. 1991). KDM5B, first named PLU-1, was discovered as a novel gene that is downregulated in HER2-overexpressed breast cancer cells

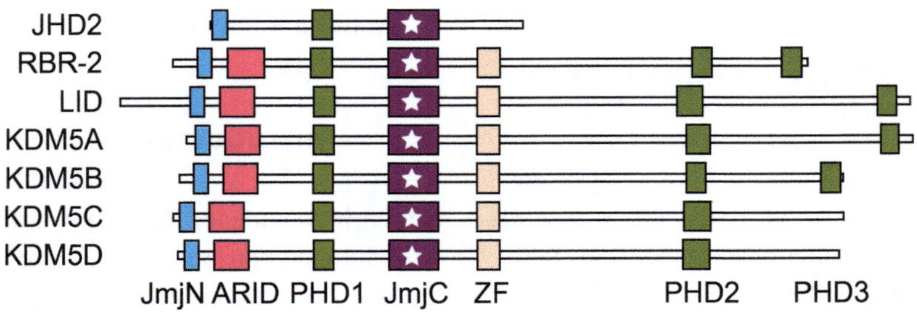

Fig. 6.1 Domain structure of KDM5 proteins from yeast (JHD2), worm (RBR-2), fly (LID) and mammals (KDM5A-D)

after treatment with an antibody that decreases HER2 phosphorylation (Lu et al. 1999), suggesting that KDM5B is a HER2 target gene. KDM5D was isolated as a transcript mapped on mouse Y chromosome and named selected mouse cDNA on Y (SMCY) (Agulnik et al. 1994a), and KDM5C was soon cloned from mouse and human cDNA library by the same group and named SMCX because of its X chromosome location and homology to SMCY (Agulnik et al. 1994b). All four members of KDM5 contain Jumonji AT-Rich Interactive Domain (Wilsker et al. 2002), thus they were also called JARID1A, B, C, and D, respectively. The complicated and noncoherent nomenclature of KDM5s used to confuse many scientists. In 2007, a common nomenclature for histone modifying enzymes was proposed (Allis et al. 2007). According to this nomenclature, histone demethylase was renamed to Lysine (K) Demethylase (KDM) to reflect their enzymatic activity, residue specificity, and existing of non-histone substrates. Therefore, RBP2/JARID1A, PLU-1/JARID1B, SMCX/JARID1C, and SMCY/JARID1D are now named as KDM5A-D, respectively.

Only a tiny percentage of H3 is methylated at lysine 4 in live cells, compared with some other more redundant histone posttranslational modifications (Peach et al. 2012). However, the functional importance of H3K4me3 was confirmed by its restricted localization on gene promoters, tightly in association with transcriptional activation (Barski et al. 2007; Koch et al. 2007), and direct effects on transcription initiation (Lauberth et al. 2013). A recent study showed that H3K4me3 is required to release paused RNA Pol II downstream of the transcription initiation site, indicating its function in transcription elongation (Wang et al. 2023). On the other hand, H3K4me1 shows a strong association with active enhancers (Heintzman et al. 2007, 2009). As the enzymes that remove H3K4me3 and could regulate H3K4me1 in both directions, KDM5 family histone demethylases play key roles to establish, maintain, and dynamically regulate development- and tissue-specific gene expression. Dysregulation of KDM5 or its regulated processes were found to contribute to human diseases, including various types of cancer, making them attractive drug targets for therapies.

This chapter reviews our current knowledge of KDM5 demethylases and their functions in physiological and pathological conditions, especially in cancer, and also discusses small molecule inhibitors of KDM5 and their potential applications in the clinic.

6.2 Structure and Activity of KDM5 Demethylases

The four family members of mammalian KDM5 demethylase share a high degree of homology in sequence and structural domain organization, which is also conserved from their homologs in yeast, worm, and fruit fly (Fig. 6.1). KDM5 family demethylases contain a JmjC domain as their catalytic core, which is the signature motif shared by all known histone demethylases except KDM1A and KDM1B (Klose et al. 2006). A related JmjN (Jumonji N) domain localizes at the N-terminus of all KDM5 homologs and is separated from JmjC by a PHD finger (plant homeobox domain) in JHD2 or by an ARID (AT-rich interacting domain; also known as BRIGHT domain) plus a PHD finger in Rbr-2, Lid, and mammalian KDM5s. The existence of JmjN and an atypical insertion between two Jumonji domains make the KDM5 family structurally unique among JmjC-containing histone demethylases. The second half of KDM5, except in yeast, contains a C_5HC_2-type zinc finger domain and one or two additional PHD domains (Fig. 6.1).

Different from KDM1s but similar to other JmjC domain-containing KDMs, KDM5 catalyzes hydroxylation on methylated lysine with iron and α-ketoglutarate (α-KG, also known as 2-oxoglutarate or 2-OG) as cofactors, resulting in hydroxylated methyl-lysine, a thermodynamically unstable intermediate (Klose et al. 2006). Then the hydroxylated methyl group is released in the form of formaldehyde, leaving a demethylated lysine residue (Klose et al. 2006).

Successful reconstitution of demethylase activity in vitro by combining directly-linked JmjN and JmjC, and the zinc finger domains suggests that these are the minimal domains required for the enzymatic activity of KDM5 (Horton et al. 2016a). The crystal structures of the JmjN-JmjC catalytic core of KDM5A, KDM5B, and KDM5C, in the presence of substrates or diverse inhibitors, have been solved by multiple groups (Horton et al. 2016a, b; Johansson et al. 2016; Vinogradova et al. 2016; Wu et al. 2018).

The ARID domain is a helix–turn–helix motif-based DNA-binding domain found in more than a dozen distinct human proteins. Early studies showed ARID's selective binding to AT-rich sequences, as indicated by its name (Patsialou et al. 2005). However, ARID domains in KDM5 bind preferentially to GC-rich motifs (Scibetta et al. 2007; Tu et al. 2008; Yao et al. 2010), also shown by the crystal structures (Tu et al. 2008; Yao et al. 2010). Although it is not required for the demethylase activity in vitro, the DNA-binding ARID domain may be involved in anchoring KDM5 onto nucleic acid wrapped around its substrate nucleosome (Yao et al. 2010).

The PHD finger, typically with 50–80 amino acid residues, is a small protein domain-containing a zinc-binding motif (Aasland et al. 1995). Found in many chromatin-associated proteins, it can bind histone tails with diverse posttranslational modifications, making it a perfect epigenome reader (Sanchez and Zhou 2011). Indeed, the binding affinity of PHD fingers in KDM5 to histone H3 tail depends on the methylation status of lysine 4. The first PHD domain (PHD1) of KDM5A and KDM5B is highly specific for histone H3 with unmodified lysine 4 (H3K4me0) (Wang et al. 2009; Klein et al. 2014; Zhang et al. 2014b; Torres et al. 2015), while PHD1 of KDM5C binds H3K9me3 (Iwase et al. 2007). While KDM5A demethylase activity can be stimulated when PHD1 is occupied by H3K4me0 (Torres et al. 2015), PHD1 domain of KDM5C inhibits its demethylase activity (Ugur et al. 2023). The third PHD domain (PHD3), which does not exist in KDM5C or KDM5D, shows a preference for H3K4me3/2 (Wang et al. 2009; Klein et al. 2014). The second PHD domain (PHD2) of KDM5 apparently does not recognize the H3 tail, as suggested by pull down experiments (Iwase et al. 2007). A similar observation was reported for Lid, in which PHD1 and PHD3 bind to unmethylated and tri-methylated H3K4, respectively, while PHD2 does not show interaction with histone (Li et al. 2010). The structures of some PHD domains in KDM5 have been reported and are consistent with their specificities (Wang et al. 2009; Zhang et al. 2014b). The binding of KDM5A and KDM5B PHD domains to both the substrate (H3K4me3) and the product (H3K4me0) of its demethylase reaction may anchor the enzyme to the boundaries of H3K4me3-enriched promoters and prevent the spreading of H3K4me3 to nearby histones to ensure the precision initiation of gene transcription. However, this does not apply to other family members since JHD2 only has PHD1, and KDM5C and KDM5D do not have PHD3 (Fig. 6.1).

6.3 KDM5 and Gene Regulation

6.3.1 Transcriptional Regulation

The KDM5 family enzymes are often regarded as transcriptional repressors as they demethylate H3K4me3 (Fig. 6.2a). This histone modification marks promoters/transcription start sites of actively transcribed genes from yeast to mammals (Santos-Rosa et al. 2002; Koch et al. 2007; Consortium 2012). Additionally, the levels of H3K4me3 occupancy are strongly associated with gene expression levels (Barski et al. 2007; Koch et al. 2007; Consortium 2012). Methylated H3K4 recruits a number of factors involved in transcription (Ruthenburg et al. 2007; Vermeulen et al. 2007) and facilitates preinitiation complex assembly and postinitiation processes (Sims et al. 2007; Lauberth et al. 2013).

At the enhancers, KDM5 enzymes were reported to act both as transcription activators and repressors. Enhancers are classically defined as cis-acting DNA sequences that can induce transcription (Pennacchio et al. 2013).

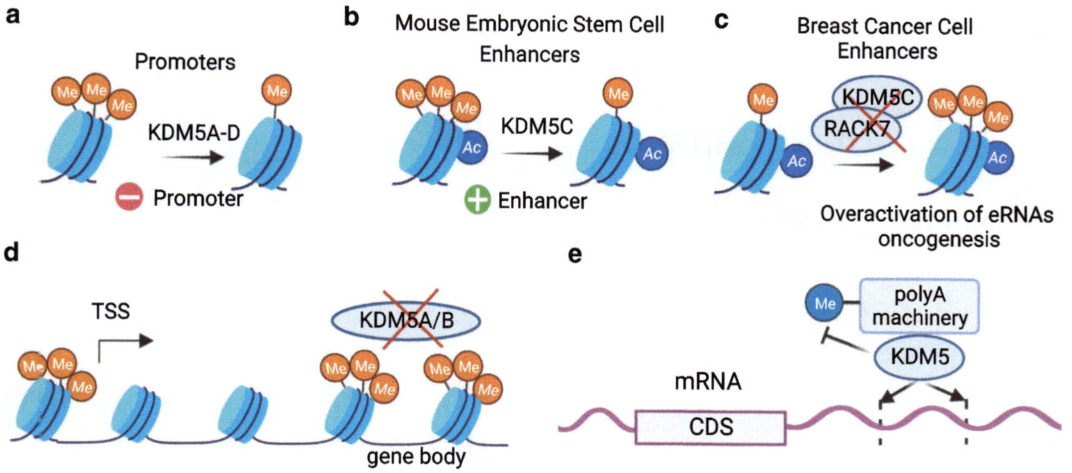

Fig. 6.2 KDM5 demethylases regulate gene expression in multiple ways. **a** KDM5 demethylates H3K4me3 at the promoters to repress gene expression. **b** KDM5C activates the enhancers by generating H3K4me1, which in combination with H3K27Ac, mark active enhancers. **c** KDM5C is recruited by RACK7 to the enhancers to remove H3K4me3. Loss of KDM5C or RACK7 leads to increased H3K4me3 and eRNA expression, resulting in activation of oncogenes regulated by these enhancers. **d** KDM5A/B repress spurious transcription initiation in the gene body by removing H3K4me3. TSS, transcriptional start site. **e** KDM5 recruits the polyadenylation (polyA) machinery to regulate alternative polyadenylation of mRNA, potentially by demethylating the components of polyA machinery. Dotted lines indicate polyadenylation sites on the nascent transcript. CDS, coding sequence. Created with BioRender.com

Genome-wide profiling of histone modifications found that H3K4me1 defines active enhancers (Heintzman et al. 2009; Consortium 2012). Because KDM5 demethylases can demethylate all three levels of H3K4 methylation (H3K4me3, H3K4me2, and H3K4me1) with more robust activity on H3K4me3/2, they it can theoretically decrease or increase H3K4me1, therefore regulating the enhancer activity in both directions. In fact, KDM5C can be recruited to the enhancers in mouse embryonic stem cells and stimulate enhancer activity by increasing the H3K4me1 level (Outchkourov et al. 2013) (Fig. 6.2b). In human breast cancer cells, KDM5C was also shown to be recruited by RACK7 to enhancers to remove enhancer H3K4me3, leading to decreased transcription of eRNAs and nearby genes (Shen et al. 2016; Scandaglia et al. 2017) (Fig. 6.2c).

In addition, KDM5 proteins interact with a large number of transcriptional repressors to maintain gene silencing (Fig. 6.3), e.g., KDM5A binds to the SIN3/HDAC complex (Hayakawa et al. 2007; van Oevelen et al. 2008), the Polycomb-Repressive Complex 2 (PRC2) complex (Pasini et al. 2008), MAD1 (Ge et al. 2010), RBP-J (Liefke et al. 2010), the G9A-GLP complex (Chaturvedi et al. 2012), and NuRD complex (Nishibuchi et al. 2014). Similarly, KDM5B interacts with the LSD1/NuRD complex (Li et al. 2011), HP1γ-LSD1-HDAC1/2 and CoREST complex (Vicent et al. 2013), the PRC2 complex (Zhang et al. 2014a), and SETDB1 (Zhang et al. 2021). KDM5C interacts with G9A, HDAC1/2, and the transcription repressor REST complex (Iwase et al. 2007; Tahiliani et al. 2007). Lastly, KDM5D forms a complex with RING6A (polycomb-like) (Lee et al. 2007). In all these cases, the removal of KDM5 led to reactivation of target genes.

Although KDM5 enzymes are more well-known as transcriptional suppressors due to their H3K4 demethylase activity, many studies suggest that KDM5 demethylases are also capable of activating gene expression. Several mechanisms have been proposed: (1) as discussed above, KDM5 demethylases activate enhancers by demethylating H3K4me3/2 to set up active

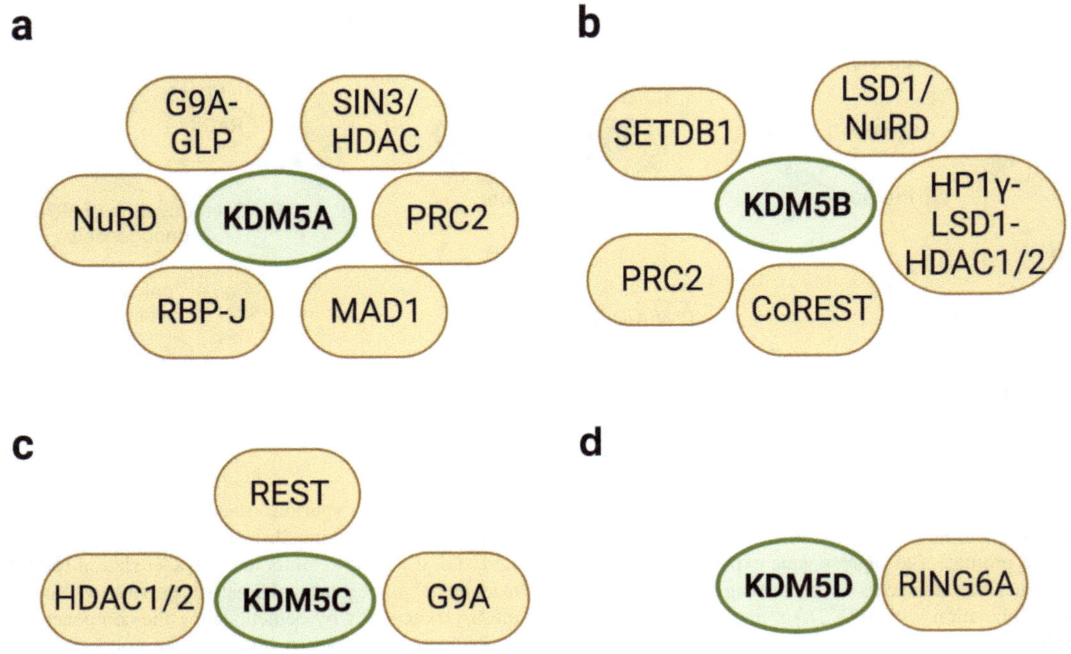

Fig. 6.3 KDM5 proteins bind many transcriptional repressors to silence gene expression. **a–d**. KDM5A-D interacting proteins. Created with BioRender.com

enhancer mark H3K4me1 (Outchkourov et al. 2013); (2) KDM5 proteins function as epigenetic "readers" instead of "erasers" by binding to chromatin and recruiting co-activators (Liu and Secombe 2015); (3) KDM5 enzymes ensure transcription by reducing spurious transcription initiation (Hayakawa et al. 2007; Xie et al. 2011; Kidder et al. 2014).

KDM5 is a multi-domain protein (Fig. 6.1). Two PHD domains in KDM5A and KDM5B, as well as in Lid and Rbr-2, recognize unmethylated and tri-methylated H3K4, respectively. Other domains in KDM5 may mediate additional protein–protein interactions. Thus, KDM5 may carry demethylation-independent functions, such as recruiting transcriptional co-activators, e.g., Lid activates genes required for mitochondrial function in flies in its demethylase activity-independent manner (Liu and Secombe 2015). Lid is also necessary for dMyc-induced cell growth by recruiting c-Myc to H3K4me3 occupied promoters (Secombe et al. 2007). Similar co-activator functions have been discovered on KDM5A and KDM5B (Chan and Hong 2001; Benevolenskaya et al. 2005; Lee et al. 2009; Loft et al. 2016). Proximity labeling reveals additional KDM5-interacting proteins, such as chromatin remodeling complexes SWI/SNF and NURF, the NSL complex, mediator, and insulator proteins (Yheskel et al. 2023).

KDM5A was shown to maintain reduced H3K4 methylation at the transcribed regions, which could facilitate transcriptional elongation (Hayakawa et al. 2007). In addition, hydroxylation of proline at residue 16 (H3P16oh) of histone H3, catalyzed by the proline hydroxylase EGLN2, has been shown to enhance chromatin recruitment of KDM5A to target genes and a corresponding decrease of H3K4me3 (Liu et al. 2022b). KDM5B was shown to co-localize to H3K4me3 and prevents H3K4 methylation from spreading out of promoters and enhancers regions (Kidder et al. 2014). KDM5B was also found to bind to gene-body regions to remove intragenic H3K4me3 (Xie et al. 2011). Thus, KDM5 enzymes activate gene expression by ensuring precise transcription initiation and preventing cryptic intragenic transcription (Hayakawa et al. 2007; Xie et al. 2011; Kidder et al. 2014) (Fig. 6.2d).

6.3.2 Other Gene Regulation Processes

Besides controlling transcriptional activities, KDM5 is also involved in other aspects of gene regulation. Emerging evidence supports functions of KDM5 after transcriptional initiation, such as regulating mRNA through 3′ untranslated region (UTR) length (Blair et al. 2016) (Fig. 6.2e) as well as alternative splicing (He and Kidder 2017). Both polyadenylation and splicing are transcription-coupled. Blair et al. have shown that Jhd2 recruits 3′ UTR processing machinery, thus regulating the alteration of 3′ UTR length by alternative polyadenylation for some genes in a demethylase-dependent manner (Blair et al. 2016). Moreover, KDM5B promotes the shortening of oncogene CCND1 transcript in breast cancer cells (Blair et al. 2016). He et al. have shown that KDM5B is enriched at nearby alternatively spliced sites and KDM5B depletion results in differential expression of transcript isoforms (He and Kidder 2017).

The involvement of KDM5A and KDM5B in site-specific genomic amplification mediated by KDM4 enzymes was a surprising finding (Mishra et al. 2018). Depletion or inhibition of KDM5A causes replication-derived, transient, but significant 1q12h copy gains. On the other hand, KDM5B suppresses the gain-of-copy number in 1p32.3 (Mishra et al. 2018). However, the detailed mechanism responsible for the locus-specificity is still unclear.

6.4 Biological Function of KDM5

6.4.1 KDM5 Gene Expression and Knockout Animals

KDM5 demethylases play pivotal roles during normal development. KDM5A is ubiquitously expressed, while KDM5B is mainly expressed during development and in limited adult tissues. KDM5C shows the highest expression level in the neuronal system. KDM5D is expressed in all male tissues (Tumber et al. 2017).

Yeasts lacking Jhd2 are viable and healthy (Liang et al. 2007). They showed increased H3K4me3, reduced H3K4me2, no change of H3K4me1, and increased telomeric silencing (Liang et al. 2007). A *C. elegans* mutant strain rbr-2(tm1231) has been isolated carrying an in-frame deletion of the JmjC domain. The global level of H3K4me3 increased significantly in all developmental stages and most animals showed moderate development defects (Christensen et al. 2007). Knockout of Lid, the only copy of KDM5 in flies, leads to embryonic lethality (Gildea et al. 2000; Secombe et al. 2007; Drelon et al. 2018).

Kdm5a knockout model was generated before the discovery of the demethylase activity of KDM5A, and is the first knockout model of genes encoding the KDM enzymes. *Kdm5a* knockout mice are viable and grossly normal in a mixed background, but die right after birth in the C57BL/6 background (Klose et al. 2007; Lin et al. 2011; Cao et al. 2014). Although it was reported that replacing *Kdm5b* exon 1 with the neomycin gene results in early embryonic lethality (Catchpole et al. 2011), *Kdm5b* knockout mice created with two different strategies can be obtained with relatively minor developmental delay, and at less than Mendelian ratio (Schmitz et al. 2011; Albert et al. 2013; Zou et al. 2014). *Kdm5c* knockout mice are viable, but are smaller and weigh less, with behavioral defects related to intellectual disability (Iwase et al. 2016; Scandaglia et al. 2017). Since there are six copies of *KDM5* genes (two *KDM5A*, two *KDM5B*, and two *KDM5C* in females or one *KDM5C* plus one *KDM5D* in males) in mammals, there may be some functional redundancy. However, the effects of deleting three or more copies of *Kdm5* genes in mice remain to be determined.

6.4.2 Pluripotency and Differentiation

In embryonic stem cells (ESCs), KDM5A loss leads to the activation of differentiation genes (Lin et al. 2011). When ESCs are induced to differentiate, although downregulation of KDM5A causes premature downregulation of stem cell markers OCT4 and NANOG, it only leads to partial activation of differentiation-related genes (Lin et al. 2011). These results suggest that KDM5A is essential for both the maintenance and differentiation of ESCs. KDM5A was discovered in a yeast two-hybrid screen for binding partners of mutant pRB that fails to bind to E2Fs but retains the ability to induce differentiation (Benevolenskaya et al. 2005). The pRB mutants that failed to bind KDM5A lose the ability to control differentiation (Benevolenskaya et al. 2005). In *Rb1*-deficient cells, KDM5A loss can rescue the differentiation defect but not permanent cell cycle withdrawal (Varaljai et al. 2015). These results suggest that KDM5A is a downstream target of pRB, and regulates differentiation independent of cell cycle regulation (Varaljai et al. 2015). The roles of KDM5A in myogenic differentiation partially depends on its ability to control mitochondrial function through PGC-1α (Varaljai et al. 2015).

The roles of KDM5B in ESCs have been controversial. Using an siRNA knockown strategy, Xie et al. showed that KDM5B is a target of NANOG and critical for the self-renewal of ESCs (Xie et al. 2011). On the other hand, using both shRNA knockdown and cre-mediated knockout techniques, Schmitz et al. showed that depletion of KDM5B does not affect the growth or morphology of ESC, and KDM5B is dispensable for ESC self-renewal, but KDM5B depletion blocks differentiation along the neural lineage, due to global increase of H3K4me3 levels and failure to silence stem- and germ-cell related genes (Schmitz et al. 2011). Similarly, depletion of KDM5B using shRNA impairs ESC differentiation to embryoid bodies, leading to partial retention in a self-renewal stage (Kidder et al. 2013).

6.4.3 Tissue-Specific Development

KDM5s have tissue-specific roles in development. A major development phenotype associated with KDM5 is the regulation of neuronal development by KDM5C. KDM5C is mainly expressed in neuronal tissues with critical functions in neuronal development (Jensen et al. 2005). Genetic mutations in KDM5C cause Claes-Jensen-type X-linked intellectual disability (XLID) (Claes et al. 2000; Jensen et al. 2005). It was estimated that mutations in KDM5C account for 0.7–3% of males with XLID (Goncalves et al. 2014; Zamurrad et al. 2018). In neural maturation, KDM5C controls the induction of genes invovled in synaptic plasticity and memory consolidation, by regulating their enhancers (Scandaglia et al. 2017). Out of neuronal cells, KDM5C binds to the REST complex to suppress gene neuron-restrictive silencing elements (Tahiliani et al. 2007). KDM5A and KDM5B mutations were also identified in mental disorders (Najmabadi et al. 2011; Iossifov et al. 2012, 2014; De Rubeis et al. 2014; Al-Mubarak et al. 2017; Lebrun et al. 2018). The function of KDM5 in neuronal development was further shown by a *Drosophila* model, in which the fly carrying a human disease causal KDM5C mutation displayed impaired learning and memory (Zamurrad et al. 2018).

Besides neuronal/mental functions, KDM5A has been shown to control bone morphogenic protein 2-induced osteogenic differentiation of bone mesenchymal stem cells during osteoporosis (Wang et al. 2016a). KDM5B loss decreases the expression of key regulators of mammary morphogenesis and luminal lineage specification and delays mammary gland development (Zou et al. 2014). These results are consistent with the phenotype caused by ARID domain deletion in KDM5B, which also leads to delayed terminal end bud development and side branching (Catchpole et al. 2011). KDM5B also regulates the proliferation of vascular smooth muscle cells under chronic hypoxia-induced pulmonary hypertension conditions (Li et al. 2018). Overexpression of KDM5B increases the proliferation and migration of pulmonary artery smooth muscle cells through vascular endothelial growth factor via the NFκB pathway (Li et al. 2018). Knockdown of all expressed KDM5 in white and brown preadipocytes blocks differentiation to mature adipocytes in an adipocyte differentiation assay (Brier et al. 2016). KDM5D, located in Y chromosome, is critical for male spermatogenesis (Akimoto et al. 2008).

6.4.4 Immune Regulation

KDM5 proteins were shown to regulate immune responses in multiple cell types. KDM5A regulates the innate immune response of natural killer (NK) cells and is requied for NK cell activation through interacting with p50 to repress the expression of suppressor of cytokine signaling 1 (SOCS1) (Zhao et al. 2016). KDM5A deletion in mice makes them more susceptible to Listeria monocytogenes infection with reduced IFN-γ production (Zhao et al. 2016). Phosphorylation and nuclear localization of STAT4 are profoundly impaired by KDM5A loss, leading to increased SOCS1 expression (Zhao et al. 2016). Mechasnistic studies further showed that KDM5A and p50 bind to the *Socs1* promoter, remove H3K4me3 and repress SOCS1 signaling (Zhao et al. 2016) (Fig. 6.4a). This study highlights the critical functions of KDM5A in regulating the innate immune system. KDM5A has also been shown to interact with PIASy, a protein inhibitor of activated signal transducer and activator of transcription (PIAS) family member to repress IFN-β through its H3K4me3 demethylase activities in mouse embryonic fibroblasts (MEFs) (Yu et al. 2017).

Similarly, KDM5B has been shown to repress type I IFN and other innate cytokines to promote Th2 response after respiratory syncytial virus (RSV) infection (Fig. 6.4b), which contributes to chronic disease development (Ptaschinski et al. 2015). KDM5B can be upregulated in RSV-infected bone marrow-derived DCs (BMDCs). Inhibition of KDM5B in BMDCs leads to increased IFN-β, as well as increased IL-6 and TNF-α. In *Kdm5b*$^{f/f}$*-CD11c-Cre+* mice, KDM5B depletion resulted in higher induction of IFN-γ and decreased Th2 pathogenesis including decreased inflammation-related IL-4, IL-5, and IL-13 production and less mucus production after RSV infection in the lungs (Ptaschinski et al. 2015). Consistently, in human monocyte-derived DCs cocultured with RSV-reactivated CD4+ T cells, KDM5B inhibitor treatment leads to increased innate cytokine levels and decreased Th2 cytokines (Ptaschinski et al. 2015).

In the cancer setting, KDM5B and KDM5C can epigenetically suppress STING [cyclic GMP-AMP (cGAMP) synthase (cGAS) stimulator of interferon genes], which senses pathogen-derived or abnormal self-DNA in the cytosol and activates innate immunity (Wu et al. 2018; Zheng et al. 2023) (Fig. 6.4c). In a mouse syngeneic epithelial ovarian cancer model, it has been shown that KDM5A inhibition can reactivate antigen-presentation pathway and promote anti-tumor immunity mediated by CD8$^+$ T cells (Liu et al. 2022a). These studies highlighted the potential of KDM5 inhibition as a STING inducer to improve the efficacy of immunotherapy. Moreover, KDM5B recruits H3K9 methyltransferase SETDB1 to repress endogenous retroelements in a demethylase-independent manner in melanoma cells (Zhang et al. 2021) (Fig. 6.4d). KDM5B loss leads to de-repression of these endogenous retroelements including *MMVL30* to activate cytosolic RNA and DNA sensing pathways, leading to induced interfereon response (Zhang et al. 2021). These changes lead to the rejection of KDM5B knockout tumors and induction of immune memory response against wild type tumors (Zhang et al. 2021), suggesting that KDM5B depletion therapy could suppress tumor recurrence. On the other hand, increased KDM5A overexpression in tumors was also shown to enhance response to PD-1 antibody treatment in mouse cancer models (Wang et al. 2020), suggesting that KDM5A level needs to be maintained at a certain range to avoid immune responses.

6.4.5 Aging

Loss of KDM5A in MEFs leads to cellular senescence (Lin et al. 2011), but the fundamental studies that connect KDM5 and aging

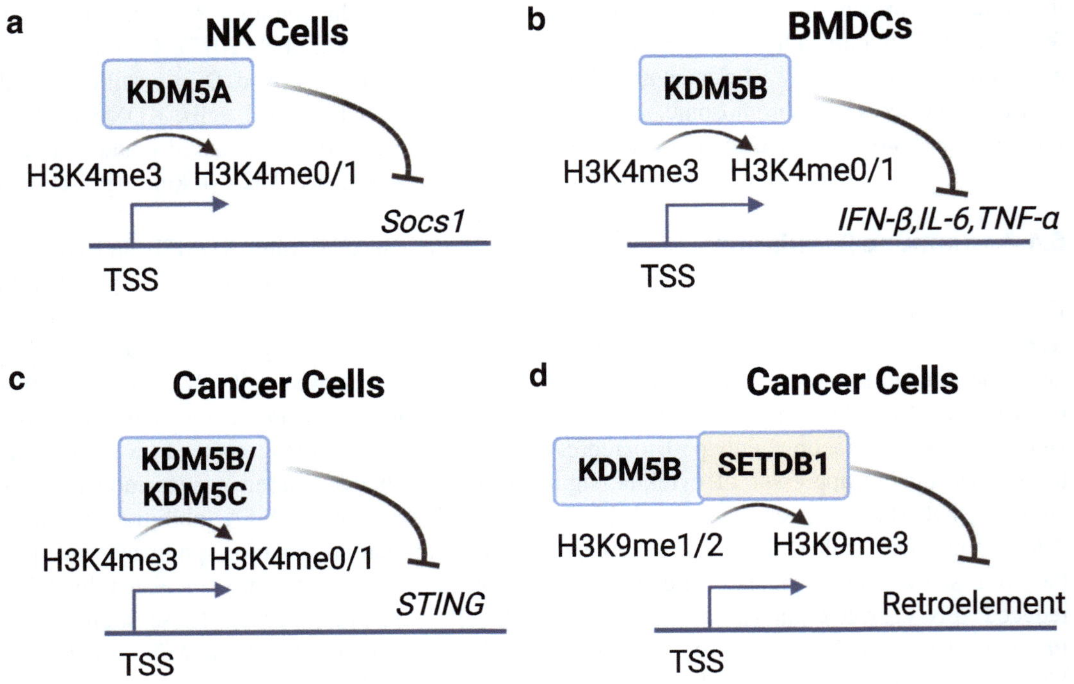

Fig. 6.4 Epigenetic regulation of immune responses by KDM5A/B. **a** KDM5A demethylates H3K4me3 at the *Socs1* promoter to prime activation of NK cells. **b** KDM5B demethylates H4K4me3 at the promoters of proinflammatory cytokine genes in DCs to suppress Th1 response and promote Th2 response, contributing to pulmonary pathogenesis. **c** KDM5B and KDM5C demethylates H3K4me3 at the *STING* promoter to suppress interferon response. **d** KDM5B recruits SETDB1 to deposit H3K9me3 marks at the retroelements, suppressing interferon response and anti-tumor immune responses. TSS, transcriptional start site. Created with BioRender.com

were done in *C. elegans* (Greer et al. 2010, 2011). It was shown that loss of Rbr-2 shortened lifespan in warm, while loss of Ash-2 histone methytransferase complex, the counterpart of KDM5, led to longevity (Greer et al. 2010). Interestingly, a followup study published by the same group found that this H3K4me3 methylation-dependent lifespan alteration can be transgenerationally inherited. They showed that deficiencies in the Ash-2 histone methyltransferase complex in the parental warms extend the lifespan of their descendents up to the third generation, and the transgenerational inheritance depends on Rbr-2 (Greer et al. 2011). It is one of the few examples that histone modifications affect transgenerational phenotypes. It would be interesting to determine if such phenotypes can be observed in mammals.

6.5 KDM5 in Cancer

6.5.1 KDM5A

KDM5A was found to be amplified in breast cancer (Hou et al. 2012) and head and neck cancer (Li et al. 2014). Overexpression of KDM5A has been observed in many cancer types including glioblastoma (Banelli et al. 2015), gastric carcinoma (Zeng et al. 2010), hepatocellular carcinoma (Wang et al. 2017), non-small cell lung cancer (Teng et al. 2013), neuroendocrine tumors (Maggi et al. 2016), ovarian cancer (Feng et al. 2017), highly metastatic breast cancer (Cao et al. 2014), and osteosarcoma (Peng et al. 2021). KDM5A was shown to drive cell growth, survival, angiogenesis, invasion, migration, and inhibit differentiation and senescence (Yang et al. 2021).

Using genetically engineered mouse models, it has been shown that deletion of the *Kdm5a* gene suppressed tumor initiation and growth caused by loss of tumor suppressor genes, such as *Rb1* and *Men1* (Lin et al. 2011; McBrayer et al. 2018; Oser et al. 2019) or by amplification of oncogenes, such as *Neu* (rat *Her2*) (Cao et al. 2014), suggesting that KDM5A targeted therapy is effective in the related settings in patients.

Knockdown of *KDM5A* in cancer cells with increased KDM5A expression usually leads to growth arrest, senescence, apoptosis, or differentiation (Zeng et al. 2010; Hou et al. 2012; Ohguchi et al. 2021; Xu et al. 2021). Mechanically, KDM5A loss induced upregulation of cyclin-dependent kinase inhibitors, such as p16, p21, p27, and p57 (Zeng et al. 2010; Hou et al. 2012; Teng et al. 2013; Maggi et al. 2016; Peng et al. 2021), some of which were shown as direct targets of KDM5A. Furthermore, KDM5A promotes metastasis in multiple cancer types. The expression level of KDM5A is associated with poor survival of estrogen receptor (ER) negative breast patients (Cao et al. 2014). Loss of KDM5A suppressed metastasis in animal models of breast (Cao et al. 2014), lung (Teng et al. 2013; Oser et al. 2019), and ovarian cancers (Feng et al. 2017).

6.5.2 KDM5B

KDM5B has more restricted expression in normal human adult tissues (Barrett et al. 2002). Similar to KDM5A, KDM5B is upregulated and contributes to tumor growth in multiple cancer types, including gastric cancer (Wang et al. 2015c; Zheng et al. 2019), lung cancer (Shen et al. 2015), prostate cancer (Xiang et al. 2007), hepatocellular carcinoma (Wang et al. 2016b), glioma (Dai et al. 2014; Fang et al. 2016), head and neck cancer (Cui et al. 2015; Facompre et al. 2016), and chronic myeloid leukemia (Xue et al. 2020).

The studies in breast cancer and melanoma have built up the foundations for the oncogenic function of KDM5B. KDM5B controls mammary gland development by regulating lineage specification genes (Catchpole et al. 2011; Zou et al. 2014). In breast tumors, copy number gain of the *KDM5B* gene and upregulation of KDM5B expression is commonly found (Lu et al. 1999; Barrett et al. 2002; Yamamoto et al. 2014). The increased activity of KDM5B in tumor tissues is associated with poor prognosis in ER+ breast cancer (Yamamoto et al. 2014; Hinohara et al. 2018). KDM5B promotes tumor growth by suppressing tumor suppressive microRNA let-7e (Mitra et al. 2011), and CDK inhibitor p21 (Cip) (Wong et al. 2012), and shortening 3′UTR of the cyclin D1 gene (Blair et al. 2016). Thus, downregulation of KDM5B restores these anti-tumor mechanisms and induces growth arrest. Specifically, KDM5B was shown as a luminal lineage-specific oncogenic driver (Yamamoto et al. 2014). Loss of KDM5B switched gene expression profile from luminal-like to basal-like programs (Yamamoto et al. 2014). Additionally, high KDM5B expression is linked to cellular transcriptomic heterogeneity, as shown by single-cell RNA sequencing (Hinohara et al. 2018). These findings highlight KDM5B as an important oncogene in breast cancer.

In melanoma, KDM5B has been found to regulate cellular heterogeneity. KDM5B defines a small subpopulation of slow-cycling melanoma cells (Roesch et al. 2010). Although these KDM5B^{high} cells grow extremely slowly, they are required for the continuous tumor growth of melanoma (Roesch et al. 2010). On the other hand, this subpopulation is temporarily distinct and dynamic and does not follow a unidirectional cancer stem cell hierarchy (Roesch et al. 2010). Interestingly, the KDM5B^{high} cells express different cell surface markers (Liu et al. 2019), and are resistant to chemo and targeted drugs (Roesch et al. 2013; Liu et al. 2019). Targeting this population by inhibiting KDM5B directly or mitochondrial respiration, which is dysregulated in this population, sensitizes melanoma to treatment (Roesch et al. 2013; Liu et al. 2019). In addition, enforced KDM5B expression can induce cell cycle arrest, direct melanoma cells toward into a persister state, promote lineage reprograming and thus lead to a lineage-directed vulnerability (Chauvistre et al. 2022).

In acute myeloid leukemia, KDM5B directly binds and represses AML stemness genes in a demethylase-independent manner. More specifically, depending on its chromatin association and/or scaffold functions, KDM5B targets "bivalent" chromatin domains, which are directly repressed by PRC2 (Ren et al. 2022).

6.5.3 KDM5C

KDM5C has been associated with oncogenesis, such as in breast and prostate cancer (Stein et al. 2014; Wang et al. 2015b). However, unlike KDM5A and KDM5B, which are generally considered oncogenes, the tumor suppressive function of KDM5C has been more well-established, especially in kidney cancer.

In clear cell renal cell carcinoma (ccRCC), KDM5C is among the most frequently mutated genes, with a significant percentage of truncation mutations (Dalgliesh et al. 2010). It was reported that dysfunction of KDM5C in ccRCC leads to heterochromatin disruption and genomic instability (Rondinelli et al. 2015). In $VHL^{-/-}$ ccRCC cells, knockdown of *KDM5C* significantly enhanced tumor growth, because it releases the suppressive effects of some HIF-induced genes (Niu et al. 2011; Liao et al. 2018). In addition, KDM5C inactivation is associated with poor prognosis in ccRCC patients (Rondinelli et al. 2015).

6.5.4 KDM5D

The functions of KDM5D in cancer are understudied compared with the other KDM5 members. Frequently loss of the *KDM5D* gene, which is localized on the Y chromosome, in prostate cancer and ccRCC, suggested its potential tumor suppressive functions (Perinchery et al. 2000; Komura et al. 2016; Li et al. 2016; Arseneault et al. 2017). In fact, KDM5D represses metastasis-associated genes including MMPs and SLUG to inhibit invasion of prostate cancer cells (Li et al. 2016).

6.5.5 KDM5 and Drug Resistance

Resistance to chemo and targeted therapeutics is the major challenge in treating cancer. Various mechanisms of resistance, such as block of drug-target interaction, activation of alternative pathways, or increased drug efflux or metabolism, have been characterized (Workman and Travers 2010). However, recent studies highlighted that epigenetic mechanisms, including KDM5-mediated histone demethylation, contribute to the development of drug resistance in various models (Plch et al. 2019) (Fig. 6.5).

A landmark study in 2010 reported that KDM5A is required for a reversible gefitinib-tolerant state in lung cancer cells (Sharma et al. 2010), linking an epigenetic mechanism to drug resistance for the first time. Since then, KDM5A has been shown as a critical factor for the resistance to temozolomide in glioblastoma (Banelli et al. 2015) and erlotinib in breast cancer (Hou et al. 2012). Similarly, KDM5B contributes to the resistance to endocrine therapy in breast cancer (Hinohara et al. 2018), cisplatin in neuroblastoma (Kuo et al. 2015), cisplatin, BRAF inhibitor, and MEK inhibitor in melanoma (Roesch et al. 2013; Liu et al. 2019; Shannan et al. 2019), and cisplatin in gastric cancer (Xu et al. 2018). In these studies, KDM5A or KDM5B was found to be upregulated in drug-tolerant cells, while in vitro knockdown of KDM5A or KDM5B in drug-tolerant cells re-sensitized them to drug treatment. Additional associations in clinical data between KDM5 and drug resistance have been observed, such as KDM5B and chemotherapy in ovarian cancer (Wang et al. 2015a), KDM5C and anti-VEGFR therapies in ccRCC (Ho et al. 2016), KDM5C and sunitinib in ccRCC (Hsieh et al. 2017), and KDM5C and radical prostatectomy in prostate cancer (Stein et al. 2014). On the other hand, KDM5C mutation and loss of KDM5D were associated with resistance to chemo in AML (Zhan et al. 2018) and docetaxel in prostate cancer (Komura et al. 2016), respectively.

Context-dependent mechanisms have been suggested in these studies to explain

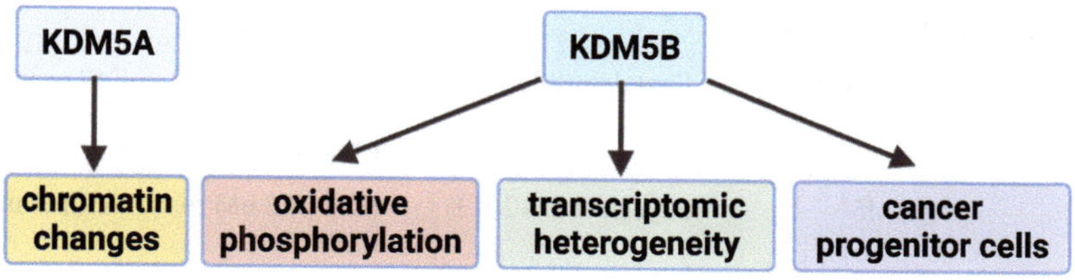

Fig. 6.5 The mechanisms by which KDM5A/B promote resistance to anti-cancer drugs. Created with BioRender.com

KDM5-mediated resistance, e.g., the insulin-like growth factor 1 receptor (IGF1R) kinase and histone deacetylases (HDACs) are involved in KDM5A-mediated gefitinib resistance (Sharma et al. 2010). Mitochondrial oxidative phosphorylation is related to KDM5B-high, slow-growing, and drug-resistant melanoma cells (Roesch et al. 2013). The impact of KDM5, particularly KDM5A and KDM5B, in promoting drug resistance appears to be consistent across multiple cancer types and with various chemotherapy or targeted drugs. These results suggest the existence of common molecular mechanisms. In ER+ breast cancer, KDM5B was shown to promote cellular transcriptomic heterogeneity and therefore increases the probability of therapeutic resistance (Hinohara et al. 2018). It is unclear yet whether this finding is a common mechanism behind most KDM5-mediated drug resistance. However, such an explanation is not against specific signal pathways discovered in the other KDM5/drug resistance studies. Most importantly, biochemical inhibition of KDM5 directly, or KDM5-associated HDACs prevents drug resistance emerging or inhibits the growth of drug resistance cells (Sharma et al. 2010; Gale et al. 2016; Vinogradova et al. 2016; Dalvi et al. 2017), highlighting KDM5 inhibitors as a potential therapeutic strategy to treat or prevent drug resistance.

6.6 KDM5 Inhibitors

Although the pivotal roles of KDM5 in cancer have been well-documented, the development of KDM5 inhibitors for investigating and potential clinical applications progresses relatively slowly, compared with other suppressive epigenetic targets, such as LSD1 and EZH2. One of the reasons is the structural similarity of the catalytic domains between KDM5 and other KDM families, especially KDM4 and KDM6 (Johansson et al. 2016; Taylor-Papadimitriou and Burchell 2017). The major KDM5 selective inhibitors are summarized in Table 6.1.

KDM5 family demethylases require 2-oxoglutarate (2-OG) as a co-substrate and could be inhibited by structurally related tricarboxylic acid (TCA) cycle metabolites, e.g., oxaloacetate and succinate, which can compete for 2-OG binding (Tarhonskaya et al. 2017). The activities of KDM5 family demethylases can be inhibited by fumarate, which has a similar molecular structure to α-ketoglutarate, acting as an antagonizing factor, thereby inhibiting demethylase activity (Lu et al. 2012; Xiao et al. 2012). In fact, many reported inhibitors for the KDM5 family are analogs of its co-factor 2-OG, such as N-oxalyl glycine (NOG), 2,4-pyridine dicarboxylic acid (2,4-PDA), or compounds with strong metal chelators, such as 2,2-bipyridines or hydroxyquinolines (Gehling et al. 2016). Although these compounds have potent biochemical inhibitory activity, they have limited selectivity and cell permeability. Several pan-inhibitors of the jumonji family of histone demethylases have been identified. Using a cell-based screen for epigenetic modulators of a GFP-linked transgene, JIB-04 was identified as a pan-inhibitor targeting jumonji family histone demethylases (Wang et al. 2013). GSK-J1, initially identified as a selective inhibitor for KDM6/JMJD3/UTX, can also inhibit KDM5 family demethylases in vitro (Kruidenier et al. 2012; Heinemann et al. 2014). Initially

Table 6.1 Selective KDM5 inhibitors

Compound name	Selectivity	First described	Best biochemical activity against KDM5	Cell or in vivo experiments
PBIT	KDM5	Sayegh et al. (2013)	IC50 of 3 μM for KDM5B	Cell permeable
YUKA1	KDM5A/C but not KDM5B	Gale et al. (2016)	IC50 of 2.7 μM for KDM5A	Cell permeable
GSK-J1	KDM6, KDM5	Kruidenier et al. (2012)	IC50 of 0.17 μM for KDM5B	Low cellular permeability
GSK-J4	KDM6, KDM5	Kruidenier et al. (2012)	IC50 of 1 μM for KDM5B	Cell permeable, used in mouse work
GSK-467	KDM6, KDM4, KDM5	Westaway et al. (2016b)	IC50 of 26 nM for KDM5B	Cell permeable
KDM5-C49 (GS-080)	KDM5, KDM4	Horton et al. (2016b), Johansson et al. (2016)	IC50 of 25 nM for KDM5A	Low cellular permeability
KDM5-C70 (GS-5801)	KDM5, KDM4	Horton et al. (2016b), Johansson et al. (2016)	IC50 of 0.3 μM for KDM5A	Cell permeable, used in mouse work and human trial
KDOAM-25	KDM5	Tumber et al. (2017)	IC50 of 19 nM for KDM5B	Cell permeable
JQKD82	KDM5	Ohguchi et al. (2021)	IC50 of ~ 0.3 μM for KDM5A	Cell permeable, used in mouse work
CPI-455	KDM5	Vinogradova et al. (2016)	IC50 of ~ 10 nM for KDM5A-C	Cell permeable, used in mouse work
CPI-48	KDM5	Liang et al. (2016)	IC50 of 15 nM for KDM5A	Cell permeable, used in mouse work
GDC-50	KDM5	Liang et al. (2017)	IC50 of 45 nM for KDM5A	Cell permeable, used in mouse work
Dong-A-167	KDM5	Wu et al. (2018)	IC50 of 0.2 μM for KDM5B	Cell permeable

IC50, half maximal inhibitory concentration

developed against KDM4, Westaway et al. reported cell permeable inhibitors with efficacy against KDM5, including GSK-467 (also called compound 41) (Westaway et al. 2016a, b).

The first KDM5 selective inhibitor PBIT was identified using a biochemical screen against recombinant full-length KDM5B (Sayegh et al. 2013). This cell permeable inhibitor is capable of inhibiting KDM5A-C at low micromolar concentration. Similar approach identified another cell permeable compound YUKA1 as an inhibitor of KDM5A, which also inhibits KDM5C with lower potency, but does not inhibit KDM5B (Gale et al. 2016), suggesting that it is possible to identify KDM5 family member-specific inhibitors.

KDM5-C49 (also known as GS-080), a 2,4-pyridinedicarboxylic acid analog, is a potent pan-KDM5 inhibitor with some activity against KDM4 enzymes in biochemical assays (Horton et al. 2016b; Johansson et al. 2016; Gilmore et al. 2022). Several derivatives of KDM5-C49 have been developed for cellular assays and animal experiments, including KDM5-C70, the ester pro-drug derived from KDM5-C49 (Horton et al. 2016b; Johansson et al. 2016); JQKD82, a phenol ester derivative of KDM5-C49 (Tumber et al. 2017); and KDOAM-25, the amide analog of KDM5-C70 (Ohguchi et al. 2021). These compounds can specifically increase cellular H3K4me3 levels (Horton et al. 2016b; Johansson et al. 2016; Tumber et al. 2017; Wu et al. 2018). KDOAM-25 was shown to have no off-target activity on a panel of 55 receptors and enzymes (Tumber et al. 2017). JQKD82 was shown to suppress the growth of myeloma in mouse xenografts (Ohguchi et al. 2021). Of note, KDM5-C70 (also known as GS-5801) has been tested in a clinical trial to treat chronic hepatitis B, but could not achieve the needed dose before liver toxicity occurred (Gilmore et al. 2022). In addition, despite strong in vitro effects, it has limited antiviral activity in humanized mouse model of hepatitis B, highlighting the challenge of translating these findings into the clinic (Gilmore et al. 2022).

CPI-455 was developed from a compound identified from a screen of KDM4C inhibitor but showed higher efficacy against KDM5A (Gehling et al. 2016; Vinogradova et al. 2016). CPI-455 is about 200-fold selective for KDM5 over KDM4, and inhibits KDM5A, KDM5B, and KDM5C with around 10 nM IC50s (Vinogradova et al. 2016). Although CPI-455 showed high cellular activity, low plasma clearance, and high oral exposure in mice, the relatively high plasma protein binding in vivo led to the unbound concentration of CPI-455 lower than its EC50 (Liang et al. 2016). A series of rationale-directed modifications were performed to generate additional derivatives. One of these derivatives is compound 48 (CPI-48), which showed high potency in vitro and good pharmacokinetics in vivo (Liang et al. 2016; Wu et al. 2018; Zheng et al. 2023). Indeed, when orally dosed twice a day at 50 mg/kg, the unbound maximal concentration is more than 15 times higher than its cellular potency, making it available for meaningful in vivo studies (Liang et al. 2016). Further development from the CPI-455, based on the structure of enzyme-inhibitor interaction, led to two covalent inhibitors of KDM5, which showed cellular activity of suppressing KDM5 (Vazquez-Rodriguez et al. 2019).

An independent compound that is selective for KDM5 inhibition was identified in another high-throughput screening. Structural analysis by NMR showed that it is competitive with histone tails to bind KDM5. This hit is structurally and mechanistically distinct from CPI-455. After several rounds of structure–activity relationship study guided by structure biology to further improve the biochemical and cellular potency, compound 50 (GDC-50) was obtained with promising in vivo pharmacokinetics profiles (Liang et al. 2017). Using a structure-based design, Nie et al. also discovered potent and selective KDM5 inhibitor compound 33, which has potent cellular activity in breast cancer cell line ZR-75-1 (Nie et al. 2018).

More than 30 KDM5 inhibitors have been systematically examined for their binding to KDM5 and ability to inhibit KDM5 (Horton et al. 2016b, 2018b; Wu et al. 2018; Gilmore et al. 2022; Tang et al. 2022). In addition to CPI-48, GDC-50, and KDM5-C70, Dong-A-167 was also shown to be a cell permeable KDM5 inhibitor that selectively induces global H3K4me3 level in cells (Wu et al. 2018). Among these inhibitors, more potent enzyme inhibition of KDM5A by the R-isoform of the cell permeable N54/N55 enantiomers correlates with their ability to inhibit cell growth (Horton et al. 2018a). Furthermore, protein degradation strategies have been explored to inhibit both catalytic function and scaffolding functions of KDM5C (Iida et al. 2021). These studies provide novel insights into further development of more potent and specific cell permeable KDM5 inhibitors for clinical applications.

6.7 Summary

In this chapter, we reviewed the recent advances in KDM5 family histone demethylases and their functions in gene regulation, development, and cancer. We also discussed available KDM5 inhibitory tool compounds. As the major demethylases in the human genome that remove

H3K4me3, a crucial transcriptional activation mark, KDM5s are involved in precise control of gene expression, thus playing key roles in cell fate determination and development. On the other hand, cancers commonly adapt KDM5-mediated mechanisms to promote tumor growth and to develop resistance to treatment, nominating KDM5s as ideal therapeutic targets. However, there are still unfilled knowledge gaps about the roles of KDM5 functions, e.g., why does loss or inhibition of KDM5, a general epigenetic regulator, only affect a limited number of genes while inducing global H3K4me3 changes, as shown in almost all the studies? On the flip side, this provides an optimal therapeutic strategy that only targets a subset of genes, thus could have fewer unintended side effects. Why are KDM5 enzymes oncogenic in one cell type, but tumor suppressive in another? What are their roles in tumor microenvironment? We expected that more potent and specific KDM5 inhibitors or degraders, especially individual KDM5 family member-specific compounds, will advance as anti-cancer drugs for clinical applications in the coming years.

Acknowledgements This work was partially supported by a start-up package from ShanghaiTech University (to S.M.Z.), Shanghai Pujiang Talent Program (No. 22PJ1411100) (to S.M.Z.), a start-up fund provided by Rutgers Cancer Institute of New Jersey and Cancer Center Support Grant P30CA072720 (to J.C.), and National Institutes of Health Awards R01CA272578 (to J.C.), R01CA237586 (to Q.Y.) and P50CA121974 (to Q.Y.).

References

Aasland R, Gibson TJ, Stewart AF (1995) The PHD finger: implications for chromatin-mediated transcriptional regulation. Trends Biochem Sci 20:56–59

Agulnik AI, Mitchell MJ, Lerner JL, Woods DR, Bishop CE (1994a) A mouse Y chromosome gene encoded by a region essential for spermatogenesis and expression of male-specific minor histocompatibility antigens. Hum Mol Genet 3:873–878

Agulnik AI, Mitchell MJ, Mattei MG, Borsani G, Avner PA, Lerner JL, Bishop CE (1994b) A novel X gene with a widely transcribed Y-linked homologue escapes X-inactivation in mouse and human. Hum Mol Genet 3:879–884

Akimoto C, Kitagawa H, Matsumoto T, Kato S (2008) Spermatogenesis-specific association of SMCY and MSH5. Genes Cells 13:623–633

Al-Mubarak B, Abouelhoda M, Omar A, AlDhalaan H, Aldosari M, Nester M, Alshamrani HA, El-Kalioby M, Goljan E, Albar R, Subhani S, Tahir A, Asfahani S, Eskandrani A, Almusaiab A, Magrashi A, Shinwari J, Monies D, Al TN (2017) Whole exome sequencing reveals inherited and de novo variants in autism spectrum disorder: a trio study from Saudi families. Sci Rep 7:5679

Albert M, Schmitz SU, Kooistra SM, Malatesta M, Morales Torres C, Rekling JC, Johansen JV, Abarrategui I, Helin K (2013) The histone demethylase Jarid1b ensures faithful mouse development by protecting developmental genes from aberrant H3K4me3. PLoS Genet 9:e1003461

Allis CD, Berger SL, Cote J, Dent S, Jenuwien T, Kouzarides T, Pillus L, Reinberg D, Shi Y, Shiekhattar R, Shilatifard A, Workman J, Zhang Y (2007) New nomenclature for chromatin-modifying enzymes. Cell 131:633–636

Arseneault M, Monlong J, Vasudev NS, Laskar RS, Safisamghabadi M, Harnden P, Egevad L, Nourbehesht N, Panichnantakul P, Holcatova I, Brisuda A, Janout V, Kollarova H, Foretova L, Navratilova M, Mates D, Jinga V, Zaridze D, Mukeria A, Jandaghi P, Brennan P, Brazma A, Tost J, Scelo G, Banks RE, Lathrop M, Bourque G, Riazalhosseini Y (2017) Loss of chromosome Y leads to down regulation of KDM5D and KDM6C epigenetic modifiers in clear cell renal cell carcinoma. Sci Rep 7:44876

Banelli B, Carra E, Barbieri F, Wurth R, Parodi F, Pattarozzi A, Carosio R, Forlani A, Allemanni G, Marubbi D, Florio T, Daga A, Romani M (2015) The histone demethylase KDM5A is a key factor for the resistance to temozolomide in glioblastoma. Cell Cycle (Georgetown, TX) 14:3418–3429

Barrett A, Madsen B, Copier J, Lu PJ, Cooper L, Scibetta AG, Burchell J, Taylor-Papadimitriou J (2002) PLU-1 nuclear protein, which is upregulated in breast cancer, shows restricted expression in normal human adult tissues: a new cancer/testis antigen? Int J Cancer 101:581–588

Barski A, Cuddapah S, Cui K, Roh T-Y, Schones DE, Wang Z, Wei G, Chepelev I, Zhao K (2007) High-resolution profiling of histone methylations in the human genome. Cell 129:823–837

Benevolenskaya EV, Murray HL, Branton P, Young RA, Kaelin WG Jr (2005) Binding of pRB to the PHD protein RBP2 promotes cellular differentiation. Mol Cell 18:623–635

Berger SL (2007) The complex language of chromatin regulation during transcription. Nature 447:407–412

Blair LP, Yan Q (2012) Epigenetic mechanisms in commonly occurring cancers. DNA Cell Biol 31(Suppl 1):S49-61

Blair LP, Cao J, Zou MR, Sayegh J, Yan Q (2011) Epigenetic regulation by lysine demethylase 5 (KDM5) enzymes in cancer. Cancers 3:1383–1404

Blair LP, Liu Z, Labitigan RL, Wu L, Zheng D, Xia Z, Pearson EL, Nazeer FI, Cao J, Lang SM, Rines RJ, Mackintosh SG, Moore CL, Li W, Tian B, Tackett AJ, Yan Q (2016) KDM5 lysine demethylases are involved in maintenance of 3′UTR length. Sci Adv 2:e1501662

Brier AB, Loft A, Madsen JG, Rosengren T, Nielsen R, Schmidt SF, Liu Z, Yan Q, Gronemeyer H, Mandrup S (2016) The KDM5 family is required for activation of pro-proliferative cell cycle genes during adipocyte differentiation. Nucleic Acids Res 45:1743–1759

Campos EI, Reinberg D (2009) Histones: annotating chromatin. Annu Rev Genet 43:559–599.

Cao J, Liu Z, Cheung William KC, Zhao M, Chen Sophia Y, Chan Siew W, Booth Carmen J, Nguyen Don X, Yan Q (2014) Histone demethylase RBP2 is critical for breast cancer progression and metastasis. Cell Rep 6:868–877

Catchpole S, Spencer-Dene B, Hall D, Santangelo S, Rosewell I, Guenatri M, Beatson R, Scibetta AG, Burchell JM, Taylor-Papadimitriou J (2011) PLU-1/JARID1B/KDM5B is required for embryonic survival and contributes to cell proliferation in the mammary gland and in ER+ breast cancer cells. Int J Oncol 38:1267–1277

Chan SW, Hong W (2001) Retinoblastoma-binding protein 2 (Rbp2) potentiates nuclear hormone receptor-mediated transcription. J Biol Chem 276:28402–28412

Chaturvedi CP, Somasundaram B, Singh K, Carpenedo RL, Stanford WL, Dilworth FJ, Brand M (2012) Maintenance of gene silencing by the coordinate action of the H3K9 methyltransferase G9a/KMT1C and the H3K4 demethylase Jarid1a/KDM5A. Proc Natl Acad Sci USA 109:18845–18850

Chauvistre H, Shannan B, Daignault-Mill SM, Ju RJ, Picard D, Egetemaier S, Varaljai R, Gibhardt CS, Sechi A, Kaschani F, Keminer O, Stehbens SJ, Liu Q, Yin X, Jeyakumar K, Vogel FCE, Krepler C, Rebecca VW, Kubat L, Lueong SS, Forster J, Horn S, Remke M, Ehrmann M, Paschen A, Becker JC, Helfrich I, Rauh D, Kaiser M, Gul S, Herlyn M, Bogeski I, Rodriguez-Lopez JN, Haass NK, Schadendorf D, Roesch A (2022) Persister state-directed transitioning and vulnerability in melanoma. Nat Commun 13:3055

Christensen J, Agger K, Cloos PA, Pasini D, Rose S, Sennels L, Rappsilber J, Hansen KH, Salcini AE, Helin K (2007) RBP2 belongs to a family of demethylases, specific for tri-and dimethylated lysine 4 on histone 3. Cell 128:1063–1076

Claes S, Devriendt K, Van Goethem G, Roelen L, Meireleire J, Raeymaekers P, Cassiman JJ, Fryns JP (2000) Novel syndromic form of X-linked complicated spastic paraplegia. Am J Med Genet 94:1–4

Consortium EP (2012) An integrated encyclopedia of DNA elements in the human genome. Nature 489:57–74

Cui Z, Song L, Hou Z, Han Y, Hu Y, Wu Y, Chen W, Mao L (2015) PLU-1/JARID1B overexpression predicts proliferation properties in head and neck squamous cell carcinoma. Oncol Rep 33:2454–2460

Dai B, Hu Z, Huang H, Zhu G, Xiao Z, Wan W, Zhang P, Jia W, Zhang L (2014) Overexpressed KDM5B is associated with the progression of glioma and promotes glioma cell growth via down regulating p21. Biochem Biophys Res Commun 454:221–227

Dalgliesh GL, Furge K, Greenman C, Chen L, Bignell G, Butler A, Davies H, Edkins S, Hardy C, Latimer C, Teague J, Andrews J, Barthorpe S, Beare D, Buck G, Campbell PJ, Forbes S, Jia M, Jones D, Knott H, Kok CY, Lau KW, Leroy C, Lin ML, McBride DJ, Maddison M, Maguire S, McLay K, Menzies A, Mironenko T, Mulderrig L, Mudie L, O'Meara S, Pleasance E, Rajasingham A, Shepherd R, Smith R, Stebbings L, Stephens P, Tang G, Tarpey PS, Turrell K, Dykema KJ, Khoo SK, Petillo D, Wondergem B, Anema J, Kahnoski RJ, Teh BT, Stratton MR, Futreal PA (2010) Systematic sequencing of renal carcinoma reveals inactivation of histone modifying genes. Nature 463:360–363

Dalvi MP, Wang L, Zhong R, Kollipara RK, Park H, Bayo J, Yenerall P, Zhou Y, Timmons BC, Rodriguez-Canales J, Behrens C, Mino B, Villalobos P, Parra ER, Suraokar M, Pataer A, Swisher SG, Kalhor N, Bhanu NV, Garcia BA, Heymach JV, Coombes K, Xie Y, Girard L, Gazdar AF, Kittler R, Wistuba II, Minna JD, Martinez ED (2017) Taxane-platin-resistant lung cancers co-develop hypersensitivity to JumonjiC demethylase inhibitors. Cell Rep 19:1669–1684

De Rubeis S, He X, Goldberg AP, Poultney CS, Samocha K, Cicek AE, Kou Y, Liu L, Fromer M, Walker S, Singh T, Klei L, Kosmicki J, Shih-Chen F, Aleksic B, Biscaldi M, Bolton PF, Brownfeld JM, Cai J, Campbell NG, Carracedo A, Chahrour MH, Chiocchetti AG, Coon H, Crawford EL, Curran SR, Dawson G, Duketis E, Fernandez BA, Gallagher L, Geller E, Guter SJ, Hill RS, Ionita-Laza J, Jimenz Gonzalez P, Kilpinen H, Klauck SM, Kolevzon A, Lee I, Lei I, Lei J, Lehtimaki T, Lin CF, Ma'ayan A, Marshall CR, McInnes AL, Neale B, Owen MJ, Ozaki N, Parellada M, Parr JR, Purcell S, Puura K, Rajagopalan D, Rehnstrom K, Reichenberg A, Sabo A, Sachse M, Sanders SJ, Schafer C, Schulte-Ruther M, Skuse D, Stevens C, Szatmari P, Tammimies K, Valladares O, Voran A, Li-San W, Weiss LA, Willsey AJ, Yu TW, Yuen RK, Cook EH, Freitag CM, Gill M, Hultman CM, Lehner T, Palotie A, Schellenberg GD, Sklar P, State MW, Sutcliffe JS, Walsh CA, Scherer SW, Zwick ME, Barett JC, Cutler DJ, Roeder K, Devlin B, Daly MJ, Buxbaum JD (2014) Synaptic, transcriptional and chromatin genes disrupted in autism. Nature 515:209–215

Defeo-Jones D, Huang PS, Jones RE, Haskell KM, Vuocolo GA, Hanobik MG, Huber HE, Oliff A (1991) Cloning of cDNAs for cellular proteins that bind to the retinoblastoma gene product. Nature 352:251–254

Drelon C, Belalcazar HM, Secombe J (2018) The histone demethylase KDM5 is essential for larval growth in *Drosophila*. Genetics 209:773–787

Facompre ND, Harmeyer KM, Sole X, Kabraji S, Belden Z, Sahu V, Whelan K, Tanaka K, Weinstein GS, Montone KT, Roesch A, Gimotty PA, Herlyn M, Rustgi AK, Nakagawa H, Ramaswamy S, Basu D (2016) JARID1B enables transit between distinct states of the stem-like cell population in oral cancers. Can Res 76:5538–5549

Fang L, Zhao J, Wang D, Zhu L, Wang J, Jiang K (2016) Jumonji AT-rich interactive domain 1B overexpression is associated with the development and progression of glioma. Int J Mol Med 38:172–182

Feng T, Wang Y, Lang Y, Zhang Y (2017) KDM5A promotes proliferation and EMT in ovarian cancer and closely correlates with PTX resistance. Mol Med Rep 16:3573–3580

Gale M, Sayegh J, Cao J, Norcia M, Gareiss P, Hoyer D, Merkel JS, Yan Q (2016) Screen-identified selective inhibitor of lysine demethylase 5A blocks cancer cell growth and drug resistance. Oncotarget 7:39931–39944

Ge Z, Li W, Wang N, Liu C, Zhu Q, Bjorkholm M, Gruber A, Xu D (2010) Chromatin remodeling: recruitment of histone demethylase RBP2 by Mad1 for transcriptional repression of a Myc target gene, telomerase reverse transcriptase. FASEB J Off Publ Fed Am Soc Exp Biol 24:579–586

Gehling VS, Bellon SF, Harmange JC, LeBlanc Y, Poy F, Odate S, Buker S, Lan F, Arora S, Williamson KE, Sandy P, Cummings RT, Bailey CM, Bergeron L, Mao W, Gustafson A, Liu Y, VanderPorten E, Audia JE, Trojer P, Albrecht BK (2016) Identification of potent, selective KDM5 inhibitors. Bioorg Med Chem Lett 26:4350–4354

Gildea JJ, Lopez R, Shearn A (2000) A screen for new trithorax group genes identified little imaginal discs, the *Drosophila melanogaster* homologue of human retinoblastoma binding protein 2. Genetics 156:645–663

Gilmore SA, Tam D, Cheung TL, Snyder C, Farand J, Dick R, Matles M, Feng JY, Ramirez R, Li L, Yu H, Xu Y, Barnes D, Czerwieniec G, Brendza KM, Appleby TC, Birkus G, Willkom M, Kobayashi T, Paoli E, Labelle M, Boesen T, Tay CH, Delaney WE, Notte GT, Schmitz U, Feierbach B (2022) Characterization of a KDM5 small molecule inhibitor with antiviral activity against hepatitis B virus. PloS One 17:e0271145

Goncalves TF, Goncalves AP, Fintelman Rodrigues N, dos Santos JM, Pimentel MM, Santos-Reboucas CB (2014) KDM5C mutational screening among males with intellectual disability suggestive of X-linked inheritance and review of the literature. Eur J Med Genet 57:138–144

Greer EL, Maures TJ, Hauswirth AG, Green EM, Leeman DS, Maro GS, Han S, Banko MR, Gozani O, Brunet A (2010) Members of the H3K4 trimethylation complex regulate lifespan in a germline-dependent manner in *C. elegans*. Nature 466:383–387

Greer EL, Maures TJ, Ucar D, Hauswirth AG, Mancini E, Lim JP, Benayoun BA, Shi Y, Brunet A (2011) Transgenerational epigenetic inheritance of longevity in *Caenorhabditis elegans*. Nature 479:365–371

Hayakawa T, Ohtani Y, Hayakawa N, Shinmyozu K, Saito M, Ishikawa F, Nakayama J (2007) RBP2 is an MRG15 complex component and down-regulates intragenic histone H3 lysine 4 methylation. Genes Cells 12:811–826

He R, Kidder BL (2017) H3K4 demethylase KDM5B regulates global dynamics of transcription elongation and alternative splicing in embryonic stem cells. Nucleic Acids Res. 45:6427–6441

Heinemann B, Nielsen JM, Hudlebusch HR, Lees MJ, Larsen DV, Boesen T, Labelle M, Gerlach LO, Birk P, Helin K (2014) Inhibition of demethylases by GSK-J1/J4. Nature 514:E1-2

Heintzman ND, Stuart RK, Hon G, Fu Y, Ching CW, Hawkins RD, Barrera LO, Van Calcar S, Qu C, Ching KA, Wang W, Weng Z, Green RD, Crawford GE, Ren B (2007) Distinct and predictive chromatin signatures of transcriptional promoters and enhancers in the human genome. Nat Genet 39:311

Heintzman ND, Hon GC, Hawkins RD, Kheradpour P, Stark A, Harp LF, Ye Z, Lee LK, Stuart RK, Ching CW, Ching KA, Antosiewicz-Bourget JE, Liu H, Zhang X, Green RD, Lobanenkov VV, Stewart R, Thomson JA, Crawford GE, Kellis M, Ren B (2009) Histone modifications at human enhancers reflect global cell-type-specific gene expression. Nature 459:108–112

Hinohara K, Wu HJ, Vigneau S, McDonald TO, Igarashi KJ, Yamamoto KN, Madsen T, Fassl A, Egri SB, Papanastasiou M, Ding L, Peluffo G, Cohen O, Kales SC, Lal-Nag M, Rai G, Maloney DJ, Jadhav A, Simeonov A, Wagle N, Brown M, Meissner A, Sicinski P, Jaffe JD, Jeselsohn R, Gimelbrant AA, Michor F, Polyak K (2018) KDM5 histone demethylase activity links cellular transcriptomic heterogeneity to therapeutic resistance. Cancer Cell 34:939-953. e939

Ho TH, Choueiri TK, Wang K, Karam JA, Chalmers Z, Frampton G, Elvin JA, Johnson A, Liu X, Lin Y, Joseph RW, Stanton ML, Miller VA, Stephens PJ, Ross JS, Ali SM, Pal SK (2016) Correlation between molecular subclassifications of clear cell renal cell carcinoma and targeted therapy response. Eur Urol Focus 2:204–209

Horton JR, Engstrom A, Zoeller EL, Liu X, Shanks JR, Zhang X, Johns MA, Vertino PM, Fu H, Cheng X (2016a) Characterization of a linked jumonji domain of the KDM5/JARID1 family of histone H3 lysine 4 demethylases. J Biol Chem 291:2631–2646

Horton JR, Liu X, Gale M, Wu L, Shanks JR, Zhang X, Webber PJ, Bell JSK, Kales SC, Mott BT, Rai G, Jansen DJ, Henderson MJ, Urban DJ, Hall MD, Simeonov A, Maloney DJ, Johns MA, Fu H, Jadhav A, Vertino PM, Yan Q, Cheng X (2016b) Structural basis for KDM5A histone lysine demethylase inhibition by diverse compounds. Cell Chem Biol 23:769–781

Horton JR, Liu X, Wu L, Zhang K, Shanks J, Zhang X, Rai G, Mott BT, Jansen DJ, Kales SC, Henderson MJ, Pohida K, Fang Y, Hu X, Jadhav A, Maloney DJ, Hall MD, Simeonov A, Fu H, Vertino PM, Yan Q, Cheng X (2018a) Insights into the action of inhibitor enantiomers against histone lysine demethylase 5A. J Med Chem 61:3193–3208

Horton JR, Woodcock CB, Chen Q, Liu X, Zhang X, Shanks J, Rai G, Mott BT, Jansen DJ, Kales SC, Henderson MJ, Cyr M, Pohida K, Hu X, Shah P, Xu X, Jadhav A, Maloney DJ, Hall MD, Simeonov A, Fu H, Vertino PM, Cheng X (2018b) Structure-based engineering of irreversible inhibitors against histone lysine demethylase KDM5A. J Med Chem 61:10588–10601

Hou J, Wu J, Dombkowski A, Zhang K, Holowatyj A, Boerner JL, Yang ZQ (2012) Genomic amplification and a role in drug-resistance for the KDM5A histone demethylase in breast cancer. Am J Transl Res 4:247–256

Hsieh JJ, Chen D, Wang PI, Marker M, Redzematovic A, Chen YB, Selcuklu SD, Weinhold N, Bouvier N, Huberman KH, Bhanot U, Chevinsky MS, Patel P, Pinciroli P, Won HH, You D, Viale A, Lee W, Hakimi AA, Berger MF, Socci ND, Cheng EH, Knox J, Voss MH, Voi M, Motzer RJ (2017) Genomic biomarkers of a randomized trial comparing first-line everolimus and sunitinib in patients with metastatic renal cell carcinoma. Eur Urol 71:405–414

Iida T, Itoh Y, Takahashi Y, Yamashita Y, Kurohara T, Miyake Y, Oba M, Suzuki T (2021) Design, synthesis, and biological evaluation of lysine demethylase 5 C degraders. ChemMedChem 16:1609–1618

Iossifov I, Ronemus M, Levy D, Wang Z, Hakker I, Rosenbaum J, Yamrom B, Lee YH, Narzisi G, Leotta A, Kendall J, Grabowska E, Ma B, Marks S, Rodgers L, Stepansky A, Troge J, Andrews P, Bekritsky M, Pradhan K, Ghiban E, Kramer M, Parla J, Demeter R, Fulton LL, Fulton RS, Magrini VJ, Ye K, Darnell JC, Darnell RB, Mardis ER, Wilson RK, Schatz MC, McCombie WR, Wigler M (2012) De novo gene disruptions in children on the autistic spectrum. Neuron 74:285–299

Iossifov I, O'Roak BJ, Sanders SJ, Ronemus M, Krumm N, Levy D, Stessman HA, Witherspoon KT, Vives L, Patterson KE, Smith JD, Paeper B, Nickerson DA, Dea J, Dong S, Gonzalez LE, Mandell JD, Mane SM, Murtha MT, Sullivan CA, Walker MF, Waqar Z, Wei L, Willsey AJ, Yamrom B, Lee YH, Grabowska E, Dalkic E, Wang Z, Marks S, Andrews P, Leotta A, Kendall J, Hakker I, Rosenbaum J, Ma B, Rodgers L, Troge J, Narzisi G, Yoon S, Schatz MC, Ye K, McCombie WR, Shendure J, Eichler EE, State MW, Wigler M (2014) The contribution of de novo coding mutations to autism spectrum disorder. Nature 515:216–221

Iwase S, Lan F, Bayliss P, de la Torre-Ubieta L, Huarte M, Qi HH, Whetstine JR, Bonni A, Roberts TM, Shi Y (2007) The X-linked mental retardation gene SMCX/JARID1C defines a family of histone H3 lysine 4 demethylases. Cell 128:1077–1088

Iwase S, Brookes E, Agarwal S, Badeaux AI, Ito H, Vallianatos CN, Tomassy GS, Kasza T, Lin G, Thompson A, Gu L, Kwan KY, Chen C, Sartor MA, Egan B, Xu J, Shi Y (2016) A mouse model of X-linked intellectual disability associated with impaired removal of histone methylation. Cell Rep 14:1000–1009

Jensen LR, Amende M, Gurok U, Moser B, Gimmel V, Tzschach A, Janecke AR, Tariverdian G, Chelly J, Fryns JP, Van Esch H, Kleefstra T, Hamel B, Moraine C, Gecz J, Turner G, Reinhardt R, Kalscheuer VM, Ropers HH, Lenzner S (2005) Mutations in the JARID1C gene, which is involved in transcriptional regulation and chromatin remodeling, cause X-linked mental retardation. Am J Hum Genet 76:227–236

Johansson C, Velupillai S, Tumber A, Szykowska A, Hookway ES, Nowak RP, Strain-Damerell C, Gileadi C, Philpott M, Burgess-Brown N, Wu N, Kopec J, Nuzzi A, Steuber H, Egner U, Badock V, Munro S, LaThangue NB, Westaway S, Brown J, Athanasou N, Prinjha R, Brennan PE, Oppermann U (2016) Structural analysis of human KDM5B guides histone demethylase inhibitor development. Nat Chem Biol 12:539–545

Kidder BL, Hu G, Yu ZX, Liu C, Zhao K (2013) Extended self-renewal and accelerated reprogramming in the absence of Kdm5b. Mol Cell Biol 33:4793–4810

Kidder BL, Hu G, Zhao K (2014) KDM5B focuses H3K4 methylation near promoters and enhancers during embryonic stem cell self-renewal and differentiation. Genome Biol 15:R32

Klein BJ, Piao L, Xi Y, Rincon-Arano H, Rothbart SB, Peng D, Wen H, Larson C, Zhang X, Zheng X, Cortazar MA, Pena PV, Mangan A, Bentley DL, Strahl BD, Groudine M, Li W, Shi X, Kutateladze TG (2014) The histone-H3K4-specific demethylase KDM5B binds to its substrate and product through distinct PHD fingers. Cell Rep 6:325–335

Klose RJ, Kallin EM, Zhang Y (2006) JmjC-domain-containing proteins and histone demethylation. Nat Rev Genet 7:715–727

Klose RJ, Yan Q, Tothova Z, Yamane K, Erdjument-Bromage H, Tempst P, Gilliland DG, Zhang Y, Kaelin WG (2007) The retinoblastoma binding protein RBP2 is an H3K4 demethylase. Cell 128:889–900

Koch CM, Andrews RM, Flicek P, Dillon SC, Karaoz U, Clelland GK, Wilcox S, Beare DM, Fowler JC,

Couttet P, James KD, Lefebvre GC, Bruce AW, Dovey OM, Ellis PD, Dhami P, Langford CF, Weng Z, Birney E, Carter NP, Vetrie D, Dunham I (2007) The landscape of histone modifications across 1% of the human genome in five human cell lines. Genome Res 17:691–707

Komura K, Jeong SH, Hinohara K, Qu F, Wang X, Hiraki M, Azuma H, Lee GS, Kantoff PW, Sweeney CJ (2016) Resistance to docetaxel in prostate cancer is associated with androgen receptor activation and loss of KDM5D expression. Proc Natl Acad Sci USA 113:6259–6264

Kruidenier L, Chung CW, Cheng Z, Liddle J, Che K, Joberty G, Bantscheff M, Bountra C, Bridges A, Diallo H, Eberhard D, Hutchinson S, Jones E, Katso R, Leveridge M, Mander PK, Mosley J, Ramirez-Molina C, Rowland P, Schofield CJ, Sheppard RJ, Smith JE, Swales C, Tanner R, Thomas P, Tumber A, Drewes G, Oppermann U, Patel DJ, Lee K, Wilson DM (2012) A selective jumonji H3K27 demethylase inhibitor modulates the proinflammatory macrophage response. Nature 488:404–408

Kuo YT, Liu YL, Adebayo BO, Shih PH, Lee WH, Wang LS, Liao YF, Hsu WM, Yeh CT, Lin CM (2015) JARID1B expression plays a critical role in chemoresistance and stem cell-like phenotype of neuroblastoma cells. PLoS ONE 10:e0125343

Lauberth SM, Nakayama T, Wu X, Ferris AL, Tang Z, Hughes SH, Roeder RG (2013) H3K4me3 interactions with TAF3 regulate preinitiation complex assembly and selective gene activation. Cell 152:1021–1036

Lebrun N, Mehler-Jacob C, Poirier K, Zordan C, Lacombe D, Carion N, Billuart P, Bienvenu T (2018) Novel KDM5B splice variants identified in patients with developmental disorders: functional consequences. Gene 679:305–313

Lee MG, Norman J, Shilatifard A, Shiekhattar R (2007) Physical and functional association of a trimethyl H3K4 demethylase and Ring6a/MBLR, a polycomb-like protein. Cell 128:877–887

Lee N, Erdjument-Bromage H, Tempst P, Jones RS, Zhang Y (2009) The H3K4 demethylase lid associates with and inhibits histone deacetylase Rpd3. Mol Cell Biol 29:1401–1410

Li L, Greer C, Eisenman RN, Secombe J (2010) Essential functions of the histone demethylase lid. PLoS Genet 6:e1001221–e1001221

Li Q, Shi L, Gui B, Yu W, Wang J, Zhang D, Han X, Yao Z, Shang Y (2011) Binding of the JmjC demethylase JARID1B to LSD1/NuRD suppresses angiogenesis and metastasis in breast cancer cells by repressing chemokine CCL14. Can Res 71:6899–6908

Li H, Wawrose JS, Gooding WE, Garraway LA, Lui VW, Peyser ND, Grandis JR (2014) Genomic analysis of head and neck squamous cell carcinoma cell lines and human tumors: a rational approach to preclinical model selection. Mol Cancer Res MCR 12:571–582

Li N, Dhar SS, Chen TY, Kan PY, Wei Y, Kim JH, Chan CH, Lin HK, Hung MC, Lee MG (2016) JARID1D is a suppressor and prognostic marker of prostate cancer invasion and metastasis. Can Res 76:831–843

Li Y, Liu S, Zhang Y, Gao Q, Sun W, Fu L, Cao J (2018) Histone demethylase JARID1B regulates proliferation and migration of pulmonary arterial smooth muscle cells in mice with chronic hypoxia-induced pulmonary hypertension via nuclear factor-kappa B (NFkB). Cardiovasc Pathol 37:8–14

Liang G, Klose RJ, Gardner KE, Zhang Y (2007) Yeast Jhd2p is a histone H3 Lys4 trimethyl demethylase. Nat Struct Mol Biol 14:243–245

Liang J, Zhang B, Labadie S, Ortwine DF, Vinogradova M, Kiefer JR, Gehling VS, Harmange JC, Cummings R, Lai T, Liao J, Zheng X, Liu Y, Gustafson A, Van der Porten E, Mao W, Liederer BM, Deshmukh G, Classon M, Trojer P, Dragovich PS, Murray L (2016) Lead optimization of a pyrazolo[1,5-a]pyrimidin-7(4H)-one scaffold to identify potent, selective and orally bioavailable KDM5 inhibitors suitable for in vivo biological studies. Bioorg Med Chem Lett 26:4036–4041

Liang J, Labadie S, Zhang B, Ortwine DF, Patel S, Vinogradova M, Kiefer JR, Mauer T, Gehling VS, Harmange J-C, Cummings R, Lai T, Liao J, Zheng X, Liu Y, Gustafson A, Van der Porten E, Mao W, Liederer BM, Deshmukh G, An L, Ran Y, Classon M, Trojer P, Dragovich PS, Murray L (2017) From a novel HTS hit to potent, selective, and orally bioavailable KDM5 inhibitors. Bioorg Med Chem Lett 27:2974–2981

Liao L, Liu ZZ, Langbein L, Cai W, Cho E-A, Na J, Niu X, Jiang W, Zhong Z, Cai WL, Jagannathan G, Dulaimi E, Testa JR, Uzzo RG, Wang Y, Stark GR, Sun J, Peiper S, Xu Y, Yan Q, Yang H (2018) Multiple tumor suppressors regulate a HIF-dependent negative feedback loop via ISGF3 in human clear cell renal cancer. eLife 7:e37925

Liefke R, Oswald F, Alvarado C, Ferres-Marco D, Mittler G, Rodriguez P, Dominguez M, Borggrefe T (2010) Histone demethylase KDM5A is an integral part of the core Notch-RBP-J repressor complex. Genes Dev 24:590–601

Lin W, Cao J, Liu J, Beshiri ML, Fujiwara Y, Francis J, Cherniack AD, Geisen C, Blair LP, Zou MR, Shen X, Kawamori D, Liu Z, Grisanzio C, Watanabe H, Minamishima YA, Zhang Q, Kulkarni RN, Signoretti S, Rodig SJ, Bronson RT, Orkin SH, Tuck DP, Benevolenskaya EV, Meyerson M, Kaelin WG, Yan Q (2011) Loss of the retinoblastoma binding protein 2 (RBP2) histone demethylase suppresses tumorigenesis in mice lacking Rb1 or Men1. Proc Natl Acad Sci 108:13379–13386

Liu X, Secombe J (2015) The histone demethylase KDM5 activates gene expression by recognizing chromatin context through its PHD reader motif. Cell Rep 13:2219–2231

Liu X, Zhang SM, McGeary MK, Krykbaeva I, Lai L, Jansen DJ, Kales SC, Simeonov A, Hall MD, Kelly DP, Bosenberg MW, Yan Q (2019) KDM5B promotes drug resistance by regulating melanoma-propagating cell subpopulations. Mol Cancer Ther 18:706–717

Liu H, Lin J, Zhou W, Moses R, Dai Z, Kossenkov AV, Drapkin R, Bitler BG, Karakashev S, Zhang R (2022a) KDM5A inhibits antitumor immune responses through down regulation of the antigen-presentation pathway in ovarian cancer. Cancer Immunol Res 10:1028–1038

Liu X, Wang J, Boyer JA, Gong W, Zhao S, Xie L, Wu Q, Zhang C, Jain K, Guo Y, Rodriguez J, Li M, Uryu H, Liao C, Hu L, Zhou J, Shi X, Tsai YH, Yan Q, Luo W, Chen X, Strahl BD, von Kriegsheim A, Zhang Q, Wang GG, Baldwin AS, Zhang Q (2022b) Histone H3 proline 16 hydroxylation regulates mammalian gene expression. Nat Genet 54:1721–1735

Lloret-Llinares M, Carré C, Vaquero A, de Olano N, Azorín F (2008) Characterization of Drosophila melanogaster JmjC+N histone demethylases. Nucleic Acids Res 36:2852–2863

Loft A, Brier A-SB, Nielsen R, Schmidt SF, Rosengren T, Mandrup S, Madsen Jesper GS, Yan Q, Liu Z, Cronemeyer H (2016) The KDM5 family is required for activation of pro-proliferative cell cycle genes during adipocyte differentiation. Nucleic Acids Res 45:1743–1759

Lu PJ, Sundquist K, Baeckstrom D, Poulsom R, Hanby A, Meier-Ewert S, Jones T, Mitchell M, Pitha-Rowe P, Freemont P, Taylor-Papadimitriou J (1999) A novel gene (PLU-1) containing highly conserved putative DNA/chromatin binding motifs is specifically up-regulated in breast cancer. J Biol Chem 274:15633–15645

Lu C, Ward PS, Kapoor GS, Rohle D, Turcan S, Abdel-Wahab O, Edwards CR, Khanin R, Figueroa ME, Melnick A, Wellen KE, O'Rourke DM, Berger SL, Chan TA, Levine RL, Mellinghoff IK, Thompson CB (2012) IDH mutation impairs histone demethylation and results in a block to cell differentiation. Nature 483:474–478

Maggi EC, Trillo-Tinoco J, Struckhoff AP, Vijayaraghavan J, Del Valle L, Crabtree JS (2016) Retinoblastoma-binding protein 2 (RBP2) is frequently expressed in neuroendocrine tumors and promotes the neoplastic phenotype. Oncogenesis 5:e257

McBrayer SK, Olenchock BA, DiNatale GJ, Shi DD, Khanal J, Jennings RB, Novak JS, Oser MG, Robbins AK, Modiste R, Bonal D, Moslehi J, Bronson RT, Neuberg D, Nguyen QD, Signoretti S, Losman JA, Kaelin WG Jr (2018) Autochthonous tumors driven by Rb1 loss have an ongoing requirement for the RBP2 histone demethylase. Proc Natl Acad Sci USA 115:E3741-e3748

Mishra S, Van Rechem C, Pal S, Clarke TL, Chakraborty D, Mahan SD, Black JC, Murphy SE, Lawrence MS, Daniels DL, Whetstine JR (2018) Cross-talk between lysine-modifying enzymes controls site-specific DNA amplifications. Cell 174:803-817.e816

Mitra D, Das PM, Huynh FC, Jones FE (2011) Jumonji/ARID1 B (JARID1B) protein promotes breast tumor cell cycle progression through epigenetic repression of microRNA let-7e. J Biol Chem 286:40531–40535

Najmabadi H, Hu H, Garshasbi M, Zemojtel T, Abedini SS, Chen W, Hosseini M, Behjati F, Haas S, Jamali P, Zecha A, Mohseni M, Puttmann L, Vahid LN, Jensen C, Moheb LA, Bienek M, Larti F, Mueller I, Weissmann R, Darvish H, Wrogemann K, Hadavi V, Lipkowitz B, Esmaeeli-Nieh S, Wieczorek D, Kariminejad R, Firouzabadi SG, Cohen M, Fattahi Z, Rost I, Mojahedi F, Hertzberg C, Dehghan A, Rajab A, Banavandi MJ, Hoffer J, Falah M, Musante L, Kalscheuer V, Ullmann R, Kuss AW, Tzschach A, Kahrizi K, Ropers HH (2011) Deep sequencing reveals 50 novel genes for recessive cognitive disorders. Nature 478:57–63

Nie Z, Shi L, Lai C, O'Connell SM, Xu J, Stansfield RK, Hosfield DJ, Veal JM, Stafford JA (2018) Structure-based design and discovery of potent and selective KDM5 inhibitors. Bioorg Med Chem Lett 28:1490–1494

Nishibuchi G, Shibata Y, Hayakawa T, Hayakawa N, Ohtani Y, Sinmyozu K, Tagami H, Nakayama J (2014) Physical and functional interactions between the histone H3K4 demethylase KDM5A and the nucleosome remodeling and deacetylase (NuRD) complex. J Biol Chem 289:28956–28970

Niu X, Zhang T, Liao L, Zhou L, Lindner DJ, Zhou M, Rini B, Yan Q, Yang H (2011) The von Hippel-Lindau tumor suppressor protein regulates gene expression and tumor growth through histone demethylase JARID1C. Oncogene 31:776

Nowak RP, Tumber A, Johansson C, Che KH, Brennan P, Owen D, Oppermann U (2016) Advances and challenges in understanding histone demethylase biology. Curr Opin Chem Biol 33:151–159

Ohguchi H, Park PMC, Wang T, Gryder BE, Ogiya D, Kurata K, Zhang X, Li D, Pei C, Masuda T, Johansson C, Wimalasena VK, Kim Y, Hino S, Usuki S, Kawano Y, Samur MK, Tai YT, Munshi NC, Matsuoka M, Ohtsuki S, Nakao M, Minami T, Lauberth S, Khan J, Oppermann U, Durbin AD, Anderson KC, Hideshima T, Qi J (2021) Lysine demethylase 5A is required for MYC driven transcription in multiple myeloma. Blood Cancer Discov 2:370–387

Oser MG, Sabet AH, Gao W, Chakraborty AA, Schinzel AC, Jennings RB, Fonseca R, Bonal DM, Booker MA, Flaifel A, Novak JS, Christensen CL, Zhang H, Herbert ZT, Tolstorukov MY, Buss EJ, Wong KK, Bronson RT, Nguyen QD, Signoretti S, Kaelin WG Jr (2019) The KDM5A/RBP2 histone demethylase represses NOTCH signaling to sustain neuroendocrine differentiation and promote small cell lung cancer tumorigenesis. Genes Dev 33:1718–1738

Outchkourov NS, Muino JM, Kaufmann K, van Ijcken WF, Groot Koerkamp MJ, van Leenen D, de Graaf P, Holstege FC, Grosveld FG, Timmers HT (2013) Balancing of histone H3K4 methylation states by the Kdm5c/SMCX histone demethylase modulates promoter and enhancer function. Cell Rep 3:1071–1079

Pasini D, Hansen KH, Christensen J, Agger K, Cloos PA, Helin K (2008) Coordinated regulation of transcriptional repression by the RBP2 H3K4 demethylase and polycomb-repressive complex 2. Genes Dev 22:1345–1355

Patsialou A, Wilsker D, Moran E (2005) DNA-binding properties of ARID family proteins. Nucleic Acids Res 33:66–80

Peach SE, Rudomin EL, Udeshi ND, Carr SA, Jaffe JD (2012) Quantitative assessment of chromatin immuno precipitation grade antibodies directed against histone modifications reveals patterns of co-occurring marks on histone protein molecules. Mol Cell Proteomics MCP 11:128–137

Peng D, Lin B, Xie M, Zhang P, Guo Q, Li Q, Gu Q, Yang S, Sen L (2021) Histone demethylase KDM5A promotes tumorigenesis of osteosarcoma tumor. Cell Death Discov 7:9

Pennacchio LA, Bickmore W, Dean A, Nobrega MA, Bejerano G (2013) Enhancers: five essential questions. Nat Rev Genet 14:288–295

Perinchery G, Sasaki M, Angan A, Kumar V, Carroll P, Dahiya R (2000) Deletion of Y-chromosome specific genes in human prostate cancer. J Urol 163:1339–1342

Plch J, Hrabeta J, Eckschlager T (2019) KDM5 demethylases and their role in cancer cell chemoresistance. Int J Cancer 144:221–231

Ptaschinski C, Mukherjee S, Moore ML, Albert M, Helin K, Kunkel SL, Lukacs NW (2015) RSV-induced H3K4 demethylase KDM5B leads to regulation of dendritic cell-derived innate cytokines and exacerbates pathogenesis in vivo. PLoS Pathog 11:e1004978

Ren Z, Kim A, Huang YT, Pi WC, Gong W, Yu X, Qi J, Jin J, Cai L, Roeder RG, Chen WY, Wang GG (2022) A PRC2-Kdm5b axis sustains tumorigenicity of acute myeloid leukemia. Proc Natl Acad Sci USA 119:e2122940119

Roesch A, Fukunaga-Kalabis M, Schmidt EC, Zabierowski SE, Brafford PA, Vultur A, Basu D, Gimotty P, Vogt T, Herlyn M (2010) A temporarily distinct subpopulation of slow-cycling melanoma cells is required for continuous tumor growth. Cell 141:583–594

Roesch A, Vultur A, Bogeski I, Wang H, Zimmermann KM, Speicher D, Korbel C, Laschke MW, Gimotty PA, Philipp SE, Krause E, Patzold S, Villanueva J, Krepler C, Fukunaga-Kalabis M, Hoth M, Bastian BC, Vogt T, Herlyn M (2013) Overcoming intrinsic multidrug resistance in melanoma by blocking the mitochondrial respiratory chain of slow-cycling JARID1B(high) cells. Cancer Cell 23:811–825

Rondinelli B, Rosano D, Antonini E, Frenquelli M, Montanini L, Huang D, Segalla S, Yoshihara K, Amin SB, Lazarevic D, The BT, Verhaak RG, Futreal PA, Di Croce L, Chin L, Cittaro D, Tonon G (2015) Histone demethylase JARID1C inactivation triggers genomic instability in sporadic renal cancer. J Clin Investig 125:4625–4637

Ruthenburg AJ, Allis CD, Wysocka J (2007) Methylation of lysine 4 on histone H3: intricacy of writing and reading a single epigenetic mark. Mol Cell 25:15–30

Sanchez R, Zhou M-M (2011) The PHD finger: a versatile epigenome reader. Trends Biochem Sci 36:364–372

Santos-Rosa H, Schneider R, Bannister AJ, Sherriff J, Bernstein BE, Emre NC, Schreiber SL, Mellor J, Kouzarides T (2002) Active genes are tri-methylated at K4 of histone H3. Nature 419:407–411

Sayegh J, Cao J, Zou MR, Morales A, Blair LP, Norcia M, Hoyer D, Tackett AJ, Merkel JS, Yan Q (2013) Identification of small molecule inhibitors of Jumonji AT-rich interactive domain 1B (JARID1B) histone demethylase by a sensitive high throughput screen. J Biol Chem 288:9408–9417

Scandaglia M, Lopez-Atalaya JP, Medrano-Fernandez A, Lopez-Cascales MT, Del Blanco B, Lipinski M, Benito E, Olivares R, Iwase S, Shi Y, Barco A (2017) Loss of Kdm5c causes spurious transcription and prevents the fine-tuning of activity-regulated enhancers in neurons. Cell Rep 21:47–59

Schmitz SU, Albert M, Malatesta M, Morey L, Johansen JV, Bak M, Tommerup N, Abarrategui I, Helin K (2011) Jarid1b targets genes regulating development and is involved in neural differentiation. EMBO J 30:4586–4600

Scibetta AG, Santangelo S, Coleman J, Hall D, Chaplin T, Copier J, Catchpole S, Burchell J, Taylor-Papadimitriou J (2007) Functional analysis of the transcription repressor PLU-1/JARID1B. Mol Cell Biol 27:7220–7235

Secombe J, Li L, Carlos L, Eisenman RN (2007) The trithorax group protein lid is a trimethyl histone H3K4 demethylase required for dMyc-induced cell growth. Genes Dev 21:537–551

Seward DJ, Cubberley G, Kim S, Schonewald M, Zhang L, Tripet B, Bentley DL (2007) Demethylation of trimethylated histone H3 Lys4 in vivo by JARID1 JmjC proteins. Nat Struct Mol Biol 14:240–242

Shannan B, Matschke J, Chauvistre H, Vogel F, Klein D, Meier F, Westphal D, Bruns J, Rauschenberg R, Utikal J, Forschner A, Berking C, Terheyden P, Dabrowski E, Gutzmer R, Rafei-Shamsabadi D, Meiss F, Heinzerling L, Zimmer L, Livingstone E, Varaljai R, Hoewner A, Horn S, Klode J, Stuschke M, Scheffler B, Marchetto A, Sannino G, Grunewald TGP, Schadendorf D, Jendrossek V, Roesch A (2019) Sequence-dependent cross-resistance of combined radiotherapy plus BRAF(V600E) inhibition in melanoma. Eur J Cancer (Oxford, England, 1990) 109:137–153

Sharma SV, Lee DY, Li B, Quinlan MP, Takahashi F, Maheswaran S, McDermott U, Azizian N, Zou L, Fischbach MA, Wong KK, Brandstetter K, Wittner B, Ramaswamy S, Classon M, Settleman J (2010) A chromatin-mediated reversible drug-tolerant state in cancer cell subpopulations. Cell 141:69–80

Shen X, Zhuang Z, Zhang Y, Chen Z, Shen L, Pu W, Chen L, Xu Z (2015) JARID1B modulates lung cancer cell proliferation and invasion by regulating p53 expression. Tumour Biol J Int Soc Oncodev Biol Med 36:7133–7142

Shen H, Xu W, Guo R, Rong B, Gu L, Wang Z, He C, Zheng L, Hu X, Hu Z, Shao ZM, Yang P, Wu F, Shi YG, Shi Y, Lan F (2016) Suppression of enhancer overactivation by a RACK7-histone demethylase complex. Cell 165:331–342

Shi Y, Lan F, Matson C, Mulligan P, Whetstine JR, Cole PA, Casero RA, Shi Y (2004) Histone demethylation mediated by the nuclear amine oxidase homolog LSD1. Cell 119:941–953

Sims RJ, Millhouse S, Chen C-F, Lewis BA, Erdjument-Bromage H, Tempst P, Manley JL, Reinberg D (2007) Recognition of trimethylated histone H3 lysine 4 facilitates the recruitment of transcription postinitiation factors and pre-mRNA splicing. Mol Cell 28:665–676

Stein J, Majores M, Rohde M, Lim S, Schneider S, Krappe E, Ellinger J, Dietel M, Stephan C, Jung K, Perner S, Kristiansen G, Kirfel J (2014) KDM5C is overexpressed in prostate cancer and is a prognostic marker for prostate-specific antigen-relapse following radical prostatectomy. Am J Pathol 184:2430–2437

Tahiliani M, Mei P, Fang R, Leonor T, Rutenberg M, Shimizu F, Li J, Rao A, Shi Y (2007) The histone H3K4 demethylase SMCX links REST target genes to X-linked mental retardation. Nature 447:601–605

Tang K, Jiao LM, Qi YR, Wang TC, Li YL, Xu JL, Wang ZW, Yu B, Liu HM, Zhao W (2022) Discovery of novel pyrazole-based KDM5B inhibitor TK-129 and its protective effects on myocardial remodeling and fibrosis. J Med Chem 65:12979–13000

Tarhonskaya H, Nowak RP, Johansson C, Szykowska A, Tumber A, Hancock RL, Lang P, Flashman E, Oppermann U, Schofield CJ, Kawamura A (2017) Studies on the interaction of the histone demethylase KDM5B with tricarboxylic acid cycle intermediates. J Mol Biol 429:2895–2906

Taylor-Papadimitriou J, Burchell J (2017) JARID1/KDM5 demethylases as cancer targets? Expert Opin Ther Targets 21:5–7

Teng YC, Lee CF, Li YS, Chen YR, Hsiao PW, Chan MY, Lin FM, Huang HD, Chen YT, Jeng YM, Hsu CH, Yan Q, Tsai MD, Juan LJ (2013) Histone demethylase RBP2 promotes lung tumorigenesis and cancer metastasis. Can Res 73:4711–4721

Torres IO, Kuchenbecker KM, Nnadi CI, Fletterick RJ, Kelly MJ, Fujimori DG (2015) Histone demethylase KDM5A is regulated by its reader domain through a positive-feedback mechanism. Nat Commun 6:6204

Trewick SC, McLaughlin PJ, Allshire RC (2005) Methylation: lost in hydroxylation? EMBO Rep 6:315–320

Tsukada Y, Fang J, Erdjument-Bromage H, Warren ME, Borchers CH, Tempst P, Zhang Y (2006) Histone demethylation by a family of JmjC domain-containing proteins. Nature 439:811–816

Tu S, Bulloch EMM, Yang L, Ren C, Huang W-C, Hsu P-H, Chen C-H, Liao C-L, Yu H-M, Lo W-S, Freitas MA, Tsai M-D (2007) Identification of histone demethylases in *Saccharomyces cerevisiae*. J Biol Chem 282:14262–14271

Tu S, Teng YC, Yuan C, Wu YT, Chan MY, Cheng AN, Lin PH, Juan LJ, Tsai MD (2008) The ARID domain of the H3K4 demethylase RBP2 binds to a DNA CCGCCC motif. Nat Struct Mol Biol 15:419–421

Tumber A, Nuzzi A, Hookway ES, Hatch SB, Velupillai S, Johansson C, Kawamura A, Savitsky P, Yapp C, Szykowska A, Wu N, Bountra C, Strain-Damerell C, Burgess-Brown NA, Ruda GF, Fedorov O, Munro S, England KS, Nowak RP, Schofield CJ, La Thangue NB, Pawlyn C, Davies F, Morgan G, Athanasou N, Muller S, Oppermann U, Brennan PE (2017) Potent and selective KDM5 inhibitor stops cellular demethylation of H3K4me3 at transcription start sites and proliferation of MM1S myeloma cells. Cell Chem Biol 24:371–380

Ugur FS, Kelly MJS, Fujimori DG (2023) Chromatin sensing by the auxiliary domains of KDM5C regulates its demethylase activity and is disrupted by X-linked intellectual disability mutations. J Mol Biol 435:167913

van Oevelen C, Wang J, Asp P, Yan Q, Kaelin WG Jr, Kluger Y, Dynlacht BD (2008) A role for mammalian Sin3 in permanent gene silencing. Mol Cell 32:359–370

Varaljai R, Islam AB, Beshiri ML, Rehman J, Lopez-Bigas N, Benevolenskaya EV (2015) Increased mitochondrial function downstream from KDM5A histone demethylase rescues differentiation in pRB-deficient cells. Genes Dev 29:1817–1834

Vazquez-Rodriguez S, Wright M, Rogers CM, Cribbs AP, Velupillai S, Philpott M, Lee H, Dunford JE, Huber KVM, Robers MB, Vasta JD, Thezenas ML, Bonham S, Kessler B, Bennett J, Fedorov O, Raynaud F, Donovan A, Blagg J, Bavetsias V, Oppermann U, Bountra C, Kawamura A, Brennan PE (2019) Design, synthesis and characterization of covalent KDM5 inhibitors. Angew Chem Int Ed Engl 58:515–519

Vermeulen M, Mulder KW, Denissov S, Pijnappel WW, van Schaik FM, Varier RA, Baltissen MP, Stunnenberg HG, Mann M, Timmers HT (2007) Selective anchoring of TFIID to nucleosomes by trimethylation of histone H3 lysine 4. Cell 131:58–69

Vicent GP, Nacht AS, Zaurin R, Font-Mateu J, Soronellas D, Le Dily F, Reyes D, Beato M (2013) Unliganded progesterone receptor-mediated targeting of an RNA-containing repressive complex silences a subset of hormone-inducible genes. Genes Dev 27:1179–1197

Vinogradova M, Gehling VS, Gustafson A, Arora S, Tindell CA, Wilson C, Williamson KE, Guler GD, Gangurde P, Manieri W, Busby J, Flynn EM, Lan F, Kim HJ, Odate S, Cochran AG, Liu Y, Wongchenko M, Yang Y, Cheung TK, Maile TM, Lau T, Costa M, Hegde GV, Jackson E, Pitti R, Arnott D, Bailey C, Bellon S, Cummings RT, Albrecht BK, Harmange JC, Kiefer JR, Trojer P, Classon M (2016) An inhibitor of KDM5 demethylases reduces survival of drug-tolerant cancer cells. Nat Chem Biol 12:531–538

Wang GG, Song J, Wang Z, Dormann HL, Casadio F, Li H, Luo JL, Patel DJ, Allis CD (2009) Haematopoietic malignancies caused by dysregulation of a chromatin-binding PHD finger. Nature 459:847–851

Wang L, Chang J, Varghese D, Dellinger M, Kumar S, Best AM, Ruiz J, Bruick R, Pena-Llopis S, Xu J, Babinski DJ, Frantz DE, Brekken RA, Quinn AM, Simeonov A, Easmon J, Martinez ED (2013) A small molecule modulates Jumonji histone demethylase activity and selectively inhibits cancer growth. Nat Commun 4:2035

Wang L, Mao Y, Du G, He C, Han S (2015a) Overexpression of JARID1B is associated with poor prognosis and chemotherapy resistance in epithelial ovarian cancer. Tumour Biol J Int Soc Oncodev Biol Med 36:2465–2472

Wang Q, Wei J, Su P, Gao P (2015b) Histone demethylase JARID1C promotes breast cancer metastasis cells via down regulating BRMS1 expression. Biochem Biophys Res Commun 464:659–666

Wang Z, Tang F, Qi G, Yuan S, Zhang G, Tang B, He S (2015c) KDM5B is overexpressed in gastric cancer and is required for gastric cancer cell proliferation and metastasis. Am J Cancer Res 5:87–100

Wang C, Wang J, Li J, Hu G, Shan S, Li Q, Zhang X (2016a) KDM5A controls bone morphogenic protein 2-induced osteogenic differentiation of bone mesenchymal stem cells during osteoporosis. Cell Death Dis 7:e2335

Wang D, Han S, Peng R, Jiao C, Wang X, Yang X, Yang R, Li X (2016b) Depletion of histone demethylase KDM5B inhibits cell proliferation of hepatocellular carcinoma by regulation of cell cycle checkpoint proteins p15 and p27. J Exp Clin Cancer Res CR 35:37

Wang Z-Y, Yang J, Liu C-K, Shen S-Q (2017) High expression of retinoblastoma-binding protein 2 (RBP2) in patients with hepatocellular carcinoma and its prognostic significance. Med Sci Monit Int Med J Exp Clin Res 23:2736–2744

Wang L, Gao Y, Zhang G, Li D, Wang Z, Zhang J, Hermida LC, He L, Wang Z, Si J, Geng S, Ai R, Ning F, Cheng C, Deng H, Dimitrov DS, Sun Y, Huang Y, Wang D, Hu X, Wei Z, Wang W, Liao X (2020) Enhancing KDM5A and TLR activity improves the response to immune checkpoint blockade. Sci Transl Med 12:eaax2282

Wang H, Fan Z, Shliaha PV, Miele M, Hendrickson RC, Jiang X, Helin K (2023) H3K4me3 regulates RNA polymerase II promoter-proximal pause-release. Nature 615:339–348

Westaway SM, Preston AG, Barker MD, Brown F, Brown JA, Campbell M, Chung CW, Diallo H, Douault C, Drewes G, Eagle R, Gordon L, Haslam C, Hayhow TG, Humphreys PG, Joberty G, Katso R, Kruidenier L, Leveridge M, Liddle J, Mosley J, Muelbaier M, Randle R, Rioja I, Rueger A, Seal GA, Sheppard RJ, Singh O, Taylor J, Thomas P, Thomson D, Wilson DM, Lee K, Prinjha RK (2016a) Cell penetrant inhibitors of the KDM4 and KDM5 families of histone lysine demethylases. 1. 3-Amino-4-pyridine carboxylate derivatives. J Med Chem 59:1357–1369

Westaway SM, Preston AG, Barker MD, Brown F, Brown JA, Campbell M, Chung CW, Drewes G, Eagle R, Garton N, Gordon L, Haslam C, Hayhow TG, Humphreys PG, Joberty G, Katso R, Kruidenier L, Leveridge M, Pemberton M, Rioja I, Seal GA, Shipley T, Singh O, Suckling CJ, Taylor J, Thomas P, Wilson DM, Lee K, Prinjha RK (2016b) Cell penetrant inhibitors of the KDM4 and KDM5 families of histone lysine demethylases. 2. Pyrido[3,4-d]pyrimidin-4(3H)-one derivatives. J Med Chem 59:1370–1387

Wilsker D, Patsialou A, Dallas PB, Moran E (2002) ARID proteins: a diverse family of DNA binding proteins implicated in the control of cell growth, differentiation, and development. Cell Growth Differ Mol Biol J Am Assoc Cancer Res 13:95–106

Wong PP, Miranda F, Chan KV, Berlato C, Hurst HC, Scibetta AG (2012) Histone demethylase KDM5B collaborates with TFAP2C and Myc to repress the cell cycle inhibitor p21(cip) (CDKN1A). Mol Cell Biol 32:1633–1644

Workman P, Travers J (2010) Drug-tolerant insurgents. Nature 464:844–845

Wu L, Cao J, Cai WL, Lang SM, Horton JR, Jansen DJ, Liu ZZ, Chen JF, Zhang M, Mott BT, Pohida K, Rai G, Kales SC, Henderson MJ, Hu X, Jadhav A, Maloney DJ, Simeonov A, Zhu S, Iwasaki A, Hall MD, Cheng X, Shadel GS, Yan Q (2018) KDM5 histone demethylases repress immune response via suppression of STING. PLoS Biol 16:e2006134

Xiang Y, Zhu Z, Han G, Ye X, Xu B, Peng Z, Ma Y, Yu Y, Lin H, Chen AP, Chen CD (2007) JARID1B is a histone H3 lysine 4 demethylase up-regulated in prostate cancer. Proc Natl Acad Sci USA 104:19226–19231

Xiao M, Yang H, Xu W, Ma S, Lin H, Zhu H, Liu L, Liu Y, Yang C, Xu Y, Zhao S, Ye D, Xiong Y, Guan KL (2012) Inhibition of alpha-KG-dependent histone and DNA demethylases by fumarate and succinate that are accumulated in mutations of FH and SDH tumor suppressors. Genes Dev 26:1326–1338

Xie L, Pelz C, Wang W, Bashar A, Varlamova O, Shadle S, Impey S (2011) KDM5B regulates embryonic stem cell self-renewal and represses cryptic intragenic transcription. EMBO J 30:1473–1484

Xu W, Zhou B, Zhao X, Zhu L, Xu J, Jiang Z, Chen D, Wei Q, Han M, Feng L, Wang S, Wang X, Zhou J, Jin H (2018) KDM5B demethylates H3K4 to recruit XRCC1 and promote chemoresistance. Int J Biol Sci 14:1122–1132

Xu S, Wang S, Xing S, Yu D, Rong B, Gao H, Sheng M, Tan Y, Sun X, Wang K, Xue K, Shi Z, Lan F (2021) KDM5A suppresses PML-RARalpha target gene expression and APL differentiation through repressing H3K4me2. Blood Adv 5:3241–3253

Xue S, Lam YM, He Z, Zheng Y, Li L, Zhang Y, Li C, Mbadhi MN, Zheng L, Cheng Z, Liu Y, Wang X, Chan LC, Ng RK, Zhang J (2020) Histone lysine demethylase KDM5B maintains chronic myeloid leukemia via multiple epigenetic actions. Exp Hematol 82:53–65

Yamamoto S, Wu Z, Russnes HG, Takagi S, Peluffo G, Vaske C, Zhao X, Moen Vollan HK, Maruyama R, Ekram MB, Sun H, Kim JH, Carver K, Zucca M, Feng J, Almendro V, Bessarabova M, Rueda OM, Nikolsky Y, Caldas C, Liu XS, Polyak K (2014) JARID1B is a luminal lineage-driving oncogene in breast cancer. Cancer Cell 25:762–777

Yang GJ, Zhu MH, Lu XJ, Liu YJ, Lu JF, Leung CH, Ma DL, Chen J (2021) The emerging role of KDM5A in human cancer. J Hematol Oncol 14:30

Yao W, Peng Y, Lin D (2010) The flexible loop L1 of the H3K4 demethylase JARID1B ARID domain has a crucial role in DNA-binding activity. Biochem Biophys Res Commun 396:323–328

Yheskel M, Sidoli S, Secombe J (2023) Proximity labeling reveals a new in vivo network of interactors for the histone demethylase KDM5. Epigenetics Chromatin 16:8

Yu X, Chen H, Zuo C, Jin X, Yin Y, Wang H, Jin M, Ozato K, Xu S (2017) Chromatin remodeling: demethylating H3K4me3 of type I IFNs gene by Rbp2 through interacting with Piasy for transcriptional attenuation. FASEB J Official Publ Fed Am Soc Exp Biol 32:552–567

Zamurrad S, Hatch HAM, Drelon C, Belalcazar HM, Secombe J (2018) A drosophila model of intellectual disability caused by mutations in the histone demethylase KDM5. Cell Rep 22:2359–2369

Zeng J, Ge Z, Wang L, Li Q, Wang N, Bjorkholm M, Jia J, Xu D (2010) The histone demethylase RBP2 Is overexpressed in gastric cancer and its inhibition triggers senescence of cancer cells. Gastroenterology 138:981–992

Zhan D, Zhang Y, Xiao P, Zheng X, Ruan M, Zhang J, Chen A, Zou Y, Chen Y, Huang G, Hu S, Wang QF, Zhu X (2018) Whole exome sequencing identifies novel mutations of epigenetic regulators in chemorefractory pediatric acute myeloid leukemia. Leuk Res 65:20–24

Zhang Y, Liang J, Li Q (2014a) Coordinated regulation of retinoic acid signaling pathway by KDM5B and polycomb repressive complex 2. J Cell Biochem 115:1528–1538

Zhang Y, Yang H, Guo X, Rong N, Song Y, Xu Y, Lan W, Zhang X, Liu M, Xu Y, Cao C (2014b) The PHD1 finger of KDM5B recognizes unmodified H3K4 during the demethylation of histone H3K4me2/3 by KDM5B. Protein Cell 5:837–850

Zhang SM, Cai WL, Liu X, Thakral D, Luo J, Chan LH, McGeary MK, Song E, Blenman KRM, Micevic G, Jessel S, Zhang Y, Yin M, Booth CJ, Jilaveanu LB, Damsky W, Sznol M, Kluger HM, Iwasaki A, Bosenberg MW, Yan Q (2021) KDM5B promotes immune evasion by recruiting SETDB1 to silence retroelements. Nature 598:682–687

Zhao D, Zhang Q, Liu Y, Li X, Zhao K, Ding Y, Li Z, Shen Q, Wang C, Li N, Cao X (2016) H3K4me3 demethylase Kdm5a Is required for NK cell activation by associating with p50 to suppress SOCS1. Cell Rep 15:288–299

Zheng YC, Chang J, Wang LC, Ren HM, Pang JR, Liu HM (2019) Lysine demethylase 5B (KDM5B): a potential anti-cancer drug target. Eur J Med Chem 161:131–140

Zheng H, Wu L, Xiao Q, Meng X, Hafiz A, Yan Q, Lu R, Cao J (2023) Epigenetically suppressed tumor cell intrinsic STING promotes tumor immune escape. Biomed Pharmacother 157:114033

Zou MR, Cao J, Liu Z, Huh SJ, Polyak K, Yan Q (2014) Histone demethylase jumonji AT-rich interactive domain 1B (JARID1B) controls mammary gland development by regulating key developmental and lineage specification genes. J Biol Chem 289:17620–17633

Context-Dependent Functions of KDM6 Lysine Demethylases in Physiology and Disease

7

Mina Masoumeh Tayari, Celestia Fang and Panagiotis Ntziachristos

Abstract

Histone lysine methylation is a major epigenetic modification that participates in several cellular processes including gene regulation and chromatin structure. This mark can go awry in disease contexts such as cancer. Two decades ago, the discovery of histone demethylase enzymes thirteen years ago sheds light on the complexity of the regulation of this mark. Here we address the roles of lysine demethylases JMJD3 and UTX in physiological and disease contexts. The two demethylases play pivotal roles in many developmental and disease contexts via regulation of di- and trimethylation of lysine 27 on histone H3 (H3K27me2/3) in repressing gene expression programs. JMJD3 and UTX participate in several biochemical settings including methyltransferase and chromatin remodeling complexes. They have histone demethylase-dependent and -independent activities and a variety of context-specific interacting factors. The structure, amounts, and function of the demethylases can be altered in disease due to genetic alterations or aberrant gene regulation. Therefore, academic and industrial initiatives have targeted these enzymes using a number of small molecule compounds in therapeutic approaches. In this chapter, we will touch upon inhibitor formulations, their properties, and current efforts to test them in preclinical contexts to optimize their therapeutic outcomes. Demethylase inhibitors are currently used in targeted therapeutic approaches that might be particularly effective when used in conjunction with systemic approaches such as chemotherapy.

M. M. Tayari and C. Fang: These authors contributed equally to this work.

M. M. Tayari
Department of Human Genetics, Sylvester Comprehensive Cancer Center, University of Miami Miller School of Medicine, Miami, FL, USA

M. M. Tayari · C. Fang
Department of Biochemistry and Molecular Genetics, Feinberg School of Medicine, Northwestern University, Chicago, IL, USA

P. Ntziachristos (✉)
Department of Biomolecular Medicine, Faculty of Medicine and Health Sciences, Center for Medical Genetics, Ghent University, Medical Research Building 2 (MRB2), Entrance 38, Corneel Heymanslaan 10, 9000 Ghent, Belgium
e-mail: pntziachr@gmail.com; panagiotis.ntziachristos@ugent.be
URL: https://ntziachristoslab.com

P. Ntziachristos
Center for Medical Genetics, Ghent University and University Hospital, Ghent, Belgium

P. Ntziachristos
Cancer Research Institute Ghent (CRIG), Ghent, Belgium

Q. Yan (ed.), *Targeting Lysine Demethylases in Cancer and Other Human Diseases*, Advances in Experimental Medicine and Biology 1433, https://doi.org/10.1007/978-3-031-38176-8_7

Keywords

Epigenetics · Demethylases · JMJD3 · UTX · UTY · Small molecule inhibitors

7.1 Introduction

7.1.1 Epigenetics and Histone Modifications

The histone N-terminus can undergo posttranslational modifications in numerous ways (Zhao and Garcia 2015; Tan et al. 2011), including acetylation and methylation (Tan et al. 2011; Jenuwein and Allis 2001; Luger et al. 1997; Kornberg 1974). The outcome of methylation is context dependent: For instance, methylation of histone H3 lysine 27 (H3K27me2/3) (Cao et al. 2002; Muller et al. 2002) or 9 (H3K9me3) (Peters et al. 2002) is a hallmark of silenced chromatin. H3K27me2/3, catalyzed by the Polycomb repressive complex 2 (PRC2), is characteristic of facultative (dynamic) heterochromatin, while H3K9 methylation is considered a mark of constitutive heterochromatin, which is present in constantly repressed areas of the genome such as centromeres or telomeres. In contrast, methylation of lysine 4 on histone 3 (H3K4me3) is an activating histone mark (Santos-Rosa et al. 2002; Schneider et al. 2004) and methylation of H3K79 (Feng et al. 2002) or H3K36 (Klose et al. 2006a) is associated with transcriptional elongation. Histone lysine modifications are enzymatically regulated by the opposing activities of enzymes known as writers, erasers, and readers that introduce, remove, and read these marks correspondingly (Allis and Jenuwein 2016) (Fig. 7.1).

Histone methylation was mainly studied on the *Homeotic* (*HOX*) locus, which exist in a bivalent state in stem cells, and is characterized by coexistence of the activating and repressive histone marks, H3K4me3 and H3K27me3, respectively (Voigt et al. 2013; Bernstein et al. 2006). These genes are present in a poised intermediate state in embryonic stem (ES) cells and resolve to become activated (mixed-lineage leukemia (MLL)/trithorax complex bound, H3K4me3 enriched) or repressed (Polycomb complex bound, H3K27me3 enriched) during differentiation (Ringrose 2007; Schuettengruber et al. 2007; Schwartz and Pirrotta 2007). As the expression levels of genes like *Hox* are stable over long periods of time (Jenuwein 2001; Byvoet et al. 1972; Duerre and Lee 1974), it was initially thought that methylation marks were only passively removed through dilution of their nucleosomal concentration via cell division.

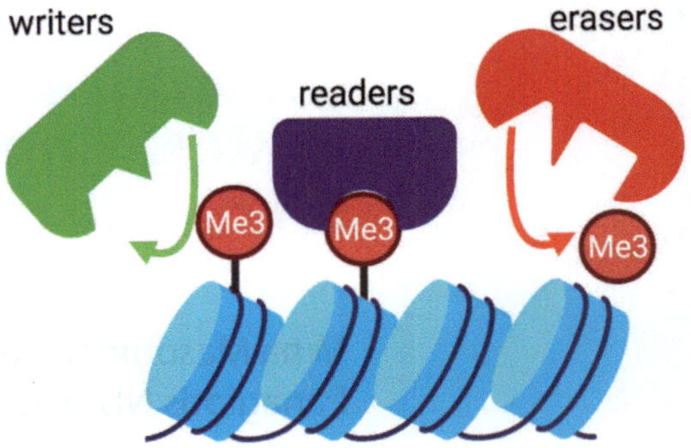

Fig. 7.1 Main categories of epigenetic regulators. Three main groups of epigenetic modulators are shown: 'writers' add the histone marks; 'readers' recognize the modifications; and 'erasers' eliminate the modifications

7.1.2 The Myth of Irreversibility for Histone Methylation

The observation that methylated histones in constitutive heterochromatin were exceedingly stable, in contrast to other histone modifications, suggested that histone methylation was irreversible. This dogma was further re-enforced by the finding that methylated lysines have the same half-life as histones (Byvoet et al. 1972; Duerre and Lee 1974).

However, in the last 20 years, two families of demethylases have been identified that can remove methylation marks through different mechanisms. It has become clear that demethylases play a multifaceted role in biology beyond their demethylase activity, as they participate in protein complexes involved in various stages of gene transcription. In this chapter, we will discuss lysine 27 demethylases as an example of demethylase biology and their diverse roles in biology.

7.1.3 Discovery of Lysine 27 Histone Demethylases

Oxidating enzymes were considered as potential demethylases, based on previous experimental evidence (Bannister et al. 2002; Borun et al. 1972; Annunziato et al. 1995; Kim et al. 1964). Lysine-specific demethylase 1 (LSD1 (Shi et al. 2004), also known as KDM1 or AOF) (Allis et al. 2007) was characterized as the first histone demethylase for H3K4me1/2 in 2004 and later as a H3K9me1/2 demethylase. LSD1/2 proteins are FAD-dependent amine oxidases that exclusively demethylate mono- and di-methylated lysine residues. They play a role in transcriptional regulation as components of corepressor complexes controlling physiological and cancer contexts (Wang et al. 2009). Rapid expansion of the demethylase field came with the identification of the Jumonji family of Fe(II)- and 2-oxoglutarate or alpha ketoglutarate (aKG)-dependent dioxygenases that demethylate trimethylated lysine residues in addition to mono and di-methyl groups (Klose et al. 2006a, b; Cloos et al. 2006; Fodor et al. 2006; Whetstine et al. 2006; Klose and Bird 2006). The family took its name from the Japanese word for cruciform, as mice with a deleted *Jarid2 gene*, a member of the family that is considered catalytically inactive, show a cross-like neural tube phenotype (Takeuchi et al. 1995). In 2006, the laboratories of Yi Zhang (Klose et al. 2006a; Yamane et al. 2006; Tsukada et al. 2006), Kristian Helin (Cloos et al. 2006), Yang Shi (Whetstine et al. 2006), and Thomas Jenuwein discovered the first Jumonji enzymes with a focus on histone H3 lysine 9 and 36 methylation. Subsequently, in 2007, the JARID1 family for H3 lysine 4 demethylases (Christensen et al. 2007; Iwase et al. 2007; Klose et al. 2007; Lee et al. 2007a; Tahiliani et al. 2007) and the JMJD3/UTX family of H3 lysine 27 demethylases (Agger et al. 2007; Santa et al. 2007; Jepsen et al. 2007; Lan et al. 2007; Lee et al. 2007b) were discovered. In addition to lysine demethylases, arginine demethylases are another family of proteins with important roles in physiology and disease (Bedford and Clarke 2009), not further discussed in this chapter.

Thirty proteins contain the Jumonji C (JMJC) catalytic domain, with about 24 of them have a documented histone demethylase activity (for an extensive overview, see Kooistra and Helin 2012). Based on the homology of the JMJC domain that determines the specificity for certain lysine residues, these histone lysine demethylases can be divided into seven subfamilies. The two H3K27me3 demethylases (Ezponda and Licht 2014), ubiquitously transcribed tetratricopeptide repeat X chromosome protein (UTX or KDM6A) and JMJD3 (KDM6B), were discovered in 2007 (Agger et al. 2007; Santa et al. 2007; Jepsen et al. 2007; Lan et al. 2007; Lee et al. 2007b; Hong et al. 2007) (Fig. 7.2). JMJD3 and UTX are essential components of regulatory transcriptional chromatin complexes. These enzymes demethylate lysine residues in histones in a sequence-specific context. UTX is encoded by the *KDM6A* gene on the short arm of chromosome X (Xp11.3), escapes X chromosome inactivation in females, and is ubiquitously expressed, whereas JMJD3 is encoded by the *KDM6B* locus on chromosome 17 and is induced by inflammatory, viral, and oncogenic stimuli (Santa et al. 2007; Anderton et al. 2011; Ntziachristos et al. 2014; Meulen et al. 2015). UTX consists of 1401 amino acids and contains the JMJC catalytic domain and six tetratricopeptide repeat (TPR) domains, which mediate protein–protein interactions (Hong et al. 2007). JMJD3 consists of 1679 amino acids, but, despite its larger size, JMJD3 does not contain any structural domains other than the JMJC catalytic domain. The JMJC domains of JMJD3 and UTX have 84% sequence similarity (Hong et al. 2007), suggesting potential differences in the strength of their catalytic activity. Other than the aforementioned two major H3K27me demethylases, UTY is a paralog of UTX located on the Y chromosome in male individuals and was originally thought to be catalytically dead due to mutations in the JMJC catalytic domain (Lan et al.

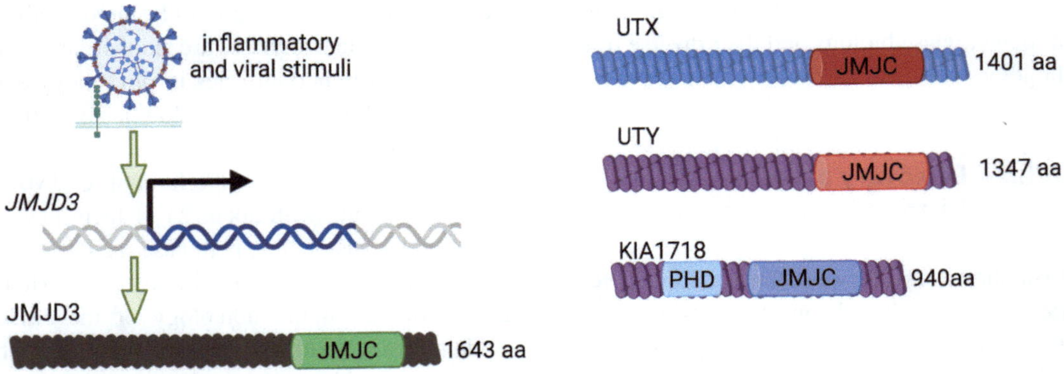

Fig. 7.2 Schematic view of the main histone H3 lysine 27 demethylase enzymes. H3K27me3 demethylases JMJD3, UTX, and the UTX paralog (UTY). KIAA1718 has demethylase activity against multiple lysine residues, including lysines 9 and 27 on histone H3. aa: amino acids, JmjC: Jumonji C domain, TPR: tetratricopeptide repeats, and PHD: plant homeodomain. Note that the JmjC domains of JMJD3, UTX, UTY, and KDM7 exhibit differences in their amino acid sequences

2007; Shpargel et al. 2012; Walport et al. 2014a). Nevertheless, UTY can partially compensate for UTX loss through its participation in biochemical complexes, and it was recently shown to retain some enzymatic activity (Walport et al. 2014a). KDM7 or KIAA1718 is a poorly characterized dual demethylase for H3 lysines 27 and 36 (Huang et al. 2010) and has been shown to interact with JMJD3 (Chen et al. 2012).

Recent studies have elucidated aspects of histone lysine demethylase biology in transcription, genome integrity, and epigenetic regulation in physiology and disease. Below, we will summarize the current understanding of JMJD3 and UTX functions in cellular biology and cancer (Klose et al. 2006b; Kooistra and Helin 2012; Hoffmann et al. 2012; Morera et al. 2016; Dawson and Kouzarides 2012; Dawson et al. 2012; Lohse et al. 2011a; Meulen et al. 2014; Arcipowski et al. 2016; Ntziachristos et al. 2016).

7.2 Demethylase-Dependent Biochemical and Physiological Roles of JMJD3 and UTX

Studies using lysine 27 as well as other lysine demethylases (Liu et al. 2010; Schmitz et al. 2011; Xie et al. 2011) suggest that these enzymes modulate subtle changes in gene expression via maintaining the methylation equilibrium on chromatin to safeguard transcription-accessible chromatin states (Kooistra and Helin 2012).The role of JMJD3 has been studied in several contexts such as development, differentiation, and inflammation (Santa et al. 2007, 2009; Shpargel et al. 2012, 2014; Dahle et al. 2010; Burgold et al. 2008; Dai et al. 2010; Shaw and Martin 2009; Sen et al. 2008; Seenundun et al. 2010; Satoh et al. 2010; Thieme et al. 2013; Welstead et al. 2012; Wang et al. 2012; Mansour et al. 2012; Zhao et al. 2013) (see Fig. 7.3 for a synopsis of JMJD3 and UTX biochemical roles).

Jmjd3 transcript is induced following lipopolysaccharide (LPS) treatment of macrophages (Santa et al. 2007, 2009) through direct transcriptional regulation by NF-kB and controls H3K27me2/3 in macrophage trans-differentiation in response to inflammatory stimuli (Santa et al. 2007, 2009). It was initially shown that the majority of JMJD3-bound loci are targets of the lysine 27 methyltransferase Polycomb group (PcG) complex. In that context, JMJD3 links epigenetic regulation to inflammation. This could be the basis for macrophage plasticity and might explain differentiation abnormalities caused by chronic inflammation. PcG proteins mediate gene silencing and repress

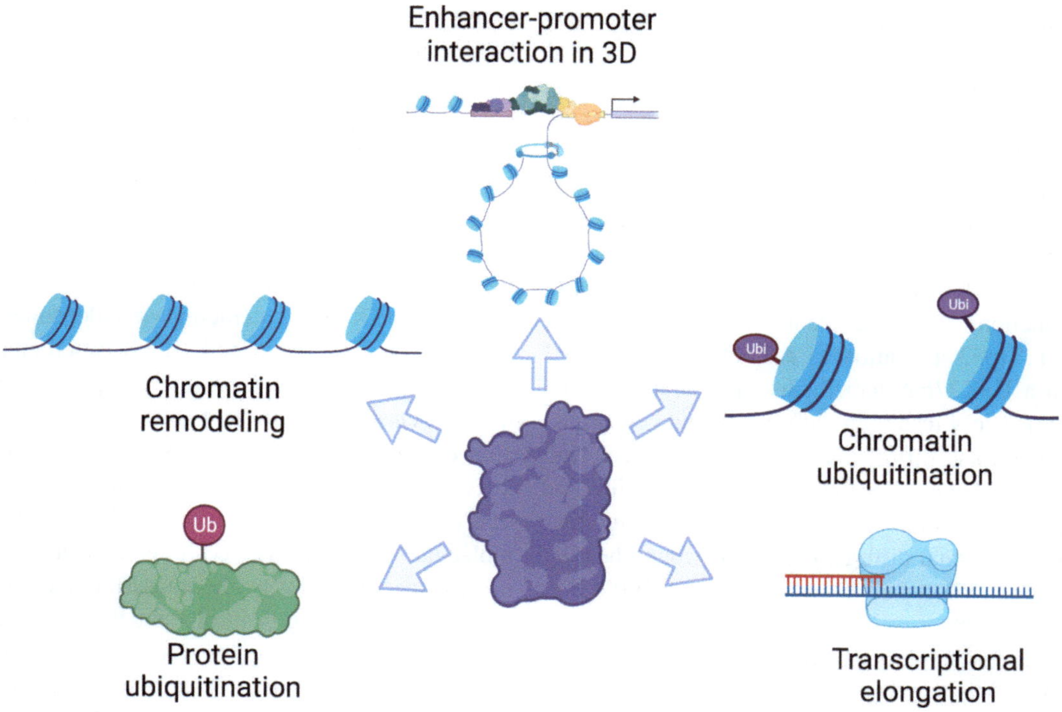

Fig. 7.3 Roles of JMJD3 and UTX in various molecular and biochemical processes. H3K27 demethylases are involved in chromatin remodeling, transcriptional elongation, protein ubiquitination, enhancer–promoter interaction, and histone ubiquitination. Lysine methylation levels can also affect genomic interactions and gene expression programs in a three-dimensional fashion. SWI/SNF: switch/sucrose non-fermentable, MLL: mixed-lineage leukemia, PRC1: Polycomb repressor complex 1

trans-differentiation in a H3K27me3-dependent manner. Further elaboration on the molecular mechanisms of inflammation showed that JMJD3 only partially depends on its demethylase activity (Agger et al. 2007). Strikingly, the majority of promoters bound by JMJD3 are not associated with H3K27me3 before JMJD3 binding, and only a minor fraction of the H3K27me3 positive promoters bound by JMJD3 show decreased levels of H3K27me3 after LPS treatment. JMJD3 preferentially binds genes with increased H3K4me3 levels. Ultimately, *Jmjd3* silencing affects the expression of relatively few genes and does not result in an increase of H3K27me3 in this context. Thus, JMJD3 activity might instead serve as a safeguard against further H3K27 methylation, thereby ensuring target gene activation in response to LPS treatment (Santa et al. 2007, 2009). This context of proinflammatory activity of JMJD3 coupled to the detrimental effects of inflammation drove the initiative for the development of a lead therapeutic tool (GSKJ4) against this demethylase by GlaxoSmithKline (GSK) in 2012 (Kruidenier et al. 2012). Indeed, treatment with GSKJ4 compound dampened the inflammatory response upon LPS in macrophages through inhibition of JMJD3 demethylase activity. Respiratory syncytial virus (RSV)-infected murine bone marrow-derived dendritic cells (BMDC) and pulmonary dendritic cells showed elevated expression of Jmjd3 and Utx expression (Malinczak et al. 2020), suggesting that Utx can be also virally induced. This demethylase upregulation strengthens cytokine production and Th2 immune response upon viral infection resulting to worse immunopathology. Although the exact role of demethylases in coronavirus infection is understudied, recent research has indicated that UTX plays a crucial part in COVID-19 infection (Wei, et al. 2021). CRISPR screens have revealed that Kdm6a is significant in viral entry, potentially by regulating receptor expression (Wei, et al. 2021).

JMJD3 also contributes to cellular and neural differentiation through Smad2/3-mediated regulation of the *Brachyury* locus and activation of *Pax6* and *Sox1* (Dahle et al. 2010; Burgold et al. 2008; Dai et al. 2010), respectively. Jmjd3 functions in cranial neural crest development, via Trp53 activation as a TFDP1 cofactor and in a H3K27me demethylase-dependent fashion. Jmjd3 loss results in cleft palate and cell proliferation and differentiation defects in mice (Guo 2022). Other demethylase-related activities of JMJD3 include activation of genes important for epidermal differentiation and wound healing during skin repair (Shaw and Martin 2009; Sen et al. 2008).

In principle, the demethylase activity of JMJD3 is regulated by its intracellular localization (Kamikawa and Donohoe 2014). The JMJD3 N-terminus contains two nuclear localization sequences (Kamikawa and Donohoe 2014). Elegant studies using forced nuclear localization of JMJD3 showed a markedly enhanced H3K27me3 demethylation, whereas cytosolic localization may lead to demethylation of non-histone proteins (Zhao et al. 2015). During senescence-associated heterochromatin foci (SAHF) formation, JMJD3 is colocalized with the Golgi protein GM130 and may demethylate non-histone proteins that undergo post-translational modifications within the Golgi, such as the retinoblastoma (RB) protein at its lysine 810 residue in the case of senescence 88.

The role of UTX in development is tied to its recruitment to and subsequent regulation of the promoters of the *HOX* cluster. The *HOX* family consists of four clusters, *HOXA* through *D*. Aberrant expression of *HOX* genes is associated with developmental disorders and diseases. Loss of *UTX* results in transcriptional repression of *HOXA* and *HOXC* clusters. UTX also occupies promoters of the *HOX* cluster leading to H3K27 demethylation and the subsequent recruitment of Polycomb repressive complex 1 and monoubiquitination of histone H2A (Lee et al. 2007b). Opposing activities of PRC2 and UTX tightly regulate *HOX* expression in order to enable context-dependent transcriptional regulation. Furthermore, UTX binds directly to the promoters of genes involved in germ layer development, including *Msi1*, *Sox1*, and *Brachyury*, leading to increased levels of H3K4me3 but no change in H3K27me3 levels (Morales Torres et al. 2013). These findings suggest that UTX has a demethylase-independent role in embryonic stem cell (ESC) differentiation. Other actions of UTX include promotion of myogenesis through activation of *myogenin* and *creatine kinase* genes (Seenundun et al. 2010). Gene regulation in the muscle tissue offers a great system to study UTX-associated molecular mechanisms: UTX is recruited to muscle-specific genes by the transcriptional regulator *Six4*, resulting in localized demethylation of the upstream transcriptional regulatory region (Seenundun et al. 2010). Once associated with a specific locus, UTX spreads into the coding region via an elongating polymerase-mediated mechanism. In natural killer T (NKT) cells, UTX mediates regulation of super-enhancer accessibility and NKT cell development (Beyaz et al. 2017). Implication of UTX in the positive or negative regulation of super-enhancers might be a recurrent theme as Andricovich and colleagues showed that in pancreatic cancer in females, loss of UTX leads to activation of disease-related superenhancers that can be targeted using bromodomain and extra-terminal domain (BET) inhibitors (Andricovich, et al. 2018). These studies provide insights into the mechanism by which UTX acts to remove the H3K27me3 mark over several kilobases of sequence at specific loci.

7.2.1 Demethylase-Independent Molecular Functions for H3K27me3 Histone Demethylases

There is cumulative evidence supports the importance of non-demethylase activities of JMJD3 and UTX. As mentioned previously, initial studies in mouse macrophages (Santa et al. 2009) showed that only a small fraction of JMJD3-occupied genes exhibited reduced levels of H3K27 methylation upon inflammation.

UTX and JMJD3 associate with the mixed-lineage leukemia (MLL, also known as COMPASS) protein complex (Fig. 7.4) (Santa et al. 2007; Ntziachristos et al. 2014; Issaeva et al. 2007), which catalyzes H3K4 methylation and contributes to gene activation. The central core common to all COMPASS and COMPASS-related complexes is composed of WDR5, ASH2, RBBP5, and DPY30 factors. The main methyltransferases include Set1A/B, the central H3K4 methyltransferases for the mammalian COMPASS (mCOMPASS), MLL1/2 (encoded by *KMT2A/B*, methylates H3K4me2), and MLL3/4 (*KMT2C/D*), which controls H3K4me1 at enhancers (Hu et al. 2013). Enhancers bearing this histone mark are active or poised for activation. There is published evidence that UTX is part of the MLL3- and MLL4-containing complexes at enhancers (Issaeva et al. 2007). Nevertheless, differences between MLL3- and MLL4-bearing complexes, as well as the exact role of UTX and its mutations on MLL localization and function, are poorly characterized. It was recently shown that the UTX-MLL4 complex leads to an increase in p300-dependent H3K27 acetylation via UTX-dependent p300 recruitment, and MLL4-mediated H3K4 monomethylation requires, in turn, p300 function (Wang et al. 2017). One speculation is that a significant part of UTX/MLL3/4 activity regulates the enhancers of tumor suppressor genes. In this case, UTX may serve as a scaffold that

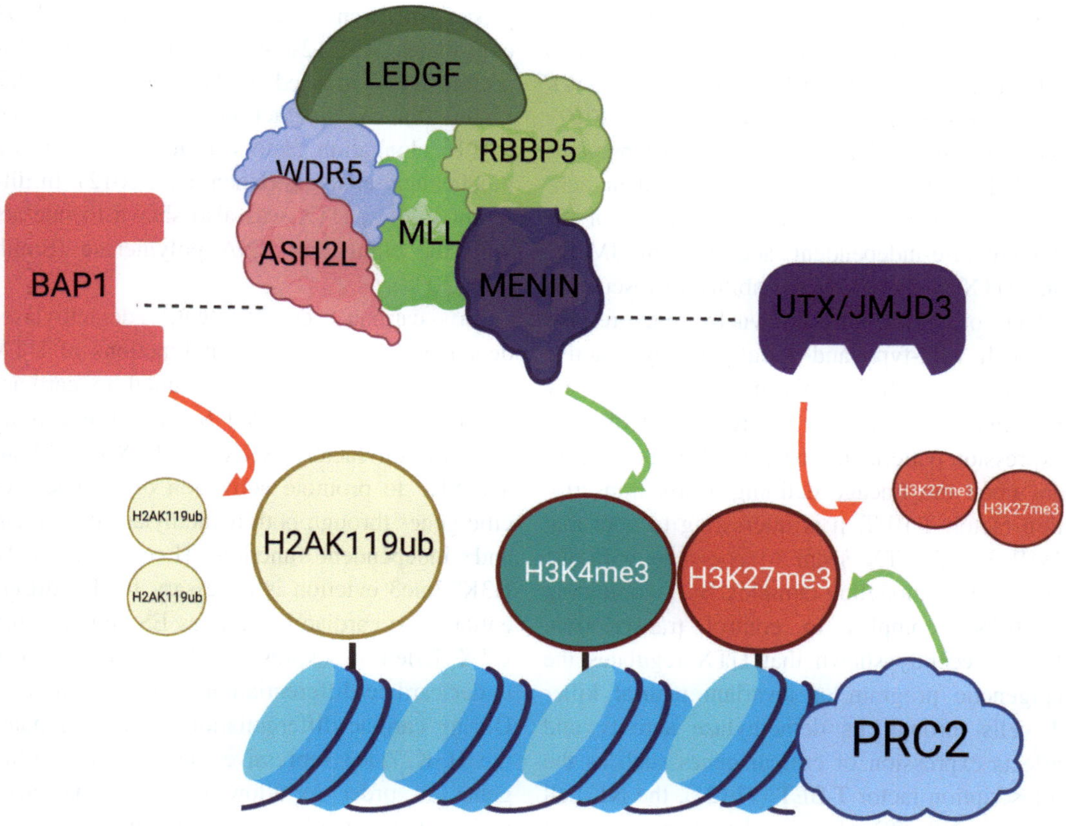

Fig. 7.4 Participation of JMJD3 and UTX in MLL lysine 4 methyltransferase complexes. Demethylase-containing MLL complexes antagonize the Polycomb complex and activate gene expression via methylation of lysine 4 and demethylation of lysine 27 on histone H3 and deubiquitination of lysine 119 on histone H2A

is required for the activity or the targeting of MLL3/MLL4 to target genes. Mutations affecting the *UTX* locus may lead to aberrant MLL localization and enhancer function on tumor suppressor genes (Herz et al. 2014). Work by Wang and Shilatifard showed that UTX/MLL3 complex associates with the BAP1 histone H2A deubiquitinase to control the balance of histone ubiquitination and methylation (Wang et al. 2018) (Fig. 7.4). The group demonstrated that the deubiquitinase activity of BAP1 and the demethylase activity of UTX are critical for MLL3 complex function. This is supported by the fact that EZH2 inhibitors can act therapeutically in cancer cases with UTX and MLL3/4 mutations (Wang et al. 2018).

JMJD3 and UTX play an important role in T cell lineage commitment by interacting with T-BET and BRG1 in a demethylase activity-independent manner (Miller et al. 2010) (Fig. 7.3). JMJD3 mediates promoter remodeling and optimal gene expression through interaction with the BRG1-containing SWI/SNF remodeling complex (Miller et al. 2010). Knockdown of UTX, JMJD3, or Brg1 prevents the T-BET transcription factor-dependent activation of several genes. The importance of the demethylase-independent activities of JMJD3 and UTX is shown by the ability to rescue the effects of JMJD3 knockdown by re-expression of both wild-type and a catalytically inactive mutant of JMJD3. This mechanistic activity for Jmjd3 is critical in the regulation of gene expression patterns in Th1 cells that are dependent upon the lineage defining T-box transcription factor, T-BET. It is interesting to note that JMJD3 and UTX seem to coevolve with the chromatin remodeling complex Brg1-containing SWI/SNF complex to control transcription. It was recently shown that UTX regulates the epigenetic program of invariant natural killer T cells through its demethylase activity and affects expression of critical genes such as the transcription factor T-BET (*Tbx21*), the NK cell receptor NKG2D (*Klrk1*), the chemokine and cytokine receptors CXCR3 (*Cxcr3*) and CD122 (*Il2rb*), the cytokine IFN-(*Ifng*), and the calcium regulator calcyclin (*S100a6*). It has been shown that UTX, BRM, and the histone acetyltransferase CREB binding protein (CBP) colocalize at many active Polycomb target genes marked by the transcriptional activation mark, acetylation of lysine 27 on histone H3 (H3K27ac) (Tie et al. 2012). UTX and BRM bind directly to conserved zinc fingers of CBP. Knockdown of UTX or BRM reduces H3K27ac levels and concomitantly increases H3K27me3 levels (Tie et al. 2012). In this biological context, the demethylases remove a repressive methyl mark and keep the promoter active through participation in chromatin remodeling complexes. This physical and functional connection between demethylases and remodelers could be evolutionarily conserved and might deserve further investigation in various developmental, physiological, and disease contexts.

Another important property of JMJD3 and UTX seems to be their participation in the process of transcriptional elongation. JMJD3 contributes to 12-O-tetradecanoylphorbol-13-acetate (TPA)-induced HL-60 (myeloid) cell differentiation via interaction with the SPT6 and SPT16 elongation factors as it was shown via biochemical analyses (Chen et al. 2012). In different studies, UTX was also shown to interact with the elongating RNA polymerase (Smith et al. 2008).

In cardiac development, demethylase-dependent and -independent functions of UTX are intertwined. UTX is recruited to cardiac-specific enhancers guided by the core cardiac transcription factors NKX2-5, TBX5, GATA4, and SRF to promote activation of cardiac-specific genes through both demethylase-dependent and -independent functions (Lee et al. 2012). H3K27me3 eviction is necessary for ES differentiation to cardiac lineage, as ES cells lacking UTX failed to express cardiac-specific genes under cardiac differentiation conditions in vitro. During cardiac differentiation, UTX eliminates the H3K27me3 repressive mark at myocardial genes in order to allow transcriptional activation. Consistently, in the absence of UTX, cardiac genes are still marked by H3K27me3 even under cardiac differentiation-promoting conditions (Lee et al. 2012). In addition, UTX and UTY facilitate the recruitment of BRG1-containing SWI/SNF chromatin remodeling complexes to cardiac-specific enhancers. The importance of UTX for cardiac differentiation is further underlined by the fact that *Utx*-null mice are embryonic lethal, with failed cardiac development (Lee et al. 2012).

7.3 Modeling JMJD3 and UTX Activity In Vivo

Numerous knockout and knockin animal models have shed light on their important biological functions. The important role for JMJD3 in development is further underlined by the perinatal death of mice bearing a germline homozygous loss of *Jmjd3* due to premature development of lung tissues leading to respiratory defects (Jepsen et al. 2007). Akira, Satoh, and colleagues showed that main hematopoietic and immune cell populations, such as T, B, dendritic, plasmacytoid dendritic natural killer cells, neutrophils, macrophages, and monocytes in the spleen were unaltered between wild-type and JMJD3 knockout background animals and the cells respond similarly to different stimuli. This included differentiation into type 1 or type 2 helper T cells (T_H1 and T_H2). Jmjd3 is dispensable for M1 macrophage polarization in response to bacterial infections, but it is essential for M2 macrophage polarization upon helminth infection (Satoh et al. 2010). Indeed, a few Jmjd3 targets, such as *Irf4*, present increased methylation of H3K27 and concomitant reduced expression. It was recently shown that production of a-ketoglutarate (aKG) via glutaminolysis is important for Jmjd3 activity and activation of M2-related genes (Liu et al. 2017). Thus, Jmjd3 and its demethylase activity is critical for the development of M2 macrophages, leading to anti-helminth host responses. The role of Jmjd33 was also studied in the worm organism *Caenorhabditis elegans*, where, surprisingly, deletion of Jmjd3-like genes has no effect on viability and fertility resulting in minor gonadal defects.

Utx plays critical roles in mouse embryonic development and homozygous Utx-deleted females and compound *Utx/Utx*-deficient male embryos showed significant growth, neural, cardiac defects, and anemia by E9.5-10.5 (Shpargel et al. 2012; Wang et al. 2012) and they die in gestation. Nevertheless, some male mice hemizygous for *Utx* that express the wild-type Uty can survive although they present with small size and reduced life span (Welstead et al. 2012). Collectively, these findings show that UTY can partially compensate for UTX. Although UTY possesses significantly lower demethylase activity (Lan et al. 2007; Walport et al. 2014b) compared to UTX, some UTX functions are demethylase independent and so UTY can compensate for UTX in demethylase-dependent and -independent manners. JMJD3 and/or UTX deletion in human embryonic stem cells (hESCs) impaired cell proliferation and neural progenitor cells differentiation to neurons and glia (Shan et al. 2020). Expression of neuron-specific chromatin remodeling BAF (nBAF) can rescue this phenotype seemingly in a demethylase-independent manner. JMJD3 and UTX are enriched in loci essential for neural development in neural progenitor cells, and JMJD3 elimination results in H3K27me3 accumulation and blockade of DNA accessibility at these genes. A recent study using *Utx* deletion in mouse neural stem/progenitor cells (NSPCs) showed that Utx regulates genes critical to proper neural development in NSPCs, and UTX loss leads to impaired cell cycle exit, reduced differentiation, and neonatal death (Koizumi et al. 2022). Male mice hemizygous for *Utx* survived postnatally and ultimately died of hydrocephalus, a manifestation of Kabuki syndrome.

Further investigation is required to elucidate unique functions of UTX compared to UTY to provide insights into the roles of histone demethylases in development and cancer. This should include generation of antibodies that can be used in characterization of biochemical complexes and chromatin topology. An important question is whether UTX and UTY are part of the same complex or complementary biochemical complexes.

7.3.1 JMJD3 and UTX: Friends or Foes?

7.3.1.1 T Cell Development: JMJD3 and UTX Collaborative Activities

Deletion of *Jmjd3* and *Utx* individually does not significantly affect T cell development (Ntziachristos et al. 2014; Satoh et al. 2010; Bosselut 2016). Nevertheless, Bosselut and colleagues generated animals with compound deletion of *Jmjd3* and *Utx* to demonstrate that the enzymes are redundantly required for H3K27me3 homeostasis and gene expression (Manna et al. 2015). The authors used non-dividing CD4, CD8 double- and single-positive T thymocyte populations to show that they are needed for the removal of H3K27me3 from the promoters of genes characteristic of mature T cells, such as *S1pr1*, needed for thymocyte egress. As a result, JMJD3 and UTX are required for the generation of a normal T cell repertoire. As this effect was not rescued by UTY, the authors concluded that the catalytic activity of UTX and not UTY is necessary for normal T cell phenotype.

7.3.1.2 Stem Cell Reprogramming and Differentiation: Contrasting Roles for UTX and JMJD3

During ESC differentiation, UTX regulates its target genes in different ways that could be dependent or independent of its H3K27me2/3 demethylation activity (Mansour et al. 2012). UTX was shown to play a critical role during reprogramming of somatic cells towards induced pluripotent stem cells (iPSCs). In this case, genome-wide changes in the transcriptome and chromatin structure are induced to achieve the switch to pluripotency. UTX has a critical role in efficient induction or re-establishment of pluripotency during the generation of iPSCs in vitro, but is dispensable for maintenance of pluripotency. The requirement for UTX to ensure correct reprogramming at least partially depends on its H3K27me3 demethylase activity. UTX target genes that are enriched in H3K4me3 in *Utx* wild-type mouse embryonic fibroblasts (MEFs) aberrantly accumulate H3K27me3 in *Utx* mutant MEFs. These loci, including the stem cell maintenance genes *Sall1*, *Sall4*, and *Utf1*, as well as validated *Klf4* and *Oct4* target genes, fail to reactivate during reprogramming due to loss of UTX. Hence, UTX seems to play a crucial role in reprogramming through its H3K27me2/3 demethylation activity for correct re-activation of essential pluripotency genes. During ESC differentiation, re-activation of developmental genes is associated with loss of H3K27me3. Loss of UTX affects the differentiation capacity of ESCs without influencing pluripotency. This is reflected by the loss of induction of a set of developmental genes including ectoderm markers (*Otx2*, *Msi1*, *Sox1*, and *Pax6*), endoderm markers (*Gata4*, *Gata6*, *Foxa2*, *Sox17*, *Gsc*, and *Ncad*), and mesoderm markers (*Vegfr2*, *Wnt3*, and *Brachyury*). UTX is required for the activation of retinoic acid (RA)-inducible bivalent genes during RA-driven differentiation of mouse embryonic stem cells (ESCs). In contrast, a decrease in H3K27me3 levels and an increase in H3K4me3 levels were noticed at the promoter of the UTX target *Hoxb1* during differentiation of wild-type ESCs. Male UTX KO ESCs that express a catalytically inactive or wild-type UTX protein could rescue the induction of expression of the mesoderm genes *Wnt3* and *Brachyury*, supporting the H3K27me3 demethylase-independent role of UTX during ESC differentiation. These findings show that UTX regulates transcriptional activity during ESC differentiation in modes both dependent and independent of its H3K27me2/3 demethylation activity.

JMJD3 modulation of iPSC formation is partially dependent on its function as a histone demethylase. The enzyme is known to target demethylation at the *INK4a/ARF* locus (Zhao et al. 2013), and it was also demonstrated to inhibit somatic cell reprogramming via regulating PHF20 ubiquitination and subsequent proteasomal degradation (Zhao et al. 2013). PHF20 plays a critical role in the maintenance of the pluripotent state. JMJD3 recruits Trim26, an E3 ligase, to PHF20 for polyubiquitination, thus blocking iPSC reprogramming. PHF20 binds to the *Oct4* promoter and specifically interacts with Wdr5. Deletion of PHF20 results in decreased Wdr5-*Oct4* promoter binding, suggesting a critical role for PHF20 in the successful re-activation of endogenous *Oct4* expression to generate fully reprogrammed iPSCs. Jmjd3 is necessary for hematopoietic stem cell (HSC) self-renewal in response to stress induced upon inflammation and proliferation in adult mice. Indeed, Jmjd3 loss in adult mice leads to a pro-differentiation poised state and HSC depletion due to induction of expression of the Fos and Jun components of the AP-1 transcription factor complex in a demethylase-independent fashion (Mallaney et al. 2019).

7.4 Roles of Lysine 27 Demethylases in Disease

There is a relatively small number of studies about lysine demethylases in diseases other than cancer with a focus on mental disorders (Pedersen and Helin 2010; Ciavatta et al. 2010; Laumonnier et al. 2005; Abidi et al. 2007; Koivisto et al. 2007; Pointon et al. 2011; Adegbola et al. 2008; Jensen et al. 2010). For instance, mutations affecting lysine 4 demethylases are found in x-linked mental retardation as it was shown in the discovery paper for JARID1C/SMCX back in 2007 (Iwase et al. 2007) and in subsequent studies (Jensen et al. 2010).

UTX and *MLL2* are frequently mutated in Kabuki syndrome (Lederer et al. 2012; Miyake et al. 2013), a rare congenital syndrome. Kabuki patients present with facial malformations and mental disorders and have a predisposition for multiple different cancers including pre-B-ALL, hepatoblastoma, neuroblastoma, Burkitt lymphoma, and fibromyxoid sarcoma. In this section, we will explore the role of lysine 27 demethylases in disease contexts using cancer as a proof-of-principle.

7.4.1 Cancer Studies Showed a Substantially Diverse Repertoire of JMJD3 Functions

Seligson et al. showed that histone modifications, methylation in particular, may predict the risk of developing prostate cancer (Seligson et al. 2005). To this end, it does not come as a surprise that epigenetic modulators might play tumor suppressor or oncogenic roles in different cancer contexts. Mechanistically, it seems that JMJD3 is highly expressed in prostate cancer and cooperates with SMAD2/3 factors to activate genes such as the *cyclin D1* locus (Cao et al. 2021). In therapy-resistant prostate cancer, inhibition of histone demethylases has been suggested as a therapeutic option (Morozov et al. 2017). Lysine 27-associated epigenetic modulators, such as the methyltransferase Polycomb complex, have been extensively studied in different cancer contexts (Ntziachristos et al. 2012; Zhang et al. 2012; Simon et al. 2012). JMJD3 was suggested to play tumor suppressor roles, as the *KDM6B* locus lies in close proximity to the well-established tumor suppressor p53, and is subject to frequent genetic lesions in cancer via allelic loss of the short arm of chromosome 17 (17p13.1) that contains both genes (Nigro et al. 1989). This loss correlates with high proliferative activity and is associated with more aggressive tumor behavior. The role of JMJD3 as a tumor suppressor is also associated with regulation of the *INK4A–ARF* locus (Barradas et al. 2009). The locus encodes for two tumor suppressor proteins, $p16^{INK4a}$ and $p14^{ARF}$ ($p19^{Arf}$ in the mouse), and is disrupted in almost 40% of human cancers. Polycomb proteins catalyze the spread of repressive H3K27me3 marks and control expression of INK4A/ARF locus (Jacobs et al. 1999; Lowe and Sherr 2003). JMJD3 plays a critical role in de-activating the *INK4A–ARF* locus through lysine demethylation, leading to senescence, and prevents reprogramming in fibroblasts (Barradas et al. 2009; Agger et al. 2009). Loss of H3K27me3 at the *INK4A–ARF* locus as a result of H3K27me3 demethylase activity, and/or loss of methyltransferase activity of the Polycomb complex, occurs in senescent cells. Inactivation of the *INK4A-ARF* locus prevents induction of cellular senescence, which occurs in a variety of cancer types. This shows that loss of activity or aberrant localization of K27 demethylases may drive cells toward a pluripotent and tumorigenic state. Several JmjC-containing genes, including *JMJD3*, *JMJD6*, and *KIAA1718 (KDM7)*, are transcriptionally induced via RAS in primary human epithelial cell lines (http://www.oncomine.org). RAS is known to trigger oncogene-induced senescence in primary mammalian cells, indicating that the three JmjC proteins may have roles in senescence induction.

Compound loss of JMJD3 and p53 may cause inactivation of both the p16 and p53 tumor suppressor pathways and likely accounts for the aggressive tumor behavior in these cancers. Moreover, p53 is one of the first non-histone substrates found to be targeted by demethylases: JMJD3 associates with and demethylates the transcriptionally active tetrameric form of p53, resulting in its stabilization and accumulation in the nucleus (Sola et al. 2011). Genome-wide mapping of JMJD3 and p53 by chromatin immunoprecipitation showed an overlap of JMJD3 and p53 target genes, which included several well-characterized p53 targets related to cell cycle, stress responses, and apoptosis (Williams et al. 2014). JMJD3 is induced by DNA damage and recruited by p53 to its target genes (Williams et al. 2014).

In colorectal carcinoma, JMJD3 expression levels are lower compared to normal tissue and correlate with increased cell cycle gene expression and lower levels of apoptosis (Tokunaga et al. 2016). JMJD3 expression is upregulated in precancerous pancreatic lesions, but is downregulated upon progression of malignant disease (Yamamoto et al. 2014). In pancreatic cancer, loss of JMJD3 augments the aggressiveness of cells and metastasis to the liver (Tokunaga et al. 2016). Moreover, leukemia cases have deletions in p53 and the *INK4A-ARF* locus, but the *KDM6B* locus is intact, seemingly decoupling JMJD3 levels and activity from p53 status. JMJD3 levels are elevated in stem and progenitor cells in patients with myelodysplastic syndrome (MDS) (Wei et al. 2013), a disease associated with abnormal hematopoietic differentiation into one or more blood cell lineages. Functional studies of JMJD3 overexpression in the hematopoietic system showed that JMJD3 can lead to MDS and CMML via modulation of H3K27me3 and H3K4me3 levels and activation of gene transcription. MDS could lead to acute myeloid leukemia (AML). In certain subtypes of AML, JMJD3 has been shown to interact with C/EBPβ to alleviate the differentiation arrest, and it thus acts as a tumor suppressor in this disease (Yu et al. 2018). These differences in JMJD3 functional role in MDS and AML further underline the context-specific role of JMJD3 in cancer.

In gastric cancer, high JMJD3 expression correlates with poor prognosis (Xu et al. 2019). Mechanistically, JMJD3 demethylates and activates control elements associated with C-X-C chemokine receptor type 4 (CXCR4) gene, facilitating proliferation and metastasis of gastric tumors (Liu et al. 2022). In breast cancer, JMJD3 is recruited to estrogen receptor-bound enhancers, leading to demethylation of H3K27 at the *BCL2* regulatory element and activation of BCL2 through formation of three-dimensional interactions with the promoter of the gene (Svotelis et al. 2011). This leads to lower ligand dependency upon estrogen receptor-mediated gene expression. JMJD3 is transcriptionally upregulated in renal cell carcinoma (Shen et al. 2012). JMJD3 facilitates TGF-β-induced epithelial–mesenchymal transition (EMT) in mammary epithelial cells through expression of the EMT-specific gene, *SNAI1*, leading to breast cancer invasion (Ramadoss et al. 2012). Similarly, in hepatocellular carcinoma upregulation of JMJD3 leads to epithelial–mesenchymal transition (EMT) and metastasis (Tang et al. 2016). In esophageal squamous cell carcinoma (ESCC), JMJD3 controls demethylation and activation of the *C/EBPβ* locus promoting metastasis, which was inhibited using the GSKJ4 compound (Qin et al. 2021). These studies suggest that JMJD3 might be a key regulator in cancer metastasis. In colon cancer, vitamin D induces expression of EMT genes such as *ZEB1*, *ZEB2*, and *SNAI1* through upregulation of JMJD3 (Pereira et al. 2012). Vitamin D regulates JMJD3 to promote gene activation by removing repressive marks in key genes associated with colon cancer cells (Pereira et al. 2012). JMJD3 promotes multiple myeloma cell survival via regulation of the MAPK pathway (Ohguchi et al. 2017), whereas, in melanoma, JMJD3 acts as a pro-oncogenic factor through its implication in NFκB and bone morphogenetic protein (BMP) pathways (Park et al. 2016).

7.4.2 The Talented Mr. JMJD3: The Role of JMJD3 in Neurogenesis and Brain Tumors

JMJD3 was shown to control brain neurogenesis through activation of neuronal gene expression (Park et al. 2014). Retinoic acid (RA)-induced neuronal differentiation in P19 cells leads to increased JMJD3, but not UTX, and subsequent expression and activation of the *Mash1/Ascl1* gene through Hes1-dependent binding to the *Mash1* promoter (Dai et al. 2010). Similarly, JMJD3 is involved in the RA- or Notch-dependent induction of differentiation along the neuronal pathway and subsequent forebrain development in the mouse (Jepsen et al. 2007). In the absence of ligand, RA-dependent differentiation along the neuronal pathway is repressed by the nuclear receptor corepressor SMRT/NCOR-2. The SMRT/NCOR-2 complex directly binds and inhibits JMJD3 transcriptional activation by promoter-mediated repression. RA-induced neuronal differentiation results in nuclear SMRT/NCOR-2 destabilization and JMJD3-dependent activation, resulting in differentiation and suppression of proliferation. This is a demethylase-mediated effect on histone methylation. JMJD3 is highly expressed in neuroblastoma compared to UTX and UTY, via super-enhancer regulation and is a critical factor for the activation of MYC, MYCN, and downstream targets of E2F transcription factor via histone demethylation and chromatin remodeling of E2F targets. JMJD3 demethylates H3K27 in enhancer areas that are bound by CTCF/BORIS and are connected in 3D with E2F-regulated promoters. JMJD3 inhibition using GSKJ4 is very efficient in targeting the activity of these enhancer areas, particularly in MYCN-amplified neuroblastoma, and yields a phenotype similar to CDK4/6 (that phosphorylate the retinoblastoma protein leading to E2F activation) inhibition.

The role of JMJD3 in glioma is of particular interest as well, as JMJD3 is highly expressed in patients with high-grade glioma (Perrigue et al. 2015). Initial studies suggested that JMJD3 is a tumor suppressor gene in glioblastoma multiforme (GBM), interacting with p53 in GBM stem cells. Furthermore, JMJD3 re-activation induces p53 nuclear accumulation, resulting in p53-mediated differentiation of glioblastoma stem cells (GSCs) via chromatin-dependent (*INK4A/ARF* locus activation) and chromatin-independent (nuclear p53 protein stabilization) mechanisms (Ene et al. 2012). Pediatric brainstem glioma often harbors the oncogenic lysine 27 to methionine mutation of histone H3.3. GSKJ4, a JMJD3 inhibitor, increases H3K27 methylation in K27M tumor cells and demonstrates potent antitumor activity in vitro and in vivo, in xenograft models. These results demonstrate that inhibition of K27 demethylase activity is a valid therapeutic strategy for treating K27M-expressing brainstem glioma.

7.4.3 UTX Mainly Acts as a Tumor Suppressor in Cancer

The histone demethylase *UTX* was the first mutated histone demethylase gene associated with cancer (Haaften et al. 2009; Wang and Shilatifard 2019; Tran et al. 2020) (also see our previous review article, ref. 64, for a summary of UTX mutations in cancer), suggesting that cancer cell growth might be regulated via H3K27 methylation levels at site-specific promoters or enhancers. UTX deletion was found to promote myelodysplastic syndrome and increase mobility of c-kit+ hematopoietic progenitors (Thieme et al. 2013), suggesting it functions as a tumor suppressor in this context. The *UTX* gene often undergoes somatic loss-of-function mutations in multiple cancers including leukemia, bladder cancer, prostate tumors, renal carcinoma, and medulloblastoma. *UTX* deletions and reduced expression were found in several mouse APL tumors (Wartman et al. 2011). Loss-of-function mutations of *UTX* were found in 5/35 T cell acute lymphoblastic leukemia (T-ALL) patient samples, three frameshift and two insertions/deletions (indels) localized within the Jumonji C catalytic domain (Meulen et al. 2015). We previously identified two patients with focal deletions of *UTX*, and six more patient cases with *UTX* mutations in T-ALL, including indels, missense, and frameshift alterations, all predicted to have an inactivating role (Ntziachristos et al. 2014). Overall *UTX* is mutated in ~5% of T-ALL cases.

In chronic myelomonocytic leukemia (CMML), a type of myeloid disease, *UTX* mutations co-occur with *ASXL1*, *TET2*, or *CBL* mutations, while in bladder cancer it co-occurs with somatic *BAP1* mutations (Nickerson et al. 2014), enhancing in vitro proliferation, in vivo tumor growth, and cell migration (Nickerson et al. 2014). Recent studies showed that loss of UTX in vivo can lead to myeloid transformation and CMML via an increase in expression of transcription factors Gata1 and Zfpm1 and aberrant hematopoietic stem cell self-renewal and differentiation (Zheng et al. 2018). Similarly, in acute myeloid leukemia, UTX acts to repress oncogenic ETS and upregulate tumor-suppressive GATA programs via modulation of the activities of the chromatin remodeling complexes and the COMPASS complex (Gozdecka et al. 2018).

Bladder cancer has one of the highest frequencies of *UTX* mutations, including truncating mutations in the JmjC domain. More than 50% of bladder cancer patients harbor genetic aberrations in a bigger set of chromatin remodeling genes including *UTX* and associated complexes, such as *CREBBP*, *EP300*, *ARID1A*, *CHD6*, *MLL1*, *MLL3*, and *NCOR1*. Analysis of noninvasive bladder cancer cohort revealed a gender bias with female patients exhibiting a higher proportion of UTX mutation compared to male ones (Hurst et al. 2017). A recent study showed that UTX interacts with FOXA1 to activate genes related to urothelial differentiation, and UTX loss leads to an epigenetic reprogramming of bladder cancer cells that promotes tumorigenesis in an ATF3-dependent manner that represses FOXA1 targets and activates cell cycle-promoting <genes (Qiu et al. 2023). Mucoadhesive nanoparticle-mediated intravesical delivery of messenger RNA (mRNA) of UTX restored the demethylase levels and exhibited therapeutic potential in treating bladder cancer metastasis (Kong 2022). This is a proof-of-principle study for therapeutic manipulation of demethylases in solid tumors.

Furthermore, multiple myeloma cases harbor mutations in *UTX* or in the trithorax complex members. The Licht laboratory demonstrated that loss of UTX promotes proliferation of multiple myeloma cells potentially via upregulation of oncogenic programs and IRF4 that stimulates MYC expression (Ezponda et al. 2017). In gastrointestinal tumors, such as liver and pancreatic cancers, UTX transcriptionally activates competitors of mTOR signaling, such as *DEPTOR*, to suppress the pathway in a demethylase-dependent fashion (Revia et al. 2022). Tumors deficient for UTX have high mTOR signaling activity and are vulnerable to mTOR targeting (Revia et al. 2022). In bladder cancer, lung cancer, multiple myeloma, as well as T-ALL, there is rationale for targeting UTX mutant using EZH2 inhibitors (Meulen et al. 2015; Ezponda et al. 2017; Ler 2017; Wu et al. 2018).

Furthermore, UTX interacts with KMT2D (*MLL4*) that is also frequently mutated in cancer (Parsons et al. 2011). *KMT2D*, but not *KMT2C (MLL3)*, was also found to be mutated and inactivated in cases of B cell lymphoma (Morin et al. 2011; Pasqualucci et al. 2011; Ortega-Molina et al. 2015; Zhang et al. 2015). *Utx* knockout in mouse B lymphocytes coupled to Eμ-Myc expression leads to aberrant expression of B Lymphocyte Kinase (Blk) and Ephrin B1 (Efnb1) genes leading to aberrant

B cell proliferation and cell adhesion and the development of lymphoma (Li et al. 2018). Characterization of the mutation status of *KMT2C/D* genes in ALL showed that *KMT2C* is mutated in both B-ALL (Mar et al. 2012; Lindqvist et al. 2015) and adult T-ALL (~10% of samples) (Wang et al. 2017). Work by the Shilatifard laboratory showed that alterations in *KTM2C* (*MLL3*) and *BAP1* in breast and other cancers affect the molecular functions of MLL complexes with regard to the control of enhancer activity and have similar molecular phenotypes as UTX mutations or deletion (Wang et al. 2018).

UTX tumor suppressor role has its molecular underpinnings in the regulation of several retinoblastoma-binding genes that mediate cell cycle arrest. Retinoblastoma (Rb) protein is a tumor suppressor that negatively regulates cell cycle progression by inhibiting the transcription factor E2F. UTX upregulates *HBP1*, a member of the HMG-box transcription factor family known to inhibit the expression of several growth regulatory genes and oncogenes. HBP1 physically interacts with RB and can enforce cell cycle arrest (Falco et al. 2006). In T-ALL, UTX controls several tumor suppressor genes, such as *Fbxw7*, *Rbbp7,* and *Suz12* (Ntziachristos et al. 2014).

dUTX, the *Drosophila* UTX homolog, is a suppressor of Notch- and Rb (Herz, et al. 2010)-dependent tumors in *Drosophila melanogaster* (Herz, et al. 2010). Notch is involved in many biological processes, including cell–cell communication, stem cell maintenance, differentiation, and proliferation. Hyperactivation of Notch in dUTX mutant cells leads to tumor-like growth when the Drosophila Rb homolog (Rbf) is mutated. Another study identified Rb-binding proteins as UTX targets and showed that, in mammalian cells, depletion of UTX resulted in increased proliferation. Thus, modulation of Rb activity by UTX appears to have distinct modes of regulation that may be tissue specific.

This antagonism between Notch and UTX potentially explains why UTX is a tumor suppressor in Notch1-expressing leukemia cases. Indeed, many UTX targets are downregulated in mouse models of UTX-deficient T-ALL. These include tumor suppressor genes, such as *FBXW7* and retinoblastoma proteins (Ntziachristos et al. 2014).

7.4.4 JMJD3 and UTX: Two Demethylases, Several Combinations

The two demethylase enzymes seem to have different behaviors in different cellular contexts and their action can be either synergistic, as we discussed the case of T cell development (Manna et al. 2015), or antagonistic, as presented below.

7.4.5 Context-Dependent Oncogenic Roles for UTX in Cancer: Leukemia and Solid Tumors

The TAL1 subgroup of T-ALL is uniquely sensitive to variations in the dosage and activity of UTX/KDM6A (Benyoucef et al. 2016). UTX is a coactivator of TAL1 and acts as a major regulator of the TAL1-positive leukemic gene expression program. Furthermore UTX, previously described as a tumor suppressor in T-ALL (Ntziachristos et al. 2014; Meulen et al. 2015), might be a pro-oncogenic cofactor essential for leukemia maintenance in the TAL1-positive subtype of T-ALL (Benyoucef et al. 2016). UTX inhibition, using the GSKJ4 compound, was proposed as a therapeutic means in TAL1-positive leukemia.

Breast cancer is another tumor type where UTX has been reported to be upregulated and play potentially pro-oncogenic roles (Kim et al. 2014; Choi, et al. 2015). UTX-regulated demethylation of H3K27 and MLL4-mediated trimethylation at H3K4 occurred interdependently on genes. In breast cancer, high levels of UTX or MLL4 were associated with poor prognosis. Furthermore, inhibition of UTX and its demethylase activity was demonstrated to increased sensitivity to radiation in cancer cell lines (Rath et al. 2018). Hypoxia is a tumor-promoting factor in breast cancer, mainly via the activation of the hypoxia-inducing factor 1 (HIF1) that orchestrates the transcription of breast cancer stem cells factors. Upon chemotherapy treatment and HIF1 activation, the HIF1 target S100A10 forms a complex with ANXA2, the nucleosomal chaperone SPT6, and UTX in OCT4-bound genomic sites, in cancer stem cell gene loci such as NANOG, SOX2, and KLF4 (Lu et al. 2020). UTX targeting KDM6A also inhibits this chemotherapy-induced phenotype. Similarly to S100A10, HIF1 targets the nuclear prelamin A recognition factor (NARF) that subsequently recruits UTX to OCT4-bound loci, such as the ones encoding the pluripotency factors (NANOG, KLF4, and SOX2), leading to H3K27 demethylation and gene activation, and maintenance of the breast cancer stem cells (Yang, et al. 2022). Thus, targeting UTX might synergize with chemotherapy to eradicate cancer stem cells in breast cancer.

In a lung cancer system, cells mutant for the SMARCA4 chromatin remodeler, presenting with accumulation of H3K27me3, are sensitive to inhibition of UTX (and JMJD3) (Romero et al. 2021). In the same study, GSKJ4-mediated inhibition of the demethylases led to a significant tumor regression in in vivo systems of lung and ovarian cancers (Romero et al. 2021). These findings point toward a context- and potentially disease stage- or treatment-specific roles for UTX.

7.4.6 Contrasting Roles for JMJD3 and UTX in T-ALL

T-ALL presents another interesting characteristic of demethylase biology: JMJD3 and UTX play contrasting roles in Notch1-positive contexts of this disease, as referred to earlier (Ntziachristos et al. 2014). Indeed, JMJD3 is a pro-oncogenic factor and is recruited by Notch1 to upregulate genes with oncogenic roles in leukemia. JMJD3 is necessary so that Notch1 expression leads to T-ALL in mice and small molecule inhibition of JMJD3 using GSKJ4 inhibits leukemia growth. In line with those findings, JMJD3 was showed to be critical for context-specific leukemogenesis for T-ALL and M5-type myeloid leukemia in mice (Mallaney et al. 2019). Further studies showed that JMJD3 prevents apoptosis induced by stress in a Notch1-expressing mouse model of T-ALL (Issa et al. 2023). In contrast to JMJD3, preliminary studies showed that UTX might control the expression of tumor suppressor genes, such as *Fbxw7* and the ones encoding for retinoblastoma-binding proteins (Ntziachristos et al. 2014). Thus, the two demethylases have the same biochemical but opposing physiological roles, potentially due to different interacting partners and ultimately different target genes (Ntziachristos et al. 2014). The exact mechanistic underpinnings of this differential behavior, including in TAL1-positive T-ALL cases (see previous paragraph and Benyoucef et al. (2016) on the context-dependent roles of UTX), remain to be characterized.

7.5 Inhibiting Histone Demethylases

Inhibition of epigenetic proteins with pro-oncogenic properties has been suggested as a targeted therapy in cancer and other diseases (Dawson and Kouzarides 2012; Dawson et al. 2012; Helin and Dhanak 2013; Hojfeldt et al. 2013). Use of DNA methylation and histone deacetylase (HDAC) inhibitors in cancer has paved the way for the use of different flavors of epigenetic therapy. Due to the role of demethylases in cancer, viral infection, and inflammation, there has been an active effort to identify specific inhibitors for these enzymes (also see Hojfeldt et al. (2013), Thinnes et al. (2014)).

7.5.1 Enzymatic Function of Lysine Demethylases

To design inhibitors against lysine 27 demethylases, one should first understand their mechanism of action. This mechanism is significantly different than the LSD family consisting of oxidases that use FAD as a cofactor, despite the fact that both reactions end up in an unstable hemiaminal intermediate that rapidly decomposes into formaldehyde and the demethylated lysine (Kooistra and Helin 2012; Hoffmann et al. 2012; Morera et al. 2016). The JMJ enzymes use two cofactors, Fe(II) and 2-oxoglutarate, which are bound to the JmjC domain; they react with dioxygen and form a highly active oxoferryl (Fe(iv)=O) intermediate that leads to hydroxylation of the ζ-methyl groups of the methylated lysine substrate. As mentioned above, this unstable lysyl hemiaminal breaks down to release the methyl group from nitrogen in the form of formaldehyde. This mechanism allows for the demethylation of lysines in all three methylation states (mono-, di-, and trimethylated lysines) (Kooistra and Helin 2012).

One main challenge related to inhibition of specific demethylases is that the JmjC domain is relatively well conserved among the 30 members of the family, which can lead to very diverse phenotypes if one takes into consideration that the enzymes participate in a wide range of reactions and aspects of gene regulation. More intriguingly, the double-stranded β-helix (DSBH) fold contained in the JmjC domain is common to a large superfamily of 2-oxoglutarate oxygenases (comprising approximately 80 human members) with a diverse substrate set. Additional sequences distinguish the different JmjC domains in various members of the Jumonji family. The active site is located at one end of the DSBH fold, where the catalytic Fe is bound by the facial triad with three conserved residues that include two histidines, and either aspartic acid or glutamic acid. The other cofactor, 2-oxoglutarate, is bound primarily through its interaction with two different residues that are also conserved among the members of the JmjC demethylase family. Mutations in the conserved three amino acids of the facial triad can be used as a predictor of inactivity, as in the case of Jumonji/ARID domain-containing protein 2 (JARID2), UTY and PHD finger protein 2 (PHF2) proteins.

7.5.2 Inhibition of JMJD3 and UTX: Challenges and Progress

7.5.2.1 Crystal Structure Analyses

Despite the presence of the conserved ARKS amino acid motif in several histones, demethylases exhibit an admirable specificity. The enzymes can discriminate between different Lys residues and their degree of methylation. The majority of the approaches for drug development focus on inhibition of substrate and/or binding of cofactors.

Initial efforts to design demethylase inhibitors were related to JMJD2A inhibition and were based on previous knowledge about known inhibitors of other iron(II) and α-KG-dependent enzymes (Rose et al. 2008). The authors took advantage of the generation of NADH from NAD in the demethylation reaction that can be measured using fluorescence and is correlated to the amount of formaldehyde produced (Rose et al. 2008; Couture et al. 2007). They showed inhibition of demethylase activity via N-oxalylglycine (NOG), an amide analog of α-KG. Nevertheless, NOG and related compounds are very polar and charged and have poor pharmacodynamics properties. At the same time, it can also inhibit the human hypoxia-inducible factor (HIF), hydroxylases (PHD1-3), and factor inhibiting HIF (FIH) (Ivan et al. 2002; McDonough et al. 2005). Newer approaches take into consideration a sub-pocket by the active site of demethylases that is larger in this family of proteins compared to FIH proteins. The most acceptable solution is to generate cell permeable drugs through generation of methyl esters. The ester group is then cleaved from the prodrug intracellularly to give rise to the active drug.

Several other types of compounds have been proposed (see Hoffmann et al. (2012), for an excellent synopsis of those compounds: These include hydroxamic acids, such as trichostatin A (TSA) and SAHA that are used as histone deacetylase (HDAC) inhibitors; pyrimidine dicarboxylic acids, such as 2,4-dicarboxylic acid (2,4-PDCA) that can inhibit Jumonji enzymes through competition with α-KG. In principle, compounds that form complexes with zinc ions can also affect demethylases, especially as some of the Jumonji demethylases have zinc-binding domains. Finally, some of the most efficient inhibitors for Jumonji family proteins can be found in nature and in pathological conditions such as isocitrate dehydrogenase (IDH) mutant tumors (McKenney and Levine 2013), including gliomas and acute myeloid leukemia. Nevertheless, the hitherto most potent class of inhibitors are iron-binding compounds, including 2,2′-bipyridines. The aforementioned inhibitors of the 2OG oxygenase enzymes (Rose et al. 2008, 2012; Hopkinson et al. 2013; Nielsen et al. 2012; Chang et al. 2011) are not specific and belong to a class of broad-spectrum inhibitors that act on several member of the JmjC domain-containing family and other oxygenases.

Clues as to what confers their substrate specificities have come from crystallographic studies. First, analysis showed that the conserved two histidine residues that position the iron ion (nickel ion: 2WWJ, 3AVR, 3U78) in an octahedral mode are conserved in the Jumonji family. The third coordination position can differ among demethylase families and alternates between aspartic acid (as in the case of JMJD3 and UTX) and glutamic acid. The cofactor α-KG and a water molecule occupy the remaining three important positions in the catalytic pocket. The JmjC domain shows a high degree of similarity among Jumonji proteins with regard to this catalytic domain. Second, the residues of the cofactor binding site are more distinct among the subfamilies and, therefore, offer the potential for a selective structure-based drug design. The co-crystallized inhibitor O-benzyl-N-(carboxycarbonyl)-D-tyrosine of 2WWJ offers a pep stacking interaction with F185 at the front part of the pocket that is only conserved within the KDM4 and KDM5 subfamilies (Lohse et al. 2011a, b). In the case of KDM6A, there is an established hydrogen bond at the back of the pocket with the carboxylic moiety of NOG and O-benzyl-N-(carboxycarbonyl)-D-tyrosine next to the Fe(II) ion.

Findings stemming from elegant analyses of the crystal structure of demethylases, such the one of UTX by Sengoku and Yokoyama (Sengoku and Yokoyama 2011), can be exploited for the design of specific inhibitors. This study delineated the structure of UTX in the free and H3 peptide-bound forms and showed that the catalytic JmjC domain binds residues 25–33 of histone H3. This includes H3R26, H3A29, and H3P30, in addition to H3K27. Moreover, UTX binds residues 17–21 of H3 using a zinc-binding domain. The zinc-binding domain recognizes the H3L20 side chain via a hydrophobic patch on its surface. Mutational analyses showcased the importance of H3R17, H3L20, H3R26, H3A29, H3P30, and H3T32 for demethylation. Similar conclusions were recently reached from crystal structure analyses for JMJD3 (Jones et al. 2018).

Another landmark study delineated the structure for the dual demethylase KDM7A, an enzyme that demethylates both lysine 27 and 9 on histone H3 (Yang et al. 2010). The authors solved the crystal structures of the free enzyme and in complex with one or two peptides containing various combinations of H3K4me3, H3K9me2, and H3K27me2 modifications. These structures showed that H3K9me2 and H3K27me2 have a similar mode of interaction with ceKDM7A. Measurement of the structures also revealed that H3K4me3 associated with the PHD finger and H3K9me2 bound to the JmjC domain are from two separate molecules, suggesting a trans-histone peptide-binding mechanism.

7.5.2.2 Inhibitors for Lysine 27 Demethylases

To date, the best described selective inhibitor of UTX and JMJD3 is GSKJ1 (Kruidenier et al. 2012). Kruidenier et al. (2012) shed light on the specificity of JMJD3 toward H3K27me compared to other histone residues (Santos-Rosa et al. 2002) using a structure–function approach. The authors solved crystal structures for 500 C-terminal amino acids of mouse and human JMJD3 fragments containing the

JmjC catalytic domain, two C helices, and a GATA-like (GATAL) motif in the presence of NOG and metal Ni(II) at 2.5 A resolution. The authors showed the importance of two particular residues on H3, proline 30 (P30), and arginine 26 (R26) as well as R1246, P1388, and glutamic acid 1244 (E1244) on JMJD3 in differentiating binding of H3 to JMJD3 compared to other demethylases (Kruidenier et al. 2012). Kruidenier et al. considered the interaction between α-KG and the P30 residue of H3 to further improve small molecules identified to a series of hits previously discovered generated using a library of 2 million compounds (Gamo et al. 2010).

This nature of the inhibitor is competitive for the two cofactors (Fe and α-KG), but not the substrate (UTX and JMJD3). GSKJ1 and its cell-active prodrug, the ethyl ester GSKJ4, show remarkable specificity for UTX and JMJD3. It has a half-maximum inhibitory concentration (IC50) of 60 nM toward JMJD3, as measured in an AlphaScreen assay (Gamo et al. 2010). GSKJ1/4 is also active against UTX (half the potency compared to JMJD3).

GSKJ4 is transformed to GSKJ1 in the first 15 min after it enters the cells, and GSKJ1 acts by chelating the Fe(II) active site and binding of a propanoic acid side chain to the 2OG binding site. Inhibition of H3K27me3 demethylases via GSKJ4 reduces Toll-like receptor-mediated proinflammatory cytokine production by human primary macrophages (Santa et al. 2007). GSKJ4 reduced the production of herpes simplex virus 1 from its latent state, which is associated with repressive marks (Messer et al. 2015). The 2,2′-bipyridine metal-binding pharmacophore utilized by GSKJ1 is a very strong metal chelator that may interact with other metalloproteins, including the Jumonji demethylases JARID1B and JMJD2C (Heinemann et al. 2014). Indeed, Helin's group recently showed that the GSK compounds are active against JARID1B/C (Heinemann et al. 2014) lysine 4 demethylases with a five–tenfold lower activity compared to JMJD3. GSK drug remains the most efficient and specific lead compound against lysine 27 demethylases.

GSKJ4 has been shown to possess antitumor activities. It was used in vitro and in vivo against pediatric brainstem gliomas harboring the oncogenic K27M mutation of histone H3.3 (Hashizume et al. 2014). These gliomas were present with significant loss of lysine 27 methylation levels, and thus inhibition of demethylases was suggested as a therapeutic tool. Indeed, GSKJ4 treatment leads to significant tumor regression in transplantation models in vivo (Hashizume et al. 2014). Treatment of T-ALL cells with GSKJ4 resulted in cell cycle arrest and increased apoptosis (Ntziachristos et al. 2014). These effects were mediated through the demethylase activity of JMJD3, since H3K27me3 levels were altered and ectopic expression of the catalytically inactive JMJD3 did not rescue the phenotype (Ntziachristos et al. 2014). Moreover, other potential targets of GSKJ1 (like JARID1B/C) (Heinemann et al. 2014) do not seem to be necessary for T-ALL progression (Ntziachristos and Aifantis, unpublished data). As JMJD3 and UTX are not required for the early stages of T cell development (to double positive (DP, for CD4/CD8) stage) (Ntziachristos et al. 2014; Satoh et al. 2010; Manna et al. 2015; Dobenecker et al. 2015; Li et al. 2014), these results might pave the way for targeted therapy in T-ALL by targeting the JMJD3 demethylase alone or in combination with other oncogenic pathways, like Notch1.

The strength of metal coordination by 2,2′-bipyridine depends on the planar orientation with respect to the Fe^{2+} ion, limiting the flexibility of the MBP for additional chemical modifications. Additional approaches have used mimetics of the α-KG co-substrate joined to a strong metal chelator. While this strategy has generated relatively potent compounds, these inhibitors do not exhibit sufficient selectivity or synthetic tractability. A persistent obstacle in the development of metalloprotein inhibitors has been the identification of diverse MBPs.

Industry and academic efforts have been focusing on alternative approaches to overcome these issues (Martin et al. 2014). Recently, Manfred Jung's group has generated substituted MBP carboxylates that can function as Jumonji inhibitors. They initially performed a virtual screen that led them to acquire and modify available compounds that had a competitive advantage in binding α-KG. It seems that compound interference with both α-KG and iron can lead to better inhibition. Finer structure analysis leading to increased structure resolution will lead to design of more specific drugs.

Nevertheless, the fact that demethylases can (a) exert their activity on non-histone substrates, such as p53 and DNMT1 (name the demethylases), E2F1 (LSD1) and many others, (b) exert different demethylase potency on different substrates or contexts, and (c) play demethylase-dependent and independent roles in several different complexes makes the design of specific inhibitors a challenging task.

7.6 Conclusions and Future Perspective

In this chapter, we discussed basic aspects of the biology of JMJD3, UTX, and UTY in normal development and disease. UTX/Y and JMJD3 participate in different complexes leading to diverse molecular and physiological outcomes. We are just in the beginning of unraveling the complexity of UTX and JMJD3 functions. More elegant tools, including specific antibodies, that can help with delineation of chromatin binding locations, intracellular localization, and in vivo models that interrogate demethylase roles in oncogenic and stress conditions are required. Finally, further understanding of the crystal structures of lysine 27-related enzymes and comparison with other Jumonji families will lead to the development of more specific inhibitors. In the era of personalized medicine, targeting JMJD3 and UTX and other related enzymes may arise as a new therapeutic intervention in a broad range of diseases.

Acknowledgements We want to thank all the members of the Ntziachristos group and especially the past laboratory members Carlos Alberto Martinez and Kelly Marie Arcipowski for critical review of the manuscript and their comments. The Ntziachristos laboratory is or has been supported by the Research Foundation Flanders (FWO, G0F4721N), a Flanders interuniversity consortium grant (BOF.IBO.2023.0006.02), a Cancer Research Institute Ghent (CRIG) partnership grant, the NCI (R00CA188293 and R01CA248770), the National Science Foundation, the Hartwell Foundation, a Gilead Research Scholarship, the American Society of Hematology, the Leukemia Research Foundation, the St. Baldrick's Foundation, the H Foundation, the Gabrielle's Angel Foundation, the Elsa Pardee Foundation, and the Zell Foundation. Figures were created using Biorender (biorender.com).

Conflict of Interest Statement The authors have no conflicts of interest.

References

Abidi F, Miano M, Murray J, Schwartz C (2007) A novel mutation in the PHF8 gene is associated with X-linked mental retardation with cleft lip/cleft palate. Clin Genet 72:19–22. https://doi.org/10.1111/j.1399-0004.2007.00817.x

Adegbola A, Gao H, Sommer S, Browning M (2008) A novel mutation in JARID1C/SMCX in a patient with autism spectrum disorder (ASD). Am J Med Genet A 146A:505–511. https://doi.org/10.1002/ajmg.a.32142

Agger K et al (2007) UTX and JMJD3 are histone H3K27 demethylases involved in HOX gene regulation and development. Nature 449:731–734. https://doi.org/10.1038/nature06145

Agger K et al (2009) The H3K27me3 demethylase JMJD3 contributes to the activation of the INK4A-ARF locus in response to oncogene- and stress-induced senescence. Genes Dev 23:1171–1176. https://doi.org/10.1101/gad.510809

Allis CD, Jenuwein T (2016) The molecular hallmarks of epigenetic control. Nat Rev Genet 17:487–500. https://doi.org/10.1038/nrg.2016.59

Allis CD et al (2007) New nomenclature for chromatin-modifying enzymes. Cell 131:633–636. https://doi.org/10.1016/j.cell.2007.10.039

Anderton JA et al (2011) The H3K27me3 demethylase, KDM6B, is induced by Epstein-Barr virus and over-expressed in Hodgkin's lymphoma. Oncogene 30:2037–2043. https://doi.org/10.1038/onc.2010.579

Andricovich J et al (2018) Loss of KDM6A activates super-enhancers to induce gender-specific squamous-like pancreatic cancer and confers sensitivity to BET inhibitors. Cancer Cell 33:512–526, e518. https://doi.org/10.1016/j.ccell.2018.02.003

Annunziato AT, Eason MB, Perry CA (1995) Relationship between methylation and acetylation of arginine-rich histones in cycling and arrested HeLa cells. Biochemistry 34:2916–2924. https://doi.org/10.1021/bi00009a023

Arcipowski KM, Martinez CA, Ntziachristos P (2016) Histone demethylases in physiology and cancer: a tale of two enzymes, JMJD3 and UTX. Curr Opin Genet Dev 36:59–67. https://doi.org/10.1016/j.gde.2016.03.010

Bannister AJ, Schneider R, Kouzarides T (2002) Histone methylation: dynamic or static? Cell 109:801–806. https://doi.org/10.1016/s0092-8674(02)00798-5

Barradas M et al (2009) Histone demethylase JMJD3 contributes to epigenetic control of INK4a/ARF by oncogenic RAS. Genes Dev 23:1177–1182. https://doi.org/10.1101/gad.511109

Bedford MT, Clarke SG (2009) Protein arginine methylation in mammals: who, what, and why. Mol Cell 33:1–13. https://doi.org/10.1016/j.molcel.2008.12.013

Benyoucef A et al (2016) UTX inhibition as selective epigenetic therapy against TAL1-driven T-cell acute lymphoblastic leukemia. Genes Dev 30:508–521. https://doi.org/10.1101/gad.276790.115

Bernstein BE et al (2006) A bivalent chromatin structure marks key developmental genes in embryonic stem cells. Cell 125:315–326. https://doi.org/10.1016/j.cell.2006.02.041

Beyaz S et al (2017) The histone demethylase UTX regulates the lineage-specific epigenetic program of invariant natural killer T cells. Nat Immunol 18:184–195. https://doi.org/10.1038/ni.3644

Borun TW, Pearson D, Paik WK (1972) Studies of histone methylation during the HeLa S-3 cell cycle. J Biol Chem 247:4288–4298

Bosselut R (2016) Pleiotropic functions of H3K27Me3 demethylases in immune cell differentiation. Trends Immunol 37:102–113. https://doi.org/10.1016/j.it.2015.12.004

Burgold T et al (2008) The histone H3 lysine 27-specific demethylase Jmjd3 is required for neural commitment. PLoS ONE 3:e3034. https://doi.org/10.1371/journal.pone.0003034

Byvoet P, Shepherd GR, Hardin JM, Noland BJ (1972) The distribution and turnover of labeled methyl groups in histone fractions of cultured mammalian cells. Arch Biochem Biophys 148:558–567

Cao R et al (2002) Role of histone H3 lysine 27 methylation in Polycomb-group silencing. Science 298:1039–1043. https://doi.org/10.1126/science.1076997

Cao Z et al (2021) KDM6B is an androgen regulated gene and plays oncogenic roles by demethylating H3K27me3 at cyclin D1 promoter in prostate cancer. Cell Death Dis 12:2. https://doi.org/10.1038/s41419-020-03354-4

Chang KH et al (2011) Inhibition of histone demethylases by 4-carboxy-2,2′-bipyridyl compounds. ChemMedChem 6:759–764. https://doi.org/10.1002/cmdc.201100026

Chen S et al (2012) The histone H3 Lys 27 demethylase JMJD3 regulates gene expression by impacting transcriptional elongation. Genes Dev 26:1364–1375. https://doi.org/10.1101/gad.186056.111

Choi HJ et al (2015) UTX inhibits EMT-induced breast CSC properties by epigenetic repression of EMT genes in cooperation with LSD1 and HDAC1. EMBO Rep 16:1288–1298. https://doi.org/10.15252/embr.201540244

Christensen J et al (2007) RBP2 belongs to a family of demethylases, specific for tri-and dimethylated lysine 4 on histone 3. Cell 128:1063–1076. https://doi.org/10.1016/j.cell.2007.02.003

Ciavatta DJ et al (2010) Epigenetic basis for aberrant upregulation of autoantigen genes in humans with ANCA vasculitis. J Clin Investig 120:3209–3219. https://doi.org/10.1172/JCI40034

Cloos PA et al (2006) The putative oncogene GASC1 demethylates tri- and dimethylated lysine 9 on histone H3. Nature 442:307–311. https://doi.org/10.1038/nature04837

Couture JF, Collazo E, Ortiz-Tello PA, Brunzelle JS, Trievel RC (2007) Specificity and mechanism of JMJD2A, a trimethyllysine-specific histone demethylase. Nat Struct Mol Biol 14:689–695. https://doi.org/10.1038/nsmb1273

Dahle O, Kumar A, Kuehn MR (2010) Nodal signaling recruits the histone demethylase Jmjd3 to counteract Polycomb-mediated repression at target genes. Sci Signal 3:ra48. https://doi.org/10.1126/scisignal.2000841

Dai JP, Lu JY, Zhang Y, Shen YF (2010) Jmjd3 activates Mash1 gene in RA-induced neuronal differentiation of P19 cells. J Cell Biochem 110:1457–1463. https://doi.org/10.1002/jcb.22703

Dawson MA, Kouzarides T (2012) Cancer epigenetics: from mechanism to therapy. Cell 150:12–27. https://doi.org/10.1016/j.cell.2012.06.013

Dawson MA, Kouzarides T, Huntly BJ (2012) Targeting epigenetic readers in cancer. N Engl J Med 367:647–657. https://doi.org/10.1056/NEJMra1112635

De Falco G, Comes F, Simone C (2006) pRb: master of differentiation. Coupling irreversible cell cycle withdrawal with induction of muscle-specific transcription. Oncogene 25:5244–5249. https://doi.org/10.1038/sj.onc.1209623

De Santa F et al (2007) The histone H3 lysine-27 demethylase Jmjd3 links inflammation to inhibition of Polycomb-mediated gene silencing. Cell 130:1083–1094. https://doi.org/10.1016/j.cell.2007.08.019

De Santa F et al (2009) Jmjd3 contributes to the control of gene expression in LPS-activated macrophages. EMBO J 28:3341–3352. https://doi.org/10.1038/emboj.2009.271

Dobenecker MW et al (2015) Coupling of T cell receptor specificity to natural killer T cell development

by bivalent histone H3 methylation. J Exp Med 212:297–306. https://doi.org/10.1084/jem.20141499
Duerre JA, Lee CT (1974) In vivo methylation and turnover of rat brain histones. J Neurochem 23:541–547
Ene CI et al (2012) Histone demethylase Jumonji D3 (JMJD3) as a tumor suppressor by regulating p53 protein nuclear stabilization. PLoS ONE 7:e51407. https://doi.org/10.1371/journal.pone.0051407
Ezponda T, Licht JD (2014) Molecular pathways: deregulation of histone h3 lysine 27 methylation in cancer-different paths, same destination. Clin Cancer Res 20:5001–5008. https://doi.org/10.1158/1078-0432.CCR-13-2499
Ezponda T et al (2017) UTX/KDM6A loss enhances the malignant phenotype of multiple myeloma and sensitizes cells to EZH2 inhibition. Cell Rep 21:628–640. https://doi.org/10.1016/j.celrep.2017.09.078
Feng Q et al (2002) Methylation of H3-lysine 79 is mediated by a new family of HMTases without a SET domain. Curr Biol 12:1052–1058. https://doi.org/10.1016/s0960-9822(02)00901-6
Fodor BD et al (2006) Jmjd2b antagonizes H3K9 trimethylation at pericentric heterochromatin in mammalian cells. Genes Dev 20:1557–1562. https://doi.org/10.1101/gad.388206
Gamo FJ et al (2010) Thousands of chemical starting points for antimalarial lead identification. Nature 465:305–310. https://doi.org/10.1038/nature09107
Gozdecka M et al (2018) UTX-mediated enhancer and chromatin remodeling suppresses myeloid leukemogenesis through noncatalytic inverse regulation of ETS and GATA programs. Nat Genet 50:883–894. https://doi.org/10.1038/s41588-018-0114-z
Guo T et al (2022) KDM6B interacts with TFDP1 to activate P53 signaling in regulating mouse palatogenesis. Elife 11. https://doi.org/10.7554/eLife.74595
Hashizume R et al (2014) Pharmacologic inhibition of histone demethylation as a therapy for pediatric brainstem glioma. Nat Med 20:1394–1396. https://doi.org/10.1038/nm.3716
Heinemann B et al (2014) Inhibition of demethylases by GSK-J1/J4. Nature 514:E1-2. https://doi.org/10.1038/nature13688
Helin K, Dhanak D (2013) Chromatin proteins and modifications as drug targets. Nature 502:480–488. https://doi.org/10.1038/nature12751
Herz HM et al (2010) The H3K27me3 demethylase dUTX is a suppressor of Notch- and Rb-dependent tumors in *Drosophila*. Mol Cell Biol 30:2485–2497. MCB.01633-09 [pii], https://doi.org/10.1128/MCB.01633-09
Herz HM, Hu D, Shilatifard A (2014) Enhancer malfunction in cancer. Mol Cell 53:859–866. https://doi.org/10.1016/j.molcel.2014.02.033
Hoffmann I et al (2012) The role of histone demethylases in cancer therapy. Mol Oncol 6:683–703. https://doi.org/10.1016/j.molonc.2012.07.004
Hojfeldt JW, Agger K, Helin K (2013) Histone lysine demethylases as targets for anticancer therapy. Nat Rev Drug Discov 12:917–930. https://doi.org/10.1038/nrd4154
Hong SH et al (2007) Identification of JmjC domain-containing UTX and JMJD3 as histone H3 lysine 27 demethylases. P Natl Acad Sci USA 104:18439–18444. https://doi.org/10.1073/pnas.0707292104
Hopkinson RJ et al (2013) 5-Carboxy-8-hydroxyquinoline is a broad spectrum 2-oxoglutarate oxygenase inhibitor which causes iron translocation. Chem Sci 4:3110–3117. https://doi.org/10.1039/c3sc51122g
Hu D et al (2013) The MLL3/MLL4 branches of the COMPASS family function as major histone H3K4 monomethylases at enhancers. Mol Cell Biol 33:4745–4754. https://doi.org/10.1128/MCB.01181-13
Huang C et al (2010) Dual-specificity histone demethylase KIAA1718 (KDM7A) regulates neural differentiation through FGF4. Cell Res 20:154–165. https://doi.org/10.1038/cr.2010.5
Hurst CD et al (2017) Genomic subtypes of non-invasive bladder cancer with distinct metabolic profile and female gender bias in KDM6A mutation frequency. Cancer Cell 32:701–715, e707. https://doi.org/10.1016/j.ccell.2017.08.005
Issa N et al (2023) KDM6B protects T-ALL cells from NOTCH1-induced oncogenic stress. Leukemia 37:728–740. https://doi.org/10.1038/s41375-023-01853-9
Issaeva I et al (2007) Knockdown of ALR (MLL2) reveals ALR target genes and leads to alterations in cell adhesion and growth. Mol Cell Biol 27:1889–1903. https://doi.org/10.1128/MCB.01506-06
Ivan M et al (2002) Biochemical purification and pharmacological inhibition of a mammalian prolyl hydroxylase acting on hypoxia-inducible factor. Proc Natl Acad Sci USA 99:13459–13464. https://doi.org/10.1073/pnas.192342099
Iwase S et al (2007) The X-linked mental retardation gene SMCX/JARID1C defines a family of histone H3 lysine 4 demethylases. Cell 128:1077–1088. https://doi.org/10.1016/j.cell.2007.02.017
Jacobs JJ, Kieboom K, Marino S, DePinho RA, van Lohuizen M (1999) The oncogene and Polycomb-group gene bmi-1 regulates cell proliferation and senescence through the ink4a locus. Nature 397:164–168. https://doi.org/10.1038/16476
Jensen LR et al (2010) A distinctive gene expression fingerprint in mentally retarded male patients reflects disease-causing defects in the histone demethylase KDM5C. PathoGenetics 3:2. https://doi.org/10.1186/1755-8417-3-2
Jenuwein T (2001) Re-SET-ting heterochromatin by histone methyltransferases. Trends Cell Biol 11:266–273. https://doi.org/10.1016/s0962-8924(01)02001-3
Jenuwein T, Allis CD (2001) Translating the histone code. Science 293:1074–1080. https://doi.org/10.1126/science.1063127
Jepsen K et al (2007) SMRT-mediated repression of an H3K27 demethylase in progression from neural

stem cell to neuron. Nature 450:415–419. https://doi.org/10.1038/nature06270

Jones SE, Olsen L, Gajhede M (2018) Structural basis of histone demethylase KDM6B histone 3 lysine 27 specificity. Biochemistry 57:585–592. https://doi.org/10.1021/acs.biochem.7b01152

Kamikawa YF, Donohoe ME (2014) The localization of histone H3K27me3 demethylase Jmjd3 is dynamically regulated. Epigenetics 9:834–841. https://doi.org/10.4161/epi.28524

Kim JH et al (2014) UTX and MLL4 coordinately regulate transcriptional programs for cell proliferation and invasiveness in breast cancer cells. Cancer Res 74:1705–1717. https://doi.org/10.1158/0008-5472.CAN-13-1896

Kim S, Benoiton L, Paik WK (1964) Epsilon-alkyllysinase. Purification and properties of the enzyme. J Biol Chem 239:3790–3796

Klose RJ, Bird AP (2006) Genomic DNA methylation: the mark and its mediators. Trends Biochem Sci 31:89–97. https://doi.org/10.1016/j.tibs.2005.12.008

Klose RJ et al (2006a) The transcriptional repressor JHDM3A demethylates trimethyl histone H3 lysine 9 and lysine 36. Nature 442:312–316. https://doi.org/10.1038/nature04853

Klose RJ, Kallin EM, Zhang Y (2006b) JmjC-domain-containing proteins and histone demethylation. Nat Rev Genet 7:715–727. https://doi.org/10.1038/nrg1945

Klose RJ et al (2007) The retinoblastoma binding protein RBP2 is an H3K4 demethylase. Cell 128:889–900. https://doi.org/10.1016/j.cell.2007.02.013

Koivisto AM et al (2007) Screening of mutations in the PHF8 gene and identification of a novel mutation in a Finnish family with XLMR and cleft lip/cleft palate. Clin Genet 72:145–149. https://doi.org/10.1111/j.1399-0004.2007.00836.x

Koizumi M et al (2022) UTX deficiency in neural stem/progenitor cells results in impaired neural development, fetal ventriculomegaly, and postnatal death. FASEB J 36:e22662. https://doi.org/10.1096/fj.202201002RR

Kong N et al (2022) Intravesical delivery of KDM6A-mRNA via mucoadhesive nanoparticles inhibits the metastasis of bladder cancer. Proc Natl Acad Sci USA 119. https://doi.org/10.1073/pnas.2112696119

Kooistra SM, Helin K (2012) Molecular mechanisms and potential functions of histone demethylases. Nat Rev Mol Cell Biol 13:297–311. https://doi.org/10.1038/nrm3327

Kornberg RD (1974) Chromatin structure—repeating unit of histones and DNA. Science 184:868–871. https://doi.org/10.1126/science.184.4139.868

Kruidenier L et al (2012) A selective jumonji H3K27 demethylase inhibitor modulates the proinflammatory macrophage response. Nature 488:404–408. https://doi.org/10.1038/nature11262

Lan F et al (2007) A histone H3 lysine 27 demethylase regulates animal posterior development. Nature 449:689–694. https://doi.org/10.1038/nature06192

Laumonnier F et al (2005) Mutations in PHF8 are associated with X linked mental retardation and cleft lip/cleft palate. J Med Genet 42:780–786. https://doi.org/10.1136/jmg.2004.029439

Lederer D et al (2012) Deletion of KDM6A, a histone demethylase interacting with MLL2, in three patients with Kabuki syndrome. Am J Hum Genet 90:119–124. https://doi.org/10.1016/j.ajhg.2011.11.021

Lee MG, Norman J, Shilatifard A, Shiekhattar R (2007a) Physical and functional association of a trimethyl H3K4 demethylase and Ring6a/MBLR, a Polycomb-like protein. Cell 128:877–887. https://doi.org/10.1016/j.cell.2007.02.004

Lee MG et al (2007b) Demethylation of H3K27 regulates Polycomb recruitment and H2A ubiquitination. Science 318:447–450. https://doi.org/10.1126/science.1149042

Lee S, Lee JW, Lee SK (2012) UTX, a histone H3-lysine 27 demethylase, acts as a critical switch to activate the cardiac developmental program. Dev Cell 22:25–37. https://doi.org/10.1016/j.devcel.2011.11.009

Ler LD et al (2017) Loss of tumor suppressor KDM6A amplifies PRC2-regulated transcriptional repression in bladder cancer and can be targeted through inhibition of EZH2. Sci Transl Med 9. https://doi.org/10.1126/scitranslmed.aai8312

Li Q et al (2014) Critical role of histone demethylase Jmjd3 in the regulation of CD4+ T-cell differentiation. Nat Commun 5:5780. https://doi.org/10.1038/ncomms6780

Li X et al (2018) UTX is an escape from X-inactivation tumor-suppressor in B cell lymphoma. Nat Commun 9:2720. https://doi.org/10.1038/s41467-018-05084-w

Lindqvist CM et al (2015) The mutational landscape in pediatric acute lymphoblastic leukemia deciphered by whole genome sequencing. Hum Mutat 36:118–128. https://doi.org/10.1002/humu.22719

Liu W et al (2010) PHF8 mediates histone H4 lysine 20 demethylation events involved in cell cycle progression. Nature 466:508–512. https://doi.org/10.1038/nature09272

Liu PS et al (2017) Alpha-ketoglutarate orchestrates macrophage activation through metabolic and epigenetic reprogramming. Nat Immunol 18:985–994. https://doi.org/10.1038/ni.3796

Liu F et al (2022) KDM6B promotes gastric carcinogenesis and metastasis via upregulation of CXCR4 expression. Cell Death Dis 13:1068. https://doi.org/10.1038/s41419-022-05458-5

Lohse B et al (2011a) Inhibitors of histone demethylases. Bioorg Med Chem 19:3625–3636. https://doi.org/10.1016/j.bmc.2011.01.046

Lohse B et al (2011b) Targeting histone lysine demethylases by truncating the histone 3 tail to obtain

selective substrate-based inhibitors. Angew Chem Int Ed Engl 50:9100–9103. https://doi.org/10.1002/anie.201101849
Lowe SW, Sherr CJ (2003) Tumor suppression by Ink4a-Arf: progress and puzzles. Curr Opin Genet Dev 13:77–83. https://doi.org/10.1016/s0959-437x(02)00013-8
Lu H et al (2020) Chemotherapy-induced S100A10 recruits KDM6A to facilitate OCT4-mediated breast cancer stemness. J Clin Invest 130:4607–4623. https://doi.org/10.1172/JCI138577
Luger K, Mader AW, Richmond RK, Sargent DF, Richmond TJ (1997) Crystal structure of the nucleosome core particle at 2.8 angstrom resolution. Nature 389:251–260. https://doi.org/10.1038/38444
Malinczak CA et al (2020) Upregulation of H3K27 demethylase KDM6 during respiratory syncytial virus infection enhances proinflammatory responses and immunopathology. J Immunol 204:159–168. https://doi.org/10.4049/jimmunol.1900741
Mallaney C et al (2019) Kdm6b regulates context-dependent hematopoietic stem cell self-renewal and leukemogenesis. Leukemia 33:2506–2521. https://doi.org/10.1038/s41375-019-0462-4
Manna S et al (2015) Histone H3 lysine 27 demethylases Jmjd3 and Utx are required for T-cell differentiation. Nat Commun 6:8152. https://doi.org/10.1038/ncomms9152
Mansour AA et al (2012) The H3K27 demethylase Utx regulates somatic and germ cell epigenetic reprogramming. Nature 488:409–413. https://doi.org/10.1038/nature11272
Mar BG et al (2012) Sequencing histone-modifying enzymes identifies UTX mutations in acute lymphoblastic leukemia. Leukemia 26:1881–1883. https://doi.org/10.1038/leu.2012.56
Martin DP et al (2014) 'Unconventional' coordination chemistry by metal chelating fragments in a metalloprotein active site. J Am Chem Soc 136:5400–5406. https://doi.org/10.1021/ja500616m
McDonough MA et al (2005) Selective inhibition of factor inhibiting hypoxia-inducible factor. J Am Chem Soc 127:7680–7681. https://doi.org/10.1021/ja050841b
McKenney AS, Levine RL (2013) Isocitrate dehydrogenase mutations in leukemia. J Clin Investig 123:3672–3677. https://doi.org/10.1172/JCI67266
Messer HG, Jacobs D, Dhummakupt A, Bloom DC (2015) Inhibition of H3K27me3-specific histone demethylases JMJD3 and UTX blocks reactivation of herpes simplex virus 1 in trigeminal ganglion neurons. J Virol 89:3417–3420. https://doi.org/10.1128/JVI.03052-14
Miller SA, Mohn SE, Weinmann AS (2010) Jmjd3 and UTX play a demethylase-independent role in chromatin remodeling to regulate T-box family member-dependent gene expression. Mol Cell 40:594–605. https://doi.org/10.1016/j.molcel.2010.10.028
Miyake N et al (2013) MLL2 and KDM6A mutations in patients with Kabuki syndrome. Am J Med Genet A 161A:2234–2243. https://doi.org/10.1002/ajmg.a.36072
Morales Torres C, Laugesen A, Helin K (2013) Utx is required for proper induction of ectoderm and mesoderm during differentiation of embryonic stem cells. PLoS ONE 8:e60020. https://doi.org/10.1371/journal.pone.0060020
Morera L, Lubbert M, Jung M (2016) Targeting histone methyltransferases and demethylases in clinical trials for cancer therapy. Clin Epigenetics 8:57. https://doi.org/10.1186/s13148-016-0223-4
Morin RD et al (2011) Frequent mutation of histone-modifying genes in non-Hodgkin lymphoma. Nature 476:298–303. https://doi.org/10.1038/nature10351
Morozov VM, Li Y, Clowers MM, Ishov AM (2017) Inhibitor of H3K27 demethylase JMJD3/UTX GSK-J4 is a potential therapeutic option for castration resistant prostate cancer. Oncotarget 8:62131–62142. https://doi.org/10.18632/oncotarget.19100
Muller J et al (2002) Histone methyltransferase activity of a *Drosophila* Polycomb group repressor complex. Cell 111:197–208. https://doi.org/10.1016/s0092-8674(02)00976-5
Nickerson ML et al (2014) Concurrent alterations in TERT, KDM6A, and the BRCA pathway in bladder cancer. Clin Cancer Res 20:4935–4948. https://doi.org/10.1158/1078-0432.Ccr-14-0330
Nielsen AL et al (2012) Identification of catechols as histone-lysine demethylase inhibitors. FEBS Lett 586:1190–1194. https://doi.org/10.1016/j.febslet.2012.03.001
Nigro JM et al (1989) Mutations in the p53 gene occur in diverse human tumour types. Nature 342:705–708. https://doi.org/10.1038/342705a0
Ntziachristos P et al (2012) Genetic inactivation of the Polycomb repressive complex 2 in T cell acute lymphoblastic leukemia. Nat Med 18:298–301. https://doi.org/10.1038/nm.2651
Ntziachristos P et al (2014) Contrasting roles of histone 3 lysine 27 demethylases in acute lymphoblastic leukaemia. Nature. https://doi.org/10.1038/nature13605
Ntziachristos P, Abdel-Wahab O, Aifantis I (2016) Emerging concepts of epigenetic dysregulation in hematological malignancies. Nat Immunol 17:1016–1024. https://doi.org/10.1038/ni.3517
Ohguchi H et al (2017) KDM6B modulates MAPK pathway mediating multiple myeloma cell growth and survival. Leukemia 31:2661–2669. https://doi.org/10.1038/leu.2017.141
Ortega-Molina A et al (2015) The histone lysine methyltransferase KMT2D sustains a gene expression program that represses B cell lymphoma development. Nat Med 21:1199–1208. https://doi.org/10.1038/nm.3943
Park DH et al (2014) Activation of neuronal gene expression by the JMJD3 demethylase is required

for postnatal and adult brain neurogenesis. Cell Rep 8:1290–1299. https://doi.org/10.1016/j.celrep.2014.07.060

Park WY, Hong BJ, Lee J, Choi C, Kim MY (2016) H3K27 demethylase JMJD3 employs the NF-kappaB and BMP signaling pathways to modulate the tumor microenvironment and promote melanoma progression and metastasis. Cancer Res 76:161–170. https://doi.org/10.1158/0008-5472.CAN-15-0536

Parsons DW et al (2011) The genetic landscape of the childhood cancer medulloblastoma. Science 331:435–439. https://doi.org/10.1126/science.1198056

Pasqualucci L et al (2011) Inactivating mutations of acetyltransferase genes in B-cell lymphoma. Nature 471:189–195. https://doi.org/10.1038/nature09730

Pedersen MT, Helin K (2010) Histone demethylases in development and disease. Trends Cell Biol 20:662–671. https://doi.org/10.1016/j.tcb.2010.08.011

Pereira F et al (2012) Vitamin D has wide regulatory effects on histone demethylase genes. Cell Cycle 11:1081–1089. https://doi.org/10.4161/cc.11.6.19508

Perrigue PM et al (2015) The histone demethylase jumonji coordinates cellular senescence including secretion of neural stem cell-attracting cytokines. Mol Cancer Res 13:636–650. https://doi.org/10.1158/1541-7786.MCR-13-0268

Peters AH et al (2002) Histone H3 lysine 9 methylation is an epigenetic imprint of facultative heterochromatin. Nat Genet 30:77–80. https://doi.org/10.1038/ng789

Pointon JJ et al (2011) The histone demethylase JARID1A is associated with susceptibility to ankylosing spondylitis. Genes Immun 12:395–398. https://doi.org/10.1038/gene.2011.23

Qin M et al (2021) KDM6B promotes ESCC cell proliferation and metastasis by facilitating C/EBPbeta transcription. BMC Cancer 21:559. https://doi.org/10.1186/s12885-021-08282-w

Qiu H et al (2023) KDM6A loss triggers an epigenetic switch that disrupts urothelial differentiation and drives cell proliferation in bladder cancer. Cancer Res 83:814–829. https://doi.org/10.1158/0008-5472.CAN-22-1444

Ramadoss S, Chen X, Wang CY (2012) Histone demethylase KDM6B promotes epithelial-mesenchymal transition. J Biol Chem 287:44508–44517. https://doi.org/10.1074/jbc.M112.424903

Rath BH, Waung I, Camphausen K, Tofilon PJ (2018) Inhibition of the histone H3K27 demethylase UTX enhances tumor cell radiosensitivity. Mol Cancer Ther 17:1070–1078. https://doi.org/10.1158/1535-7163.MCT-17-1053

Revia S et al (2022) Histone H3K27 demethylase KDM6A is an epigenetic gatekeeper of mTORC1 signalling in cancer. Gut 71:1613–1628. https://doi.org/10.1136/gutjnl-2021-325405

Ringrose L (2007) Polycomb comes of age: genome-wide profiling of target sites. Curr Opin Cell Biol 19:290–297. https://doi.org/10.1016/j.ceb.2007.04.010

Romero OA et al (2021) SMARCA4 deficient tumours are vulnerable to KDM6A/UTX and KDM6B/JMJD3 blockade. Nat Commun 12:4319. https://doi.org/10.1038/s41467-021-24618-3

Rose NR et al (2008) Inhibitor scaffolds for 2-oxoglutarate-dependent histone lysine demethylases. J Med Chem 51:7053–7056. https://doi.org/10.1021/jm800936s

Rose NR et al (2012) Plant growth regulator daminozide is a selective inhibitor of human KDM2/7 histone demethylases. J Med Chem 55:6639–6643. https://doi.org/10.1021/jm300677j

Santos-Rosa H et al (2002) Active genes are tri-methylated at K4 of histone H3. Nature 419:407–411. https://doi.org/10.1038/nature01080

Satoh T et al (2010) The Jmjd3-Irf4 axis regulates M2 macrophage polarization and host responses against helminth infection. Nat Immunol 11:936–944. https://doi.org/10.1038/ni.1920

Schmitz SU et al (2011) Jarid1b targets genes regulating development and is involved in neural differentiation. Embo J 30:4586–4600. https://doi.org/10.1038/emboj.2011.383

Schneider R et al (2004) Histone H3 lysine 4 methylation patterns in higher eukaryotic genes. Nat Cell Biol 6:73–77. https://doi.org/10.1038/ncb1076.ncb1076[pii]

Schuettengruber B, Chourrout D, Vervoort M, Leblanc B, Cavalli G (2007) Genome regulation by Polycomb and trithorax proteins. Cell 128:735–745. https://doi.org/10.1016/j.cell.2007.02.009

Schwartz YB, Pirrotta V (2007) Polycomb silencing mechanisms and the management of genomic programmes. Nat Rev Genet 8:9–22. https://doi.org/10.1038/nrg1981

Seenundun S et al (2010) UTX mediates demethylation of H3K27me3 at muscle-specific genes during myogenesis. Embo J 29:1401–1411. https://doi.org/10.1038/emboj.2010.37

Seligson DB et al (2005) Global histone modification patterns predict risk of prostate cancer recurrence. Nature 435:1262–1266. https://doi.org/10.1038/nature03672

Sen GL, Webster DE, Barragan DI, Chang HY, Khavari PA (2008) Control of differentiation in a self-renewing mammalian tissue by the histone demethylase JMJD3. Genes Dev 22:1865–1870. https://doi.org/10.1101/gad.1673508

Sengoku T, Yokoyama S (2011) Structural basis for histone H3 Lys 27 demethylation by UTX/KDM6A. Genes Dev 25:2266–2277. https://doi.org/10.1101/gad.172296.111

Shan Y et al (2020) JMJD3 and UTX determine fidelity and lineage specification of human neural progenitor cells. Nat Commun 11:382. https://doi.org/10.1038/s41467-019-14028-x

Shaw T, Martin P (2009) Epigenetic reprogramming during wound healing: loss of Polycomb-mediated silencing may enable upregulation of repair genes. EMBO Rep 10:881–886. https://doi.org/10.1038/embor.2009.102

Shen Y et al (2012) Expression and significance of histone H3K27 demethylases in renal cell carcinoma. BMC Cancer 12:470. https://doi.org/10.1186/1471-2407-12-470

Shi Y et al (2004) Histone demethylation mediated by the nuclear amine oxidase homolog LSD1. Cell 119:941–953. https://doi.org/10.1016/j.cell.2004.12.012

Shpargel KB, Sengoku T, Yokoyama S, Magnuson T (2012) UTX and UTY demonstrate histone demethylase-independent function in mouse embryonic development. PLoS Genet 8:e1002964. https://doi.org/10.1371/journal.pgen.1002964

Shpargel KB, Starmer J, Yee D, Pohlers M, Magnuson T (2014) KDM6 demethylase independent loss of histone H3 lysine 27 trimethylation during early embryonic development. PLoS Genet 10:e1004507. https://doi.org/10.1371/journal.pgen.1004507

Simon C et al (2012) A key role for EZH2 and associated genes in mouse and human adult T-cell acute leukemia. Genes Dev 26:651–656. https://doi.org/10.1101/gad.186411.111

Smith ER et al (2008) *Drosophila* UTX is a histone H3 Lys27 demethylase that colocalizes with the elongating form of RNA polymerase II. Mol Cell Biol 28:1041–1046. https://doi.org/10.1128/MCB.01504-07

Sola S et al (2011) p53 interaction with JMJD3 results in its nuclear distribution during mouse neural stem cell differentiation. PLoS ONE 6:e18421. https://doi.org/10.1371/journal.pone.0018421

Svotelis A et al (2011) H3K27 demethylation by JMJD3 at a poised enhancer of anti-apoptotic gene BCL2 determines ERalpha ligand dependency. EMBO J 30:3947–3961. https://doi.org/10.1038/emboj.2011.284

Tahiliani M et al (2007) The histone H3K4 demethylase SMCX links REST target genes to X-linked mental retardation. Nature 447:601–605. https://doi.org/10.1038/nature05823

Takeuchi T et al (1995) Gene trap capture of a novel mouse gene, jumonji, required for neural tube formation. Genes Dev 9:1211–1222. https://doi.org/10.1101/gad.9.10.1211

Tan M et al (2011) Identification of 67 histone marks and histone lysine crotonylation as a new type of histone modification. Cell 146:1016–1028. https://doi.org/10.1016/j.cell.2011.08.008

Tang B et al (2016) Aberrant JMJD3 expression upregulates slug to promote migration, invasion, and stem cell-like behaviors in hepatocellular carcinoma. Cancer Res 76:6520–6532. https://doi.org/10.1158/0008-5472.CAN-15-3029

Thieme S et al (2013) The histone demethylase UTX regulates stem cell migration and hematopoiesis. Blood 121:2462–2473. https://doi.org/10.1182/blood-2012-08-452003

Thinnes CC et al (2014) Targeting histone lysine demethylases—Progress, challenges, and the future. Biochim Biophys Acta 1839:1416–1432. https://doi.org/10.1016/j.bbagrm.2014.05.009

Tie F, Banerjee R, Conrad PA, Scacheri PC, Harte PJ (2012) Histone demethylase UTX and chromatin remodeler BRM bind directly to CBP and modulate acetylation of histone H3 lysine 27. Mol Cell Biol 32:2323–2334. https://doi.org/10.1128/MCB.06392-11

Tokunaga R et al (2016) The prognostic significance of histone lysine demethylase JMJD3/KDM6B in colorectal cancer. Ann Surg Oncol 23:678–685. https://doi.org/10.1245/s10434-015-4879-3

Tran N, Broun A, Ge K (2020) Lysine demethylase KDM6A in differentiation, development, and cancer. Mol Cell Biol 40:e00341–20. https://doi.org/10.1128/MCB.00341-20

Tsukada Y et al (2006) Histone demethylation by a family of JmjC domain-containing proteins. Nature 439:811–816. https://doi.org/10.1038/nature04433

Van der Meulen J, Speleman F, Van Vlierberghe P (2014) The H3K27me3 demethylase UTX in normal development and disease. Epigenetics 9:658–668. https://doi.org/10.4161/epi.28298

Van der Meulen J et al (2015) The H3K27me3 demethylase UTX is a gender-specific tumor suppressor in T-cell acute lymphoblastic leukemia. Blood 125:13–21. https://doi.org/10.1182/blood-2014-05-577270

van Haaften G et al (2009) Somatic mutations of the histone H3K27 demethylase gene UTX in human cancer. Nat Genet 41:521–523. https://doi.org/10.1038/ng.349

Voigt P, Tee WW, Reinberg D (2013) A double take on bivalent promoters. Genes Dev 27:1318–1338. https://doi.org/10.1101/gad.219626.113

Walport LJ et al (2014a) Human UTY(KDM6C) is a male-specific N-methyl lysyl demethylase. J Biol Chem 289:18302–18313. https://doi.org/10.1074/jbc.M114.555052

Walport LJ et al (2014b) Human UTY(KDM6C) Is a male-specific N-epsilon-methyl lysyl demethylase. J Biol Chem 289:18302–18313. https://doi.org/10.1074/jbc.M114.555052

Wang L, Shilatifard A (2019) UTX mutations in human cancer. Cancer Cell 35:168–176. https://doi.org/10.1016/j.ccell.2019.01.001

Wang Y et al (2009) LSD1 is a subunit of the NuRD complex and targets the metastasis programs in breast cancer. Cell 138:660–672. https://doi.org/10.1016/j.cell.2009.05.050

Wang C et al (2012) UTX regulates mesoderm differentiation of embryonic stem cells independent of H3K27 demethylase activity. Proc Natl Acad Sci

USA 109:15324–15329. https://doi.org/10.1073/pnas.1204166109
Wang SP et al (2017) A UTX-MLL4-p300 transcriptional regulatory network coordinately shapes active enhancer landscapes for eliciting transcription. Mol Cell 67:308–321, e306. https://doi.org/10.1016/j.molcel.2017.06.028
Wang L et al (2018) Resetting the epigenetic balance of Polycomb and COMPASS function at enhancers for cancer therapy. Nat Med 24:758–769. https://doi.org/10.1038/s41591-018-0034-6
Wartman LD et al (2011) Sequencing a mouse acute promyelocytic leukemia genome reveals genetic events relevant for disease progression. J Clin Investig 121:1445–1455. https://doi.org/10.1172/JCI45284
Wei Y et al (2013) Toll-like receptor alterations in myelodysplastic syndrome. Leukemia 27:1832–1840. https://doi.org/10.1038/leu.2013.180
Wei J et al (2021) Genome-wide CRISPR screens reveal host factors critical for SARS-CoV-2 infection. Cell 184:76–91, e13. https://doi.org/10.1016/j.cell.2020.10.028
Welstead GG et al (2012) X-linked H3K27me3 demethylase Utx is required for embryonic development in a sex-specific manner. Proc Natl Acad Sci USA 109:13004–13009. https://doi.org/10.1073/pnas.1210787109
Whetstine JR et al (2006) Reversal of histone lysine trimethylation by the JMJD2 family of histone demethylases. Cell 125:467–481. https://doi.org/10.1016/j.cell.2006.03.028
Williams K et al (2014) The histone lysine demethylase JMJD3/KDM6B is recruited to p53 bound promoters and enhancer elements in a p53 dependent manner. PLoS ONE 9:e96545. https://doi.org/10.1371/journal.pone.0096545
Wu Q et al (2018) In vivo CRISPR screening unveils histone demethylase UTX as an important epigenetic regulator in lung tumorigenesis. Proc Natl Acad Sci USA 115:E3978–E3986. https://doi.org/10.1073/pnas.1716589115
Xie L et al (2011) KDM5B regulates embryonic stem cell self-renewal and represses cryptic intragenic transcription. Embo J 30:1473–1484. https://doi.org/10.1038/emboj.2011.91
Xu Z et al (2019) Comprehensive profiling of JMJD3 in gastric cancer and its influence on patient survival. Sci Rep 9:868. https://doi.org/10.1038/s41598-018-37340-w
Yamamoto K et al (2014) Loss of histone demethylase KDM6B enhances aggressiveness of pancreatic cancer through downregulation of C/EBPalpha. Carcinogenesis 35:2404–2414. https://doi.org/10.1093/carcin/bgu136
Yamane K et al (2006) JHDM2A, a JmjC-containing H3K9 demethylase, facilitates transcription activation by androgen receptor. Cell 125:483–495. https://doi.org/10.1016/j.cell.2006.03.027
Yang Y et al (2010) Structural insights into a dual-specificity histone demethylase ceKDM7A from *Caenorhabditis elegans*. Cell Res 20:886–898. https://doi.org/10.1038/cr.2010.86
Yang Y et al (2022) NARF is a hypoxia-induced coactivator for OCT4-mediated breast cancer stem cell specification. Sci Adv 8:eabo5000. https://doi.org/10.1126/sciadv.abo5000
Yu SH et al (2018) JMJD3 facilitates C/EBPbeta-centered transcriptional program to exert oncorepressor activity in AML. Nat Commun 9:3369. https://doi.org/10.1038/s41467-018-05548-z
Zhang J et al (2012) The genetic basis of early T-cell precursor acute lymphoblastic leukaemia. Nature 481:157–163. https://doi.org/10.1038/nature10725
Zhang J et al (2015) Disruption of KMT2D perturbs germinal center B cell development and promotes lymphomagenesis. Nat Med 21:1190–1198. https://doi.org/10.1038/nm.3940
Zhao Y, Garcia BA (2015) Comprehensive catalog of currently documented histone modifications. Cold Spring Harb Perspect Biol 7:a025064. https://doi.org/10.1101/cshperspect.a025064
Zhao W et al (2013) Jmjd3 inhibits reprogramming by upregulating expression of INK4a/Arf and targeting PHF20 for ubiquitination. Cell 152:1037–1050. https://doi.org/10.1016/j.cell.2013.02.006
Zhao L et al (2015) JMJD3 promotes SAHF formation in senescent WI38 cells by triggering an interplay between demethylation and phosphorylation of RB protein. Cell Death Differ 22:1630–1640. https://doi.org/10.1038/cdd.2015.6
Zheng L et al (2018) Utx loss causes myeloid transformation. Leukemia 32:1458–1465. https://doi.org/10.1038/s41375-018-0011-6

KDM7 Demethylases: Regulation, Function and Therapeutic Targeting

8

Peng Shao, Qi Liu and Hank Heng Qi

Abstract

It was more than a decade ago that PHF8, KDM7A/JHDM1D and PHF2 were first proposed to be a histone demethylase family and were named as KDM7 (lysine demethylase) family. Since then, knowledge of their demethylation activities, roles as co-regulators of transcription and roles in development and diseases such as cancer has been steadily growing. The demethylation activities of PHF8 and KDM7A toward various methylated histones including H3K9me2/1, H3K27me2 and H4K20me1 have been identified and proven in various cell types. In contrast, PHF2, due to a mutation of a key residue in an iron-binding domain, demethylates H3K9me2 upon PKA-mediated phosphorylation. Interestingly, it was reported that PHF2 possesses an unusual H4K20me3 demethylation activity, which was not observed for PHF8 and KDM7A. PHF8 has been most extensively studied with respect to its roles in development and oncogenesis, revealing that it contributes to regulation of the cell cycle, cell viability and cell migration. Moreover, accumulating lines of evidence demonstrated that the KDM7 family members are subjected to post-transcriptional and post-translational regulations, leading to a higher horizon for evaluating their actual protein expression and functions in development and cancer. This chapter provides a general view of the current understanding of the regulation and functions of the KDM7 family and discusses their potential as therapeutic targets in cancer as well as perspectives for further studies.

Keywords

PHF8 · KDM7A · PHF2 · Histone demethylase · Cancer

The authors Peng Shao and Qi Liu contributed equally to this work

Present address: Department of Microbiology and Immunology, Carver College of Medicine, University of Iowa, 51 Newton Road, Iowa City, IA 52242, USA.

P. Shao · Q. Liu · H. H. Qi (✉)
Department of Anatomy and Cell Biology, Carver College of Medicine, University of Iowa, 51 Newton Road, Iowa City, IA 52242, USA
e-mail: hankqi168@gmail.com

P. Shao
e-mail: peng-shao@uiowa.edu

Q. Liu
e-mail: qi.liu@northwestern.edu

Q. Yan (ed.), *Targeting Lysine Demethylases in Cancer and Other Human Diseases*, Advances in Experimental Medicine and Biology 1433, https://doi.org/10.1007/978-3-031-38176-8_8

8.1 Members of the KDM7 Family: Their Demethylation Activities in Transcriptional Regulation

The first histone demethylase LSD1 was identified in 2004 (Shi et al. 2004). This was a milestone that changed the long-standing belief that histone methylation is not reversible. Soon after this discovery, the first Jumonji C (JmjC) domain-containing histone demethylase, JHDM1, was discovered by Yi Zhang's laboratory (Tsukada et al. 2006). This laboratory immediately followed up on this finding with a systematic analysis of all JmjC domain-containing proteins and hypothesized that many of them would be active histone demethylases (Klose et al. 2006). Mechanistically, JmjC domain-containing histone demethylase functions via an oxidative reaction that requires iron Fe(II), α-ketoglutarate (αKG) and oxygen as cofactors (Klose et al. 2006; Tsukada et al. 2006). PHF8/KDM7B, KIAA1718/JHDM1D/KDM7A and PHF2/KDM7C (hereafter, referred to as PHF8, KDM7A and PHF2) were proposed to be active histone demethylases based on the conserved PHD domain adjacent to the JmjC domain, despite the fact that PHF2 contains a histidine-to-tyrosine substitution within the third iron-binding residue in the JmjC domain (Klose et al. 2006). It was four years after the hypothesis was originally proposed that several studies proved the demethylase activities of PHF8 and KDM7A toward multiple methylated histones: di/mono-methylated histone 3 lysine 9 (H3K9me2/1), dimethylated histone 3 lysine 27 (H3K27me2) and monomethylated histone 4 lysine 20 (H4K20me1) (Feng et al. 2010; Fortschegger et al. 2010; Kleine-Kohlbrecher et al. 2010; Liu et al. 2010; Loenarz et al. 2010; Qi et al. 2010). PHF2 was first reported to demethylate H3K9me1 in vitro (Wen et al. 2010). However, such demethylation activity was not detected using bacterially purified PHF2 (Horton et al. 2011). Importantly, PHF2 was shown to also be capable of demethylating H3K9me2, specifically following its phosphorylation by PKA (Baba et al. 2011). Most of these initial discoveries were confirmed by following studies in cells (Table 8.1).

8.1.1 The Demethylation Activities of PHF8 and Their Roles in Transcriptional Regulation

The in vitro demethylation activity of PHF8 toward H3K9me2 is consistent throughout most of the studies that have been performed. However, such demethylation activity was not immediately proved for PHF8 target genes on which PHF8 binds to their transcription start sites (TSS) (Fortschegger et al. 2010; Kleine-Kohlbrecher et al. 2010; Liu et al. 2010; Qi et al. 2010), except the case of rRNA genes, on which PHF8 demethylates H3K9me2 and serves as a co-activator (Feng et al. 2010). Our work using H3K9me2 ChIP-seq in HeLa cells demonstrated that PHF8 knockdown elevated H3K9me2 levels on non-TSS PHF8 targets, suggesting that PHF8 may regulate H3K9me2 at yet unidentified genomic loci (Qi et al. 2010). Consistently, several studies demonstrated that PHF8 demethylates H3K9me2 on selected genes in MCF7 cells (Wang et al. 2016), mouse embryonic stem cells (ESC) (Tang et al. 2016) and human umbilical vein endothelial cells (HUVECs) (Gu et al. 2016). Our study also revealed that PHF8 knockdown in MCF10A cells increased the H3K9me2 level on *SNAI1*, not only at the TSS, but also in the gene body region (Shao et al. 2017). These observations imply that the demethylation activity of PHF8 toward H3K9me2 is highly dependent on the cellular context, gene and cell type.

PHF8 can also demethylate H3K27me2, as reported in a *C. elegans* study (Kleine-Kohlbrecher et al. 2010). Consistent with this finding, PHF8 knockdown resulted in elevated levels of H3K27me2 on NOTCH1-regulated genes (*IL7R* and *DTX1*) (Yatim et al. 2012). This elevation was not limited to NOTCH1 binding sites within these genes (Yatim et al. 2012), suggesting the involvement of additional regulatory mechanisms after PHF8 knockdown.

Table 8.1 In vitro and in vivo demethylation activities of members of the KDM7 family

KDM7 family member	In vitro demethylation activity toward	Demethylation activity in vivo**
PHF8	H3K9me1	HeLa (Liu et al. 2010; Qi et al. 2010), MC3T3-E1 (Han et al. 2015)
	H3K9me2	HeLa (Liu et al. 2010; Qi et al. 2010), MCF7 (Wang et al. 2016), MCF10A (Shao et al. 2017), HUVECs (Gu et al. 2016), primary neurons (Oey et al. 2015)
	H3K27me2	T-ALL cells (Yatim et al. 2012)
	H4K20me1*	HeLa (Liu et al. 2010; Qi et al. 2010; Asensio-Juan et al. 2012), T-ALL (Yatim et al. 2012), HUVECs (Gu et al. 2016; Hori et al. 2014)
KDM7A	H3K9me2/ H3K27me2	293F (Yokoyama et al. 2010), mESC (Huang et al. 2010), Neuro2A (Tsukada et al. 2010)
	H4K20me1*	No studies
PHF2	H3K9me1	U2OS (Wen et al. 2010)
	H3K9me2#	293F (Baba et al. 2011), N8 mesenchymal cells (Pattabiraman et al. 2016), chondrocytes (Hata et al. 2013), pre-adipocyte cells (Lee et al. 2014)
	H4K20me3*	Macrophage (Stender et al. 2012)

* On nucleosome substrate only; #: PHF2 protein complex on both bulk histones and nucleosomes; **: in vivo designated to animal models and/or cells

We (Qi et al. 2010) and the Rosenfeld laboratory (Liu et al. 2010) have also reported that PHF8 is capable of demethylating H4K20me1, in both in vitro assays (on nucleosome substrate only) and in cells, and that this demethylation activity confers the co-activator function of PHF8 in transcription regulation (Liu et al. 2010; Qi et al. 2010). Several subsequent studies support the notion that PHF8 has demethylation activity toward H4K20me1: PHF8 regulates H4K20me1 at the TSS of selected cytoskeletal genes (e.g., *RHOA*, *GSK3B* and *CTNNA1*) in HeLa cells (Asensio-Juan et al. 2012), and PHF8 overexpression downregulates global H4K20me1 in HUVECs (Gu et al. 2016). Additional supporting evidence is that PHF8 exhibited H4K20me1 demethylation activity when its expression was guided specifically to the centromere (Hori et al. 2014).

Although all of the studies above show that PHF8 serves as a transcription co-activator, a bioinformatics analysis demonstrated that PHF8 and RE-1 silencing transcription factor (REST) co-occupy genes (Wang et al. 2014). REST is a transcription repressor; thus, the co-occupancy of PHF8 and REST implies that PHF8 has an alternative function as a co-repressor on REST target genes. In light of this finding, another study showed that PHF8 forms complexes with HDAC1 and SIN3A in demethylating H4K20me1 and thus keeps the co-occupied promoters silent (Asensio-Juan et al. 2017). It is possible that a similar mechanism may apply to the co-repressor function of PHF8 in regulating REST target genes.

8.1.2 Dual Demethylation Activities of KDM7A on H3K9me2 and H3K27me2

Several groups have shown KDM7A to have dual demethylation activities toward H3K9me2 and H3K27me2, both in vitro and in cells (Huang et al. 2010; Lin et al. 2010; Tsukada et al. 2010; Yokoyama et al. 2010). Tsukada Y et al. demonstrated that KDM7A demethylates H3K9me2 and H3K27me2 on bulk histones and on the TSS of *follistatin* gene in Neuro2A cells; consequentially, KDM7A positively regulates *follistatin* expression (Tsukada et al. 2010). Huang C et al. also showed the H3K9me2 and H3K27me2 demethylation activities of KDM7A on bulk histones and on the TSS of FGF4 gene as well as the co-activator function of KDM7A in regulating FGF4 in Embryonic Stem Cells (ESCs) (Huang et al. 2010). Importantly, the *C. elegans* KDM7A (ceKDM7A) can demethylate H3K9me2/1 and H3K27me2 on bulk histones and ceKDM7A loss of function reduced the expression of its target genes and increased the levels of H3K9me2 and H3K27me2 on these genes (Lin et al. 2010). These data strongly support that KDM7A possesses dual demethylation activities on H3K9me2 and H3K27me2. Beyond these two repressive histone marks, our previous study showed that KDM7A can demethylate H4K20me1 on nucleosomes (Qi et al. 2010). However, further studies are needed to test such demethylation activity of KDM7A in cells.

8.1.3 The Induced Demethylation Activity of PHF2

Due to a mutation leading to substitution of a tyrosine for a histidine within the third iron-binding residue of the JmjC domain, the demethylation activity of PHF2 was questionable. Bacterially purified PHF2 did not show demethylation activity toward bulk histones (Horton et al. 2011). However, another study showed that bacterially purified PHF2 demethylates H3K9me1 on both histones and nucleosomes, as well as H4K20me3 on nucleosomes (Stender et al. 2012). PHF2 protein complex pulled down from HEK293T cells showed demethylation activity toward H3K9me1 (Wen et al. 2010). Further study showed that upon phosphorylation by PKA, PHF2 demethylates H3K9me2 (Baba et al. 2011). The phosphorylation sites are located at the C-terminus of PHF2 (S757, S899, S954 and S1056). The S1056 seems critical to mediate the phosphorylation by PKA. Such activity was confirmed by another group, which showed that in N8 mesenchymal cells, PHF2 occupancy is inversely correlated with the levels of H3K9me2/3 (Pattabiraman et al. 2016). In all cases, the current studies support that PHF2 executed its co-activator function by demethylating H3K9me2.

8.2 Roles of KDM7 Family Members in Development

8.2.1 Development of Craniofacial Structure, Bones and Neurons

Among the three members of the KDM7 family, PHF8 is most strongly associated with craniofacial and neuronal development. Initially, deletion of a large genomic region encompassing *PHF8* (Xp11.3-q21.3) was associated with a family in which two males were diagnosed with borderline mental retardation accompanying cleft lip/palate (CLP) (Siderius et al. 1999). Later, truncation mutations of *PHF8* resulting in expression of PHF8 with amino acids (aa) 1–211 (Laumonnier et al. 2005) or 1–177 (Abidi et al. 2007), and a point mutation (F279S), as well as a total deletion (Qiao et al. 2008; Nava et al. 2012), were identified in families in which the affected males had intellectual disability (ID), CLP, a long face, large hands and flat feet. The work of several groups demonstrated that the point mutation (F279S) abolished the demethylation activity of PHF8 (Feng et al. 2010; Kleine-Kohlbrecher et al. 2010; Qi et al. 2010). In addition, the affected males with total *PHF8* deletion also showed autism spectrum disorders (Qiao et al. 2008; Nava et al. 2012). Collectively, these findings suggest that PHF8 plays roles in development of the craniofacial structure, neurons and bones.

Following these studies, biochemical analyses revealed that PHF8 interacts with ZNF711, a gene associated with X-linked mental retardation (XLMR) syndrome, and that in HEK293 cells, PHF8 positively regulates the genes co-occupied by PHF8 and ZNF711(Kleine-Kohlbrecher et al. 2010). PHF8 positively regulates rRNA genes, implying that PHF8 could contribute to craniofacial development through general protein synthesis (Feng et al. 2010). Our previous study demonstrated that knockdown of PHF8 in zebrafish causes apoptosis in the developing brain and the neural tube, as well as developmental defects of the lower jaw and pharyngeal arches (Qi et al. 2010). In addition, PHF8 appears to be required for retinoic acid (RA)-induced neuronal differentiation of P19 cells (Qiu et al. 2010) and to interact with TIP60 in regulating the expression of *Arc*, an important mediator of synaptic plasticity, upon increased synaptic activity (Oey et al. 2015). Moreover, PHF8 expression was reported to be elevated in preosteoblasts and bone marrow stromal cells (BMSCs) and to play a role in the differentiation of osteoblasts by regulating the expression of *SATB2* (Han et al. 2015). Collectively, these data support a role for PHF8 in the development of craniofacial structures, bones and neurons. However, two studies of *Phf8* knockout mice did not reveal a defect of craniofacial development, but rather behavior problems such as anxiety and depression (Walsh et al. 2017; Chen et al. 2018). It is possible that the requirements for PHF8 differ by model system and that the defects may be compensated by a rescue by other histone demethylases. Moreover, it is possible that families with PHF8 mutations/deletion have additional genetic abnormalities, which play synergistic roles with PHF8 in these developmental processes.

KDM7A has also been recognized to play an important role in neurodevelopment. In zebrafish, this demethylase is expressed predominantly in brain, and morpholino-mediated knockdown impedes tectum development (Tsukada et al. 2010). KDM7A promotes the expression of genes that are important for neurodevelopment, such as *follistatin* in mouse Neuro2A cells (Tsukada et al. 2010), and *Fgf4* in mouse ESC cells during their differentiation into neurons (Huang et al. 2010).

Like KDM7A, PHF2 is a positive regulator of gene expression. During osteoblast differentiation, it upregulates the expression of *RUNX2* and promotes bone formation (Kim et al. 2014). In chondrocytes, PHF2 coordinates with ARID5B to regulate SOX9 target genes and stimulates H3K9me2 demethylation of these genes (Hata et al. 2013); thus, it appears to be critical for chondrogenesis.

8.2.2 Adipogenesis

Both PHF2 and KDM7A have been reported to function in adipogenesis. In the case of PHF2, knockout mice show reduced adipogenesis (Okuno et al. 2013), and under normal conditions, PHF2 interacts with C/EBPα to regulate pro-adipogenic genes (Okuno et al. 2013). Another study confirmed this interaction and showed that PHF2 interacts with C/EBPδ to regulate adipogenic genes and thus plays an essential role in the differentiation of pre-adipocytes (Lee et al. 2014). During the differentiation of brown adipocytes, expression of the KDM7A mRNA is upregulated (Son et al. 2016), consistent with a role in adipogenesis. However, further studies are needed to confirm that this is the case.

8.2.3 Development of Other Systems

In addition to regulating the development of craniofacial structures, bones and neurons, PHF8 has been reported to regulate the migration and proliferation of endothelial cells (Gu et al. 2016). Studies using a *Phf8* knockout mouse model (*Phf8*$-^{/Y}$) showed that phf8 promotes commitment to the mesodermal lineage (Tang et al. 2016). This study further showed that deletion of *Phf8* did not affect the self-renewal, proliferation or early ectodermal/endodermal differentiation of ESCs. Studies in *C. elegans* identified jmjd-1.2/PHF8 as a positive regulator of lifespan in response to mitochondrial dysfunction (Merkwirth et al. 2016). PHF8 also promotes the macrophage response to endotoxin (lipopolysaccharide, i.e., LPS) (Erdogan et al. 2016). This study also revealed that PHF8 plays roles in the activation and proliferation of T-cells in this context.

Taken together, the findings of the roles that KDM7 family members play in many processes fundamental to development and beyond indicate that caution needs to be exerted in developing therapeutics based on the manipulation of their demethylation activities.

8.3 Roles of KDM7 Family Members in Cancer

The functions of KDM7 family members in cancer quickly emerged. The mRNA expressions of KDM7A, PHF8 and PHF2 were analyzed through Gene Expression Profiling Interactive Analysis (GEPIA2) (Tang et al. 2017), which has the RNA sequencing expression data of 9736 tumor and 8587 normal samples from the Cancer Genome Atlas (TCGA) and the Genotype-Tissue Expression (GTEx) projects. As shown in Fig. 8.1a, *KDM7A* is significantly elevated in LGG and decreased in SKCM and UCS cancers compared with normal tissues. *PHF8* expression is increased in LGG and THYM cancers, while its expression is decreased in TGCT. Same as *PHF8*, *PHF2* RNA levels were also significantly elevated in LGG, THYM cancers. In contrast, the mRNA expression of *PHF2* is decreased in CESC, OV, UCEC and UCS.

The association of KDM7 family members with cancer overall survival (OS) and disease-free survival [DFS, also called relapse-free survival (RFS)] was also analyzed through GEPIA2 (Fig. 8.1b). Importantly, the expression of *KDM7A* is significantly correlated with better overall survival probability of CHOL and SKCM patients. In contrary, *PHF8* is significantly correlated with poorer overall survival of ESCA, KIRP and LGG. *PHF8* is a poor overall survival prognostic marker of ACC but good of KIRC and LGG. Disease-free survivals of KDM7 families mostly follow the same pattern of overall survival, except for PHF8 in BLCA and KDM7A in LUSC exhibiting significant opposite hazard ratio of overall survival and disease-free survival. These expression data provide a general view on the potential roles of the KDM7 family members in cancer development. Nevertheless, individual studies provided more information of their expression and functions in cancers.

Again, most of the studies addressing cancer have focused on PHF8, especially in the cases of prostate cancer and breast cancer. Nevertheless, PHF2 has been implicated as having dual roles in tumor suppression and cancer stemness. Very few studies have been performed on KDM7A (Table 8.2). In this section, we review the current findings and discuss the potential of KDM7 family members as targets for cancer therapeutics.

8.3.1 PHF8: Oncogenic Functions in Various Cancers

Although the gene expression data on mRNA expression revealed PHF8 upregulation in only a few types of cancers, individual studies showed that levels of PHF8 proteins are elevated in esophageal squamous cell carcinomas (Sun et al. 2013b), lung cancers (Shen et al. 2014), prostate cancers (Bjorkman et al. 2012; Ma et al. 2015; Maina et al. 2016), breast cancers (Shao et al. 2017; Wang et al. 2016) and hepatocellular carcinoma (Zhou et al. 2018; Ye et al. 2019). These studies revealed that PHF8 has similar roles across cell types, including promotion of proliferation, suppression of apoptosis and promotion of migration.

In the case of prostate cancers, the elevation of PHF8 protein levels is associated with disease progression (Bjorkman et al. 2012; Ma et al. 2015; Tong et al. 2016), post-castration prostate cancer (Tong et al. 2016) and castration-resistant prostate cancer (Maina et al. 2016). Most of these studies found PHF8 to promote cell proliferation and cell migration and to repress apoptosis (Bjorkman et al. 2012). From a mechanistic perspective, PHF8 was found to regulate integrin signaling to facilitate cell migration (Bjorkman et al. 2012). PHF8 was also found to be upregulated by hypoxia and to interact with androgen receptor (AR) in regulating AR target genes (Tong et al. 2016). In the context of hypoxia signaling, we have revealed that PHF8 plays an essential role in regulating hypoxia-responsive genes including a key HIF1α-co-activator, KDM3A (Maina et al. 2017). Moreover, miR-125b was identified as a direct PHF8 target in prostate cancer cells, where it mediates PHF8 cellular functions in promoting cell proliferation and repressing apoptosis (Ma et al. 2015). This study showed that knockdown of PHF8 upregulated apoptotic factors and downregulated the expression of the anti-apoptotic gene BCL-2.

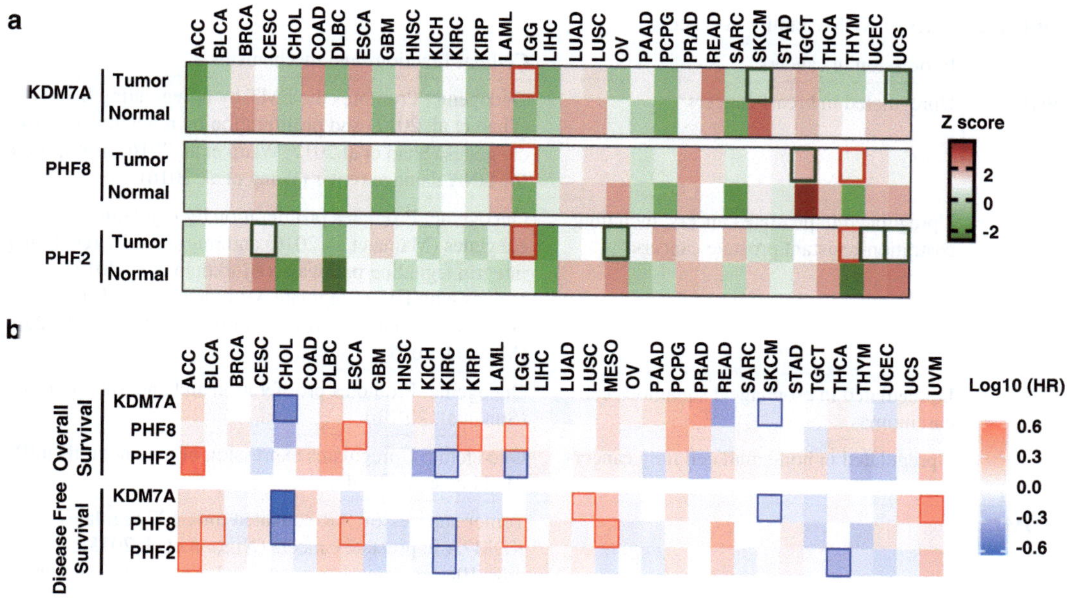

Fig. 8.1 Gene expression analysis of KDM7 family members in cancers. a Gene expression levels of KDM7 family members were evaluated by GEPIA2 on the RNA sequencing data of 9736 tumor and 8587 normal samples from the TCGA and GTEx projects, using a standard processing pipeline. Z score-transformed expression data were used for plotting. The density of color in each block represents the median expression value of a gene in a given tissue, normalized by the maximum median expression value across all blocks. Significantly upregulated expression in tumor tissues was marked as red box and downregulated expression was marked as green box. **b** Log-rank test was used for hypothesis test. The cox proportional hazard ratio (HR) and 95% confidence interval information are included. Significant correlations were marked with blue box when log10 (HR)<0 and red box when log10 (HR)>0. Median (cutoff high 50% and cutoff low 50%) is used as suitable expression threshold for splitting the high-expression and low-expression cohorts. Abbreviations: ACC: adrenocortical carcinoma; BLCA: bladder urothelial carcinoma; BRCA: breast invasive carcinoma; CESC: cervical squamous cell carcinoma and endocervical adenocarcinoma; CHOL: cholangiocarcinoma; COAD: colon adenocarcinoma; DLBC: lymphoid neoplasm diffuse large B-cell lymphoma; ESCA: esophageal carcinoma; GBM: glioblastoma multiforme; HNSC: head and neck squamous cell carcinoma; KICH: kidney chromophobe; KIRC: kidney renal clear cell carcinoma; KIRP: kidney renal papillary cell carcinoma; LAML: acute myeloid leukemia; LGG: brain lower grade glioma; LIHC: liver hepatocellular carcinoma; LUAD: lung adenocarcinoma; LUSC: lung squamous cell carcinoma; MESO: mesothelioma; OV: ovarian serous cystadenocarcinoma; PAAD: pancreatic adenocarcinoma; PCPG: pheochromocytoma and paraganglioma; PRAD: prostate adenocarcinoma; READ: rectum adenocarcinoma; SARC: sarcoma; SKCM: skin cutaneous melanoma; STAD: stomach adenocarcinoma; TGCT: testicular germ cell tumors; THCA: thyroid carcinoma; THYM: thymoma; UCEC: uterine corpus endometrial carcinoma; UCS: uterine carcinosarcoma; UVM: uveal melanoma

We reported that PHF8 is expressed in a unique pattern: It is downregulated during androgen depletion and IL-6-induced neuroendocrine differentiation (NED) and upregulated in castration-resistant prostate cancer (CRPC) cells (Maina et al. 2016). We also identified the post-transcriptional regulatory mechanisms by which c-MYC upregulates PHF8 via repression of miR-22, which targets and regulates PHF8 in prostate cancer cells (Maina et al. 2016). This c-MYC-miR-22-PHF8 axis mediates the regulation of PHF8 in NED induced by androgen depletion and IL-6 treatment. However, under hypoxia condition, this regulatory axis seems disrupted, as the upregulated PHF8 did not follow the downregulated c-MYC (Maina et al. 2016). It is likely that the transcriptional activation of PHF8 by HIF (Tong et al. 2016) bypasses that repression of PHF8 by miR-22.

Table 8.2 Roles of KDM7 family in cancers

	Expression in cancers	Cellular functions and mechanisms
PHF8	Upregulated in breast cancers*	Oncogenic: Promotes the EMT by upregulating SNAI1 (Shao et al. 2017) and proliferation by regulating cell-cycle genes (Shao et al.2017; Wang et al. 2016); is required for DNA damage repair (Wang et al. 2016)
	Upregulated in prostate cancers, including castration-resistant prostate cancers*	Oncogenic: Promotes proliferation by regulating cell-cycle genes (Maina et al. 2016) and migration by regulating integrin signaling pathways (Bjorkman et al. 2012); synergizes with HIF to regulate AR target genes (Tong et al. 2016); upregulates expression of the oncomiR miR-125b (Ma et al. 2015)
	Upregulated in esophageal squamous cell carcinomas	Oncogenic: Promotes proliferation and anti-apoptotic (Sun et al. 2013b)
	Upregulated in non-small cell lung cancers	Oncogenic: Upregulates expression of the oncomiR miR-21 (Shen et al. 2014)
KDM7A		Tumor suppressor: AR-activated miR-137 regulates KDM7A in prostate cancers (Nilsson et al. 2015); miR-10b regulates syndecan-1, whose loss of function downregulates KDM7A expression (Ibrahim et al. 2012); inhibits angiogenesis by downregulating *VEGF-B* and angiopoietin-encoding genes (Osawa et al. 2011)
PHF2	Deletions, truncations	Tumor suppressor: Interacts with p53 to regulate its target genes (Lee et al. 2015), co-repressor function downstream of PKA; plays an essential role in MET during which tumor-initiating ability is lost (Pattabiraman et al. 2016)
	Overexpression in esophageal squamous cell carcinomas#	High cytoplasmic staining is associated with decreased overall survival of esophageal squamous cell carcinomas (Sun et al. 2013a)
	Overexpression in clear cell renal cell carcinoma*	Nuclear expression of PHF2 may serve as a prognostic marker of clear cell renal cell carcinoma (Park et al. 2018)

*: IHC studies; #: conclusions drawn on basis of cytoplasmic staining for PHF2

We and another group showed that PHF8 is oncogenic in breast cancer (Shao et al. 2017; Wang et al. 2016; Liu et al. 2020). Wang et al. found that PHF8 is upregulated in breast cancer and that it is associated with disease progression (Wang et al. 2016). This study also identified the USP7-PHF8-CCNA2 axis in breast cancer cells, with the deubiquitinase USP7 stabilizing PHF8 and that in turn upregulating CCNA2. We also found that the PHF8 protein is significantly upregulated in breast cancer samples and that it promotes an EMT-like process by upregulating the expression of SNAI1 and ZEB1(Shao et al. 2017; Liu et al. 2020). Moreover, the c-MYC-miR-22-PHF8 axis is conserved in breast cancer cells and mediates the negative regulation of PHF8 by TGF-β signaling in non-malignant cell types such as the MCF10A and HaCat cell lines. Notably, when c-MYC was upregulated by TGF-β signaling in cancer cells, PHF8 failed to be downregulated by TGF-β signaling, accounting for the pro-proliferative role of PHF8 in the context of excessive TGF-β signaling in cancer cells (Shao et al. 2017). An independent study showed that PHF8 associates with c-MYC to regulate dynamics of the cytoskeleton in HeLa cells (Asensio-Juan et al. 2012). This supports the role of PHF8 in promoting cell migration. Furthermore, PHF8 promotes melanoma invasion and metastasis by controlling the TGF-β signaling pathway in its demethylase activity manner (Moubarak et al. 2022).

PHF8 has also been found to interact with RARα in sensitizing cells to all-*trans* retinoic acid (ATRA), an agent used in treating acute promyelocytic leukemia (APL) (Arteaga et al. 2013). PHF8 also activates NOTCH1 in the context of T-cell acute lymphoblastic leukemia (T-ALL), as evident from the regulation of its target genes (Yatim et al. 2012).

8.3.2 KDM7A: A Tumor Suppressor?

KDM7A has not been extensively studied. Its reduced expression in UCS and SKCM shown in gene expression analysis (Fig. 8.1) may reflect a tumor suppressor function in these malignancies. In contrast, the elevated expression of KDM7A in LGG implicates its oncogenic function in this type of cancer. In prostate cancer cells, AR-activated miR-137 downregulated KDM7A expression, implying that KDM7 and AR play antagonistic roles in prostate cancer (Nilsson et al. 2015). A deficiency for syndecan-1 or the downregulation of its expression by miR-10b leads to increased mobility of breast cancer cells; KDM7A is downregulated in this context, suggesting that it may play an anti-migratory role (Iqbal and Iqbal 2014). Moreover, KDM7A is upregulated in the context of nutrient starvation, and the overexpression of KDM7A in mouse melanoma (B16) cells and human cervical carcinoma (HeLa) cells led to significant reductions in tumor growth in vivo. Increased expression of KDM7A suppressed tumor growth by downregulating multiple proangiogenic factors such as *VEGF-B* and *Ang1* in the nutrient-starved tumor microenvironment (Osawa et al. 2011). As discussed later, KDM7A could also be heavily regulated post-transcriptionally. As such, more comprehensive profiling of KDM7A protein levels in cancer samples to complement its mRNA expression will be necessary to provide insights into its functions in cancers.

8.3.3 PHF2: Dual Roles in Cancer?

PHF2 is located at 9q22, a region that is frequently deleted, either fully or partially, in several forms of cancer including: breast cancer (Sinha et al. 2008), squamous cell carcinoma (Ghosh et al. 2012), gastric and colorectal cancers (resulting in truncation of the PHF2 protein from aa 492 or aa 954 onward) (Lee et al. 2016). This finding supports its role as a tumor suppressor. A functional study showed that PHF2 interacts with the tumor suppressor p53 and that it contributes to the regulation of p53 target genes, consistent with such a role as a tumor suppressor (Lee et al. 2015). This study also revealed that PHF2 sensitizes cells to several anti-cancer drugs that induce apoptosis, including oxaliplatin, doxorubicin and 5-fluorouracil.

On the other hand, PHF2 has been reported to be over-expressed in esophageal squamous carcinoma (Sun et al. 2013a). However, the conclusions regarding PHF2 protein expression were based on its localization to the cytoplasm, which is inconsistent with other published data (Baba et al. 2011; Lee et al. 2015) that PHF2 is nuclear. Another study showed that PHF2 acts downstream of PKA and that it plays essential roles in induction of the mesenchymal-to-epithelial transition (MET) and loss of the tumor-initiating ability of mesenchymal cells (Pattabiraman et al. 2016). The question of how PHF2 expression changes in cancer cells still remains unclear.

8.4 Regulation of KDM7 Family Members

Information about gene expression at the RNA level from individual studies as well as from TCGA has greatly advanced our understanding of the association of genes with development and disease, as well as about their potential roles in both. In addition, both post-transcriptional and post-translational modifications play important roles in the final protein levels. Without exception, the KDM7 family members are regulated at all three levels (Figs. 8.2 and 8.3), and thus, taking these regulations into consideration is critical to deduce their functions in relevant development and disease.

8.4.1 Transcriptional Regulation

Among the three members of the KDM7 family, KDM7A is most affected by transcriptional regulation. In PANC-1 pancreatic cancer cells, its expression was repressed by the H3K9me2 methyltransferase G9a, and this downregulation was critical for the repression of E-cadherin (Pan et al. 2015). In leukocytes, KDM7A expression was upregulated by TGF-α, and it functioned as a co-activator TGF-α-mediated upregulation of ICAM1 (Choi and Jo 2016). In several cancer cell lines, nutrient starvation triggered transcriptional upregulation of KDM7A (Osawa et al. 2011). In the triple-negative breast cancer cell line MDA-MB-231, KDM7A mRNA expression was downregulated by syndecan-1 depletion (Ibrahim et al. 2012). PHF8 was also reported to be transcriptionally upregulated by hypoxia in prostate cancer cells (Tong et al. 2016; Maina et al. 2017). Tong's study found that both hypoxia-inducible factors (HIFs) HIF1α and HIF2α play roles in the transcriptional regulation of PHF8 induced by hypoxia. However, such transcriptional regulation has not been observed in other cell types that have been examined, including human primary renal proximal epithelia cells (Beyer et al. 2008), RCC4 clear cell renal cell carcinoma cells (Krieg et al. 2010) and HepG2 cells (Xia et al. 2009). Moreover, HIF1α ChIP-chip analysis of HepG2 cells and RCC4 cells did not reveal binding of HIF1α to the PHF8 promoter (Xia et al. 2009; Krieg et al. 2010). Thus, it is possible that hypoxia triggers transcriptional regulation of PHF8 in cell context-dependent manner. PHF2 has not been shown to be regulated at the transcriptional level.

8.4.2 Post-transcriptional Regulation

MicroRNA-mediated post-transcriptional regulation of members of the KDM7 family has been reported. In the case of KDM7A, AR signaling has been reported to upregulate the expression of miR-137, which suppresses several transcription co-regulators including KDM7A, in androgen-sensitive prostate cancer cells (Nilsson et al. 2015) (Fig. 8.2a). We delineated the c-MYC-miR-22-PHF8 regulatory axis, in which c-MYC maintains PHF8 expression by repressing miR-22, which targets and regulates PHF8. This regulatory axis mediates the regulation of PHF8 by AR signaling in prostate cancer cells (Maina et al. 2016) and by TGF-β in both non-malignant mammary gland epithelial cells (MCF10A) and keratinocytes (HaCaT) (Shao et al. 2017) (Fig. 8.2a). This post-transcriptional regulatory axis could potentially place PHF8 in many signaling pathways in which c-MYC serves as a critical mediator or effector, such as in ER and ERBB2 signaling pathways (Hynes and Stoelzle 2009). Moreover, we have shown that other microRNAs such as miR-31 and let-7, which could potentially target and regulate PHF8, are also repressed by c-MYC overexpression in MCF10A cells (Shao et al. 2017). Beyond these reported microRNAs, analysis using TargetScanHuman (Agarwal et al. 2015) shows that many microRNAs have seed sequence in the 3′ untranslated region (UTR) of KDM7A and PHF8 (Fig. 8.2b). Further studies on whether these microRNAs directly regulate KDM7A and PHF8 are expected to shed light on the understanding of the post-transcriptional regulations of these two histone demethylases. In contrast, no microRNA target sites with higher probability of preferential conservation in PHF2 3′ UTR were found through this analysis.

a

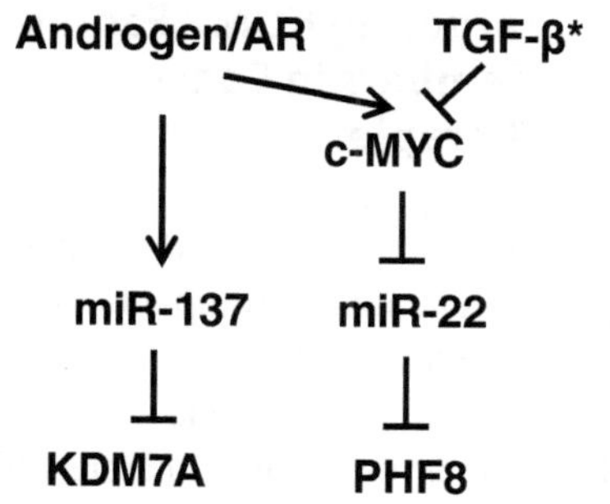

b

KDM7A:
miR-21-5p, miR-144-3p, miR-128-3p, miR-34-5p, miR-153-3p, miR-135-5p, mir-200bc-3p, miR-148-3p

PHF8:
miR-9-5p (three sites), let-7-5p

Fig. 8.2 MicroRNA-mediated regulations of KDM7A and PHF8. **a** miR-137 and miR-22 target and mediated the regulation of KDM7A and PHF8, respectively. *: TGF-β represses c-MYC in non-malignance cells. **b** Predicted microRNA target sites in the 3' UTR of KDM7A and PHF8 using TargetScanHuman. Only microRNA target sites with higher probability of preferential conservation are shown

8.4.3 Post-translational Regulation

The study of post-translational regulation of PHF8 was prompted by the discoveries that PHF8 associates with chromatin at G0/G1 phase and that it dissociates from chromatin during mitosis (Liu et al. 2010). The dissociation of PHF8 from chromatin is coincident with the accumulation of H4K20me1 and associated chromatin condensation. PHF8 re-associates with chromatin at mitotic exit, at which point H4K20me1 is reduced and the chromatin is de-condensed (Liu et al. 2010). Moreover, this study showed that PHF8 is phosphorylated at S33 and S84 of PHF8 (isoform 2 of 1024 aa in length vs. the 1060 aa isoform 1) by CCNB1/CDK1, and this phosphorylation is required for the dissociation of PHF8 from chromatin when the cells enter G2/M phase. Importantly, phosphorylation at S33 and S84 was also stimulated by ATRA, and mimics (S33D, S84D) of constitutively phosphorylated PHF8 strongly bound to the target genes of PML-RARα. These results imply that phosphorylation at S33 and S84 of PHF8 activates its transcriptional regulatory function (Arteaga et al. 2013). PHF8 was also found to be phosphorylated at S844 (of 1024 aa of isoform 2), in this case by CCNE/CDK2, and this enhanced PHF8 function in the transcriptional regulation of cell-cycle genes during the G1/S transition (Sun et al. 2015). ERK2 phosphorylation of PHF8 isoform 1 at S751 (of PHF8 isoform 1, S715 of isoform 2) was reported (Asensio-Juan et al. 2017). This phosphorylation is triggered by the immune stimulatory cytokine IFNγ and causes the dissociation of PHF8 from the promoters co-occupied by HDAC1/SIN3A/PHF8 complex. Thus, PHF8 serves as transcriptional repressor that allows accurate immune response (Asensio-Juan et al. 2017).

These individual studies shed light on the post-translational modification of PHF8, as well as on the impact of such modification on its functions and improved our understanding of the regulation and function of PHF8. However, unbiased mass-spectrometry-based analysis of global phosphorylation throughout the genome has provided additional evidence and an alternative view of PHF8 phosphorylation. An analysis using PhosphoSitePlus (http://www.phosphosite.org/homeAction.action; Cell Signaling Technology) (Hornbeck et al. 2015), which collects data from independent global phosphorylation profiling analyses, shows that PHF8 at S818 and S821 (PHF8 isoform 2) is more phosphorylated (Fig. 8.3), less frequently at S33 and S84, and not detectably at S715 (S751 of PHF8 isoform 1). Although it is likely that the cells used for the mass-spectrometry studies were all at steady state, and other states have not been sampled, antibodies recognizing the phosphorylated PHF8 at specific sites are still needed to further investigate the differential phosphorylation of PHF8 in the context of PHF8 association with and dissociation from chromatin and upon stimulations by agents such as IFNγ, or ATRA.

Moreover, the impact of the phosphorylation of PHF8 at S33 and S84 remains controversial, with one study suggesting that phosphorylation leads to the release of PHF8 from chromatin (Liu et al. 2010), and another showing that it leads to more active participation in transcriptional regulation (Asensio-Juan et al. 2017). Another key question that remains is how phosphorylation of the PHF8 C-terminus affects the demethylation activity of the N-terminal JmjC domain.

In addition to the phosphorylation, Lim et al. reported that PHF8 interacts with, and is degraded by, the APC/CDC20 complex during G2/M phase of the cell cycle (Lim et al. 2013). This study revealed that a LXPKXLF motif (aa 495–501) of PHF8 isoform 2 mediates the interaction between the demethylase and CDC20 and its degradation by the APC/CDC20 complex. The deubiquitinase USP7 was found to interact with PHF8 and to counteract the ubiquitination-mediated degradation of PHF8 (Wang et al. 2016). This interaction appeared to be mediated by the C-terminus (aa 401–1024) of PHF8 (Wang et al. 2016).

In reference to PHF2, we discussed PKA-mediated PHF2 phosphorylation, and that S1056 is likely the phosphorylation site (Baba et al. 2011). Although analysis based on PhosphoSitePlus (Hornbeck et al. 2015) shows that this serine is highly phosphorylated (Fig. 8.3), phosphorylation was also detected at many other sites. It was shown recently that AMPK phosphorylates PHF2 at S655, which enhances its demethylase activity and suppresses lung cancer metastasis (Dong et al. 2023). In the case of KDM7A, post-translational modification has not been reported. The PhosphoSitePlus-based analysis shows that KDM7A is phosphorylated at T437 and S604 (Fig. 8.3). Further studies will be required to identify the post-translational modifications of KDM7A, preferentially in cells expressing KDM7A at high levels.

8.5 Targeting KDM7 Family Members in Cancer Therapies

The discovery that histone demethylases have oncogenic functions prompted the development of inhibitors of these enzymes. As a JmjC domain-containing histone demethylases, KDM7 proteins use 2-oxoglutarate (2OG) as a cofactor, and thus, they can be inhibited by 2OG analogs. Although the field of histone demethylase inhibitors has quickly evolved, it also faces challenges. Given that progress on the mechanisms whereby histone demethylase inhibitors function has been extensively discussed in several reviews (Hojfeldt et al. 2013; McAllister et al. 2016; Song et al. 2016Thaler et al. 2016), here we focus on inhibitors of the KDM7 family and their potential uses in cancer therapy.

Daminozide (N-(dimethylamino) succinamic acid, 160 Da), a regulator of plant growth, was found to selectively inhibit PHF8 (IC_{50} = 0.55 μM by AlphaScreen), KDM7A (IC_{50} = 2.1 μM by a MALDI assay) and KDM2A (IC_{50} = 1.5 μM by AlphaScreen) (Rose et al. 2012). In B16-F1 melanoma cells, treatment with daminozide at 2 μM for 48 h elevated the levels of H3K9me2 (Tan et al. 2014). Although the authors compared the effects of this treatment with that of KDM7A knockdown, presumably, the elevation in H3K9me2 could have been caused by inhibition of both PHF8 and KDM7A. Due to the potential carcinogenicity of the metabolites of daminozide, this agent is unlikely to be usable for therapeutics. However, soon after the discovery of daminozide, compound 9 was also identified as an inhibitor of KDM2A, KDM7A and PHF8, with IC_{50}s of 6.8, 0.2 and 1.2 μM, respectively (Suzuki et al. 2013). Moreover, compound 9 inhibited the growth of both HeLa and KYSE150 cells, downregulated expression of the E2F1 gene and lengthened G0/G1 phase in both cell lines, consistent with a function for PHF8 in cell-cycle regulation (Suzuki et al. 2013). A scientific comment on patent US20160102096A1 detailed the development of additional histone demethylase

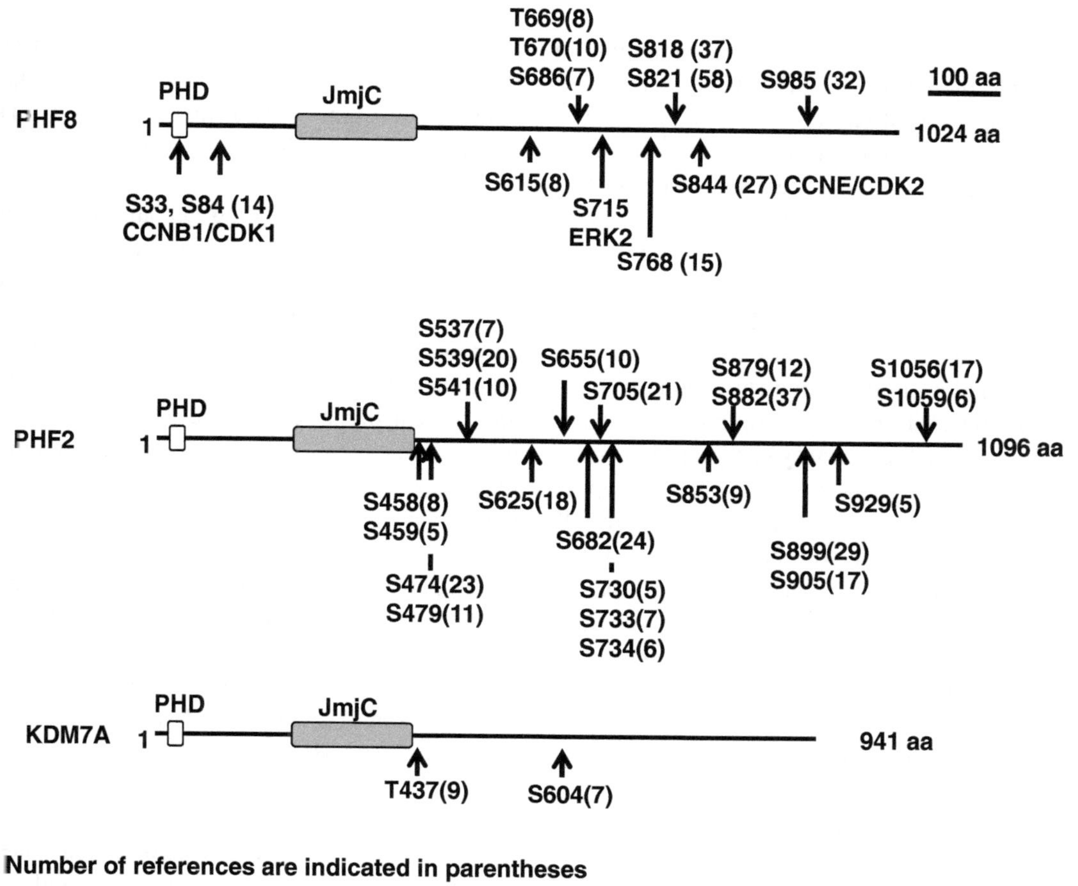

Fig. 8.3 Phosphorylation profile of KDMA7 family members. The phosphorylation data were retrieved from PhosphoSitePlus, Cell Signaling Technology. Number of references/studies is indicated in parentheses. For PHF8, the isoform 2 with 1024 aa compared with inform 2 of 1060 aa is used

inhibitors (Thaler and Mercurio 2016). Among these new derivatives, several compounds demonstrate concurrent inhibition of KDM2B and PHF8 in vitro. For example, compound 103 shows IC_{50} of 0.56 and 0.16 μM for KDM2B and PHF8, respectively (Thaler and Mercurio 2016). However, this evaluation also emphasized the need for cellular data for the effectiveness of these compounds.

The oncogenic functions of PHF8 in several types of cancer make it a good candidate target for cancer therapeutics. However, this may be a challenge given that KDM7A and PHF2 may have tumor suppressor functions or could potentially be functionally redundant. Thus, it will be critical to develop PHF8-specific inhibitors for cancer treatment. Furthermore, more systematic studies on the expression and functions of all three KDM7 family numbers within the same type of cancer and cellular context are needed. The oncogenic function of KDM2B in breast cancer (Kottakis et al. 2014) may shed light on the use of compounds that concurrently inhibit KDM2B and PHF8 in breast cancer therapy. Moreover, functions of PHF8 in normal mammary gland cells would be essential to shed light on using these inhibitors toward breast cancer therapy.

8.6 Perspectives

Since the discovery of the histone demethylation activity of KDM7 family more than a decade ago, our understanding of these proteins in development and diseases including cancer has improved significantly. Targeted inhibition of a single, if not all, KDM7 family members in a specific type of cancer such as breast cancer, seems feasible for cancer therapy. However, several questions about members of the KDM7 family remain to be solved if their inhibitors are to be applied clinically: their expression in large cohorts of patients with cancers of various types; their functions in cancer development; the mechanisms whereby they regulate gene transcription; their functions in regulating chromatin dynamics independent of their transcriptional roles; and their functional redundancy/compensation.

Due to the post-transcriptional and post-translational mechanisms that regulate KDM7 family members, it will be necessary to perform immunohistochemical staining for all three members in the same type of cancer. Such study in a large cohort of a specific cancer type at different stages with follow-up information will generate data correlating their expression with survival and drug resistance. Further characterization of their co-expression with known oncogenic signaling pathways will be useful to deduce their functions. Due to the high structural similarity between members of the KDM7 and KDM2 families, it will also be important to analyze their co-expression in the same cancer type before directing use of the inhibitors.

A common but important question that remains for all histone demethylases of the KDM7 family is how they contribute to transcriptional regulation. In the case of PHF8, the model is that it interacts with transcription factors. For example, it interacts with E2F1 and c-MYC to regulate the genes that are important for cell-cycle progression (Liu et al. 2010; Asensio-Juan et al. 2012; Shao et al. 2017). It will be necessary to perform ChIP-seq for members of the KDM7 family during a dynamic cellular process such as transformation or differentiation, followed by integrative analysis with the known transcription factors, as well as gene expression profiling. Such analyses will be essential to developing a recruitment model that is dynamic even when the protein levels are not changed.

To date, the studies of the KDM7 proteins have focused mainly on their roles in transcriptional regulation, since the PHD domains of all three proteins bind to H3K4me3. However, the majority of their binding sites is located in non-coding regions. Hence, the roles of KDM7 family in regulating non-coding genomic loci need to be clarified. Beyond, whether KDM7 family members could directly demethylate histones during cell-cycle progression remains to be addressed. This question is especially important with respect to PHF8 and KDM7A, as they are able to demethylate H4K20me1 (Qi et al. 2010), which participates not only in transcriptional regulation, but also directly contributes to chromatin condensation during mitosis, and to the response to/repair of DNA damage (Beck et al. 2012). H4K20me1 is also a precondition for the reestablishment of H4K20me2 and H4K20me3 upon mitotic exit. Thus, whether over-expressed PHF8 or KDM7A in cancer cells downregulates H4K20me1 and further affects the levels of H4K20me2 and H4K20me3 will be worth further investigation.

With respect to the post-translational regulation, many abundant phosphorylation sites on PHF8 and PHF2 have not been studied. Identification of the corresponding kinases will shed light on their involvement in signaling pathways in which the kinase(s) play a critical role. Furthermore, the roles of PHF8 and KDM7A in cancer stem cells are not known. A study of prostate cancer stem cells has demonstrated that PHF8 is one of the chromatin regulators whose expression is raised in $PSA^{-/low}$ prostate cancer stem cells (Liu et al. 2011). Thus, it is essential to study if PHF8 has alternative functions in cancer stem cells.

References

Abidi FE, Miano MG, Murray JC, Schwartz CE (2007) A novel mutation in the PHF8 gene is associated with X-linked mental retardation with cleft lip/cleft palate. Clin Genet 72:19–22

Agarwal V, Bell GW, Nam JW, Bartel DP (2015) Predicting effective microRNA target sites in mammalian mRNAs. eLife 4:e05005

Arteaga MF, Mikesch JH, Qiu J, Christensen J, Helin K, Kogan SC, Dong S, So CW (2013) The histone demethylase PHF8 governs retinoic acid response in acute promyelocytic leukemia. Cancer Cell 23:376–389

Asensio-Juan E, Fueyo R, Pappa S, Iacobucci S, Badosa C, Lois S, Balada M, Bosch-Presegue L, Vaquero A, Gutierrez S, Caelles C, Gallego C, de la Cruz X, Martinez-Balbas MA (2017) The histone demethylase PHF8 is a molecular safeguard of the IFNγ response. Nucleic Acids Res 45(7):3800–3811

Asensio-Juan E, Gallego C, Martinez-Balbas MA (2012) The histone demethylase PHF8 is essential for cytoskeleton dynamics. Nucleic Acids Res 40:9429–9440

Baba A, Ohtake F, Okuno Y, Yokota K, Okada M, Imai Y, Ni M, Meyer CA, Igarashi K, Kanno J, Brown M, Kato S (2011) PKA-dependent regulation of the histone lysine demethylase complex PHF2-ARID5B. Nat Cell Biol 13:668–675

Beck DB, Oda H, Shen SS, Reinberg D (2012) PR-Set7 and H4K20me1: at the crossroads of genome integrity, cell cycle, chromosome condensation, and transcription. Genes Dev 26:325–337

Beyer S, Kristensen MM, Jensen KS, Johansen JV, Staller P (2008) The histone demethylases JMJD1A and JMJD2B are transcriptional targets of hypoxia-inducible factor HIF. J Biol Chem 283:36542–36552

Bjorkman M, Ostling P, Harma V, Virtanen J, Mpindi JP, Rantala J, Mirtti T, Vesterinen T, Lundin M, Sankila A, Rannikko A, Kaivanto E, Kohonen P, Kallioniemi O, Nees M (2012) Systematic knockdown of epigenetic enzymes identifies a novel histone demethylase PHF8 overexpressed in prostate cancer with an impact on cell proliferation, migration and invasion. Oncogene 31:3444–3456

Chen X, Wang S, Zhou Y, Han Y, Li S, Xu Q, Xu L, Zhu Z, Deng Y, Yu L, Song L, Chen AP, Song J, Takahashi E, He G, He L, Li W, Chen CD (2018) Phf8 histone demethylase deficiency causes cognitive impairments through the mTOR pathway. Nat Commun 9:114

Choi JY, Jo SA (2016) KDM7A histone demethylase mediates TNF-alpha-induced ICAM1 protein upregulation by modulating lysosomal activity. Biochem Biophys Res Commun 478:1355–1362

Dong Y, Hu H, Zhang X, Zhang Y, Sun X, Wang H, Kan W, Tan MJ, Shi H, Zang Y, Li J (2023) Phosphorylation of PHF2 by AMPK releases the repressive H3K9me2 and inhibits cancer metastasis. Signal Transduct Target Ther 8:95

Erdogan O, Xie L, Wang L, Wu B, Kong Q, Wan Y, Chen X (2016) Proteomic dissection of LPS-inducible, PHF8-dependent secretome reveals novel roles of PHF8 in TLR4-induced acute inflammation and T cell proliferation. Sci Rep 6:24833

Feng W, Yonezawa M, Ye J, Jenuwein T, Grummt I (2010) PHF8 activates transcription of rRNA genes through H3K4me3 binding and H3K9me1/2 demethylation. Nat Struct Mol Biol 17:445–450

Fortschegger K, de Graaf P, Outchkourov NS, van Schaik FM, Timmers HT, Shiekhattar R (2010) PHF8 targets histone methylation and RNA polymerase II to activate transcription. Mol Cell Biol 30:3286–3298

Ghosh A, Ghosh S, Maiti GP, Mukherjee S, Mukherjee N, Chakraborty J, Roy A, Roychoudhury S, Panda CK (2012) Association of FANCC and PTCH1 with the development of early dysplastic lesions of the head and neck. Ann Surg Oncol 19(Suppl 3):S528–S538

Gu L, Hitzel J, Moll F, Kruse C, Malik RA, Preussner J, Looso M, Leisegang MS, Steinhilber D, Brandes RP, Fork C (2016) The histone demethylase PHF8 is essential for endothelial cell migration. PLoS ONE 11:e0146645

Han Q, Yang P, Wu Y, Meng S, Sui L, Zhang L, Yu L, Tang Y, Jiang H, Xuan D, Kaplan DL, Kim SH, Tu Q, Chen J (2015) Epigenetically modified bone marrow stromal cells in silk scaffolds promote craniofacial bone repair and wound healing. Tissue Eng Part A 21:2156–2165

Hata K, Takashima R, Amano K, Ono K, Nakanishi M, Yoshida M, Wakabayashi M, Matsuda A, Maeda Y, Suzuki Y, Sugano S, Whitson RH, Nishimura R, Yoneda T (2013) Arid5b facilitates chondrogenesis by recruiting the histone demethylase Phf2 to Sox9-regulated genes. Nat Commun 4:2850

Hojfeldt JW, Agger K, Helin K (2013) Histone lysine demethylases as targets for anticancer therapy. Nat Rev Drug Discovery 12:917–930

Hori T, Shang WH, Toyoda A, Misu S, Monma N, Ikeo K, Molina O, Vargiu G, Fujiyama A, Kimura H, Earnshaw WC, Fukagawa T (2014) Histone H4 Lys 20 monomethylation of the CENP-A nucleosome is essential for kinetochore assembly. Dev Cell 29:740–749

Hornbeck PV, Zhang B, Murray B, Kornhauser JM, Latham V, Skrzypek E (2015) PhosphoSitePlus, 2014: mutations, PTMs and recalibrations. Nucleic Acids Res 43:D512-520

Horton JR, Upadhyay AK, Hashimoto H, Zhang X, Cheng X (2011) Structural basis for human PHF2 Jumonji domain interaction with metal ions. J Mol Biol 406:1–8

Huang C, Xiang Y, Wang Y, Li X, Xu L, Zhu Z, Zhang T, Zhu Q, Zhang K, Jing N, Chen CD (2010) Dual-specificity histone demethylase KIAA1718 (KDM7A) regulates neural differentiation through FGF4. Cell Res 20:154–165

Hynes NE, Stoelzle T (2009) Key signalling nodes in mammary gland development and cancer: Myc. Breast Cancer Res: BCR 11:210

Ibrahim SA, Yip GW, Stock C, Pan JW, Neubauer C, Poeter M, Pupjalis D, Koo CY, Kelsch R, Schule R, Rescher U, Kiesel L, Gotte M (2012) Targeting of syndecan-1 by microRNA miR-10b promotes breast cancer cell motility and invasiveness via a Rho-GTPase- and E-cadherin-dependent mechanism. Int J Cancer 131:E884-896

Iqbal N, Iqbal N (2014) Human epidermal growth factor receptor 2 (HER2) in cancers: overexpression and therapeutic implications. Mol Biol Int 2014:852748

Kim HJ, Park JW, Lee KH, Yoon H, Shin DH, Ju UI, Seok SH, Lim SH, Lee ZH, Kim HH, Chun YS (2014) Plant homeodomain finger protein 2 promotes bone formation by demethylating and activating Runx2 for osteoblast differentiation. Cell Res 24:1231–1249

Kleine-Kohlbrecher D, Christensen J, Vandamme J, Abarrategui I, Bak M, Tommerup N, Shi X, Gozani O, Rappsilber J, Salcini AE, Helin K (2010) A functional link between the histone demethylase PHF8 and the transcription factor ZNF711 in X-linked mental retardation. Mol Cell 38:165–178

Klose RJ, Kallin EM, Zhang Y (2006) JmjC-domain-containing proteins and histone demethylation. Nat Rev Genet 7:715–727

Kottakis F, Foltopoulou P, Sanidas I, Keller P, Wronski A, Dake BT, Ezell SA, Shen Z, Naber SP, Hinds PW, McNiel E, Kuperwasser C, Tsichlis PN (2014) NDY1/KDM2B functions as a master regulator of polycomb complexes and controls self-renewal of breast cancer stem cells. Can Res 74:3935–3946

Krieg AJ, Rankin EB, Chan D, Razorenova O, Fernandez S, Giaccia AJ (2010) Regulation of the histone demethylase JMJD1A by hypoxia-inducible factor 1 alpha enhances hypoxic gene expression and tumor growth. Mol Cell Biol 30:344–353

Laumonnier F, Holbert S, Ronce N, Faravelli F, Lenzner S, Schwartz CE, Lespinasse J, Van Esch H, Lacombe D, Goizet C, Phan-Dinh Tuy F, van Bokhoven H, Fryns JP, Chelly J, Ropers HH, Moraine C, Hamel BC, Briault S (2005) Mutations in PHF8 are associated with X linked mental retardation and cleft lip/cleft palate. J Med Genet 42:780–786

Lee JH, Yoo NJ, Kim MS, Lee SH (2017) Histone demethylase gene PHF2 is mutated in gastric and colorectal cancers. Pathol Oncol Res 23(3):471–476

Lee KH, Ju UI, Song JY, Chun YS (2014) The histone demethylase PHF2 promotes fat cell differentiation as an epigenetic activator of both C/EBPα and C/EBPδ. Mol Cells 37:734–741

Lee KH, Park JW, Sung HS, Choi YJ, Kim WH, Lee HS, Chung HJ, Shin HW, Cho CH, Kim TY, Li SH, Youn HD, Kim SJ, Chun YS (2015) PHF2 histone demethylase acts as a tumor suppressor in association with p53 in cancer. Oncogene 34:2897–2909

Lim HJ, Dimova NV, Tan MK, Sigoillot FD, King RW, Shi Y (2013) The G2/M regulator histone demethylase PHF8 is targeted for degradation by the anaphase-promoting complex containing CDC20. Mol Cell Biol 33:4166–4180

Lin H, Wang Y, Wang Y, Tian F, Pu P, Yu Y, Mao H, Yang Y, Wang P, Hu L, Lin Y, Liu Y, Xu Y, Chen CD (2010) Coordinated regulation of active and repressive histone methylations by a dual-specificity histone demethylase ceKDM7A from Caenorhabditis elegans. Cell Res 20:899–907

Liu C, Kelnar K, Liu B, Chen X, Calhoun-Davis T, Li H, Patrawala L, Yan H, Jeter C, Honorio S, Wiggins JF, Bader AG, Fagin R, Brown D, Tang DG (2011) The microRNA miR-34a inhibits prostate cancer stem cells and metastasis by directly repressing CD44. Nat Med 17:211–215

Liu Q, Borcherding NC, Shao P, Maina PK, Zhang W, Qi HH (2020) Contribution of synergism between PHF8 and HER2 signalling to breast cancer development and drug resistance. EBioMedicine 51:102612

Liu W, Tanasa B, Tyurina OV, Zhou TY, Gassmann R, Liu WT, Ohgi KA, Benner C, Garcia-Bassets I, Aggarwal AK, Desai A, Dorrestein PC, Glass CK, Rosenfeld MG (2010) PHF8 mediates histone H4 lysine 20 demethylation events involved in cell cycle progression. Nature 466:508–512

Loenarz C, Ge W, Coleman ML, Rose NR, Cooper CD, Klose RJ, Ratcliffe PJ, Schofield CJ (2010) PHF8, a gene associated with cleft lip/palate and mental retardation, encodes for an Nepsilon-dimethyl lysine demethylase. Hum Mol Genet 19:217–222

Ma Q, Chen Z, Jia G, Lu X, Xie X, Jin W (2015) The histone demethylase PHF8 promotes prostate cancer cell growth by activating the oncomiR miR-125b. Onco Targets Ther 8:1979–1988

Maina PK, Shao P, Jia X, Liu Q, Umesalma S, Marin M, Long D, Concepcion-Roman S, Qi HH (2017) Histone demethylase PHF8 regulates hypoxia signaling through HIF1alpha and H3K4me3. Biochim Biophys Acta Gene Regul Mech 1860(9):1002–1012

Maina PK, Shao P, Liu Q, Fazli L, Tyler S, Nasir M, Dong X, Qi HH (2016) c-MYC drives histone demethylase PHF8 during neuroendocrine differentiation and in castration-resistant prostate cancer. Oncotarget 7(46):75585–75602

McAllister TE, England KS, Hopkinson RJ, Brennan PE, Kawamura A, Schofield CJ (2016) Recent progress in histone demethylase inhibitors. J Med Chem 59:1308–1329

Merkwirth C, Jovaisaite V, Durieux J, Matilainen O, Jordan SD, Quiros PM, Steffen KK, Williams EG, Mouchiroud L, Tronnes SU, Murillo V, Wolff SC, Shaw RJ, Auwerx J, Dillin A (2016) Two conserved histone demethylases regulate mitochondrial stress-induced longevity. Cell 165:1209–1223

Moubarak RS, de Pablos-Aragoneses A, Ortiz-Barahona V, Gong Y, Gowen M, Dolgalev I, Shadaloey SAA, Argibay D, Karz A, Von Itter R, Vega-Saenz de Miera EC, Sokolova E, Darvishian F, Tsirigos A, Osman I, Hernando E (2022) The histone demethylase PHF8 regulates TGFbeta signaling and promotes melanoma metastasis. Sci Adv 8:eabi7127

Nava C, Lamari F, Heron D, Mignot C, Rastetter A, Keren B, Cohen D, Faudet A, Bouteiller D, Gilleron M, Jacquette A, Whalen S, Afenjar A, Perisse D, Laurent C, Dupuits C, Gautier C, Gerard M, Huguet G, Caillet S, Leheup B, Leboyer M, Gillberg C, Delorme R, Bourgeron T, Brice A, Depienne C (2012) Analysis of the chromosome X exome in patients with autism spectrum disorders identified novel candidate genes, including TMLHE. Transl Psychiatry 2:e179

Nilsson EM, Laursen KB, Whitchurch J, McWilliam A, Odum N, Persson JL, Heery DM, Gudas LJ, Mongan NP (2015) MiR137 is an androgen regulated repressor of an extended network of transcriptional coregulators. Oncotarget 6:35710–35725

Oey NE, Leung HW, Ezhilarasan R, Zhou L, Beuerman RW, VanDongen HM, VanDongen AM (2015) A neuronal activity-dependent dual function chromatin-modifying complex regulates arc expression. eNeuro 2(1):ENEURO.0020-14.2015

Okuno Y, Ohtake F, Igarashi K, Kanno J, Matsumoto T, Takada I, Kato S, Imai Y (2013) Epigenetic regulation of adipogenesis by PHF2 histone demethylase. Diabetes 62:1426–1434

Osawa T, Muramatsu M, Wang F, Tsuchida R, Kodama T, Minami T, Shibuya M (2011) Increased expression of histone demethylase JHDM1D under nutrient starvation suppresses tumor growth via down-regulating angiogenesis. Proc Natl Acad Sci USA 108:20725–20729

Pan MR, Hsu MC, Chen LT, Hung WC (2015) G9a orchestrates PCL3 and KDM7A to promote histone H3K27 methylation. Sci Rep 5:18709

Park JH, Jung M, Moon KC (2018) The prognostic significance of nuclear expression of PHF2 and C/EBPalpha in clear cell renal cell carcinoma with consideration of adipogenic metabolic evolution. Oncotarget 9:142–151

Pattabiraman DR, Bierie B, Kober KI, Thiru P, Krall JA, Zill C, Reinhardt F, Tam WL, Weinberg RA (2016) Activation of PKA leads to mesenchymal-to-epithelial transition and loss of tumor-initiating ability. Science 351:aad3680

Qi HH, Sarkissian M, Hu GQ, Wang Z, Bhattacharjee A, Gordon DB, Gonzales M, Lan F, Ongusaha PP, Huarte M, Yaghi NK, Lim H, Garcia BA, Brizuela L, Zhao K, Roberts TM, Shi Y (2010) Histone H4K20/H3K9 demethylase PHF8 regulates zebrafish brain and craniofacial development. Nature 466:503–507

Qiao Y, Liu X, Harvard C, Hildebrand MJ, Rajcan-Separovic E, Holden JJ, Lewis ME (2008) Autism-associated familial microdeletion of Xp11.22. Clin Genet 74:134–144

Qiu J, Shi G, Jia Y, Li J, Wu M, Li J, Dong S, Wong J (2010) The X-linked mental retardation gene PHF8 is a histone demethylase involved in neuronal differentiation. Cell Res 20:908–918

Rose NR, Woon EC, Tumber A, Walport LJ, Chowdhury R, Li XS, King ON, Lejeune C, Ng SS, Krojer T, Chan MC, Rydzik AM, Hopkinson RJ, Che KH, Daniel M, Strain-Damerell C, Gileadi C, Kochan G, Leung IK, Dunford J, Yeoh KK, Ratcliffe PJ, Burgess-Brown N, von Delft F, Muller S, Marsden B, Brennan PE, McDonough MA, Oppermann U, Klose RJ, Schofield CJ, Kawamura A (2012) Plant growth regulator daminozide is a selective inhibitor of human KDM2/7 histone demethylases. J Med Chem 55:6639–6643

Shao P, Liu Q, Maina PK, Cui J, Bair TB, Li T, Umesalma S, Zhang W, Qi HH (2017) Histone demethylase PHF8 promotes epithelial to mesenchymal transition and breast tumorigenesis. Nucleic Acids Res 45(4):1687–1702

Shen Y, Pan X, Zhao H (2014) The histone demethylase PHF8 is an oncogenic protein in human non-small cell lung cancer. Biochem Biophys Res Commun 451(1):119–125

Shi Y, Lan F, Matson C, Mulligan P, Whetstine JR, Cole PA, Casero RA (2004) Histone demethylation mediated by the nuclear amine oxidase homolog LSD1. Cell 119:941–953

Siderius LE, Hamel BC, van Bokhoven H, de Jager F, van den Helm B, Kremer H, Heineman-de Boer JA, Ropers HH, Mariman EC (1999) X-linked mental retardation associated with cleft lip/palate maps to Xp11.3-q21.3. Am J Med Genet 85:216–220

Sinha S, Singh RK, Alam N, Roy A, Roychoudhury S, Panda CK (2008) Alterations in candidate genes PHF2, FANCC, PTCH1 and XPA at chromosomal 9q22.3 region: pathological significance in early- and late-onset breast carcinoma. Mol Cancer 7:84

Son MJ, Kim WK, Oh KJ, Park A, da Lee S, Han BS, Lee SC, Bae KH (2016) Methyltransferase and demethylase profiling studies during brown adipocyte differentiation. BMB Rep 49:388–393

Song Y, Wu F, Wu J (2016) Targeting histone methylation for cancer therapy: enzymes, inhibitors, biological activity and perspectives. J Hematol Oncol 9:49

Stender JD, Pascual G, Liu W, Kaikkonen MU, Do K, Spann NJ, Boutros M, Perrimon N, Rosenfeld MG, Glass CK (2012) Control of proinflammatory gene programs by regulated trimethylation and demethylation of histone H4K20. Mol Cell 48:28–38

Sun L, Huang Y, Wei Q, Tong X, Cai R, Nalepa G, Ye X (2015) Cyclin E-CDK2 protein phosphorylates plant homeodomain finger protein 8 (PHF8) and regulates its function in the cell cycle. J Biol Chem 290:4075–4085

Sun LL, Sun XX, Xu XE, Zhu MX, Wu ZY, Shen JH, Wu JY, Huang Q, Li EM, Xu LY (2013a) Overexpression of Jumonji AT-rich interactive domain 1B and PHD finger protein 2 is involved in the progression of esophageal squamous cell carcinoma. Acta Histochem 115:56–62

Sun X, Qiu JJ, Zhu S, Cao B, Sun L, Li S, Li P, Zhang S, Dong S (2013b) Oncogenic features of PHF8 histone demethylase in esophageal squamous cell carcinoma. PLoS ONE 8:e77353

Suzuki T, Ozasa H, Itoh Y, Zhan P, Sawada H, Mino K, Walport L, Ohkubo R, Kawamura A, Yonezawa M, Tsukada Y, Tumber A, Nakagawa H, Hasegawa M, Sasaki R, Mizukami T, Schofield CJ, Miyata N (2013) Identification of the KDM2/7 histone lysine demethylase subfamily inhibitor and its antiproliferative activity. J Med Chem 56:7222–7231

Tan Y, Tajik A, Chen J, Jia Q, Chowdhury F, Wang L, Chen J, Zhang S, Hong Y, Yi H, Wu DC, Zhang Y, Wei F, Poh YC, Seong J, Singh R, Lin LJ, Doganay S, Li Y, Jia H, Ha T, Wang Y, Huang B, Wang N (2014) Matrix softness regulates plasticity of tumour-repopulating cells via H3K9 demethylation and Sox2 expression. Nat Commun 5:4619

Tang Y, Hong YZ, Bai HJ, Wu Q, Chen CD, Lang JY, Boheler KR, Yang HT (2016) Plant homeo domain finger protein 8 regulates mesodermal and cardiac differentiation of embryonic stem cells through mediating the histone demethylation of pmaip1. Stem Cells 34:1527–1540

Tang Z, Li C, Kang B, Gao G, Li C, Zhang Z (2017) GEPIA: a web server for cancer and normal gene expression profiling and interactive analyses. Nucleic Acids Res 45:W98–W102

Thaler F, Mercurio C (2016) Compounds and methods for inhibiting histone demethylases: a patent evaluation of US20160102096A1. Expert Opin Ther Pat 26:1367–1370

Tong D, Liu Q, Liu G, Yuan W, Wang L, Guo Y, Lan W, Zhang D, Dong S, Wang Y, Xiao H, Mu J, Mao C, Wong J, Jiang J (2016) The HIF/PHF8/AR axis promotes prostate cancer progression. Oncogenesis 5:e283

Tsukada Y, Fang J, Erdjument-Bromage H, Warren ME, Borchers CH, Tempst P, Zhang Y (2006) Histone demethylation by a family of JmjC domain-containing proteins. Nature 439:811–816

Tsukada Y, Ishitani T, Nakayama KI (2010) KDM7 is a dual demethylase for histone H3 Lys 9 and Lys 27 and functions in brain development. Genes Dev 24:432–437

Walsh RM, Shen EY, Bagot RC, Anselmo A, Jiang Y, Javidfar B, Wojtkiewicz GJ, Cloutier J, Chen JW, Sadreyev R, Nestler EJ, Akbarian S, Hochedlinger K (2017) Phf8 loss confers resistance to depression-like and anxiety-like behaviors in mice. Nat Commun 8:15142

Wang J, Lin X, Wang S, Wang C, Wang Q, Duan X, Lu P, Wang Q, Wang C, Liu XS, Huang J (2014) PHF8 and REST/NRSF co-occupy gene promoters to regulate proximal gene expression. Sci Rep 4:5008

Wang Q, Ma S, Song N, Li X, Liu L, Yang S, Ding X, Shan L, Zhou X, Su D, Wang Y, Zhang Q, Liu X, Yu N, Zhang K, Shang Y, Yao Z, Shi L (2016) Stabilization of histone demethylase PHF8 by USP7 promotes breast carcinogenesis. J Clin Investig 126:2205–2220

Wen H, Li J, Song T, Lu M, Kan PY, Lee MG, Sha B, Shi X (2010) Recognition of histone H3K4 trimethylation by the plant homeodomain of PHF2 modulates histone demethylation. J Biol Chem 285:9322–9326

Xia X, Lemieux ME, Li W, Carroll JS, Brown M, Liu XS, Kung AL (2009) Integrative analysis of HIF binding and transactivation reveals its role in maintaining histone methylation homeostasis. Proc Natl Acad Sci USA 106:4260–4265

Yatim A, Benne C, Sobhian B, Laurent-Chabalier S, Deas O, Judde JG, Lelievre JD, Levy Y, Benkirane M (2012) NOTCH1 nuclear interactome reveals key regulators of its transcriptional activity and oncogenic function. Mol Cell 48:445–458

Ye H, Yang Q, Qi S, Li H (2019) PHF8 plays an oncogene function in hepatocellular carcinoma formation. Oncol Res 27(5):613–621

Yokoyama A, Okuno Y, Chikanishi T, Hashiba W, Sekine H, Fujiki R, Kato S (2010) KIAA1718 is a histone demethylase that erases repressive histone methyl marks. Genes Cells: Dev Mol Cell Mech 15:867–873

Zhou W, Gong L, Wu Q, Xing C, Wei B, Chen T, Zhou Y, Yin S, Jiang B, Xie H, Zhou L, Zheng S (2018) PHF8 upregulation contributes to autophagic degradation of E-cadherin, epithelial-mesenchymal transition and metastasis in hepatocellular carcinoma. J Exp Clin Cancer Res: CR 37:215

MIX
Papier aus verantwortungsvollen Quellen
Paper from responsible sources
FSC® C105338
FSC
www.fsc.org

If you have any concerns about our products,
you can contact us on
ProductSafety@springernature.com

In case Publisher is established outside the EU,
the EU authorized representative is:
Springer Nature Customer Service Center GmbH
Europaplatz 3, 69115 Heidelberg, Germany

Printed by Libri Plureos GmbH
in Hamburg, Germany